T0227023

Aneurysmal Subarachnoid Hemorrhage

Guest Editors

PAUL NYQUIST, MD, MPH
NEERAJ NAVAL, MD
RAFAEL J. TAMARGO, MD

NEUROSURGERY CLINICS OF NORTH AMERICA

www.neurosurgery.theclinics.com

Consulting Editors
ANDREW T. PARSA, MD, PhD
PAUL C. McCORMICK, MD, MPH

April 2010 • Volume 21 • Number 2

SAUNDERS an imprint of ELSEVIER, Inc.

W.B. SAUNDERS COMPANY
A Division of Elsevier Inc.

1600 John F. Kennedy Blvd. ● Suite 1800 ● Philadelphia, PA 19103-2899

http://www.theclinics.com

NEUROSURGERY CLINICS OF NORTH AMERICA Volume 21, Number 2
April 2010 ISSN 1042-3680, ISBN-13: 978-1-4377-1928-4

Editor: Ruth Malwitz
Developmental Editor: Donald Mumford

Neurosurgery Clinics of North America (ISSN 1042-3680) is published quarterly by Elsevier Inc., 360 Park Avenue South, New York, NY 10010-1710. Months of issue are January, April, July, and October. Business and Editorial Offices: 1600 John F. Kennedy Blvd., Suite 1800, Philadelphia, PA 19103-2899. Customer Service Office: 11830 Westline Industrial Drive, St. Louis, MO 63146. Periodicals postage paid at New York, NY, and additional mailing offices. Subscription prices are $296.00 per year (US individuals), $447.00 per year (US institutions), $324.00 per year (Canadian individuals), $546.00 per year (Canadian institutions), $414.00 per year (international individuals), $546.00 per year (international institutions), $149.00 per year (US students), and $204.00 per year (international students). International air speed delivery is included in all *Clinics* subscription prices. All prices are subject to change without notice. **POSTMASTER:** Send address changes to *Neurosurgery Clinics of North America*, Elsevier Periodicals Customer Service, 11830 Westline Industrial Drive, St. Louis, MO 63146. **Customer Service: 1-800-654-2452 (US and Canada). From outside the US and Canada, call: 314-447-8871. Fax: 314-447-8029. E-mail: JournalsCustomerService-usa@elsevier.com (for print support) and journalsonlinesupport-usa@elsevier.com (for online support).**

Reprints. For copies of 100 or more, of articles in this publication, please contact the Commercial Reprints Department, Elsevier Inc., 360 Park Avenue South, New York, NY 10010-1710. Tel. (212) 633-3812; Fax: (212) 462-1935; E-mail: reprints@elsevier.com.

Neurosurgery Clinics of North America is covered in *MEDLINE/PubMed (Index Medicus), EMBASE/Excerpta Medica, and Current Contents/Clinical Medicine (CC/CM).*

Printed in the United States of America.

Cover image copyright © 2010, The Johns Hopkins University. All rights reserved. Courtesy of Ian Suk, Johns Hopkins University; with permission.

Printed and bound in the United Kingdom
Transferred to Digital Print 2011

Contributors

CONSULTING EDITORS

ANDREW T. PARSA, MD, PhD
Assistant Professor, Department of
Neurological Surgery, University of California,
San Francisco, San Francisco, California

PAUL C. MCCORMICK, MD, MPH, FACS
New York Neurological Institute, New York,
New York

GUEST EDITORS

PAUL NYQUIST, MD, MPH
Assistant Professor, Departments of
Neurology, Anesthesiology/Critical Care
Medicine, and Neurosurgery, The Johns
Hopkins University School of Medicine,
Baltimore, Maryland

NEERAJ NAVAL, MD
Neurosciences ICU Fellowship Program
Director, Neurosciences ICU Associate
Director, Oregon Health & Science University
(OHSU), Portland, Oregon

RAFAEL J. TAMARGO, MD, FACS
Walter E. Dandy Professor of Neurosurgery,
Director of Cerebrovascular Neurosurgery,
Professor of Neurosurgery and
Otolaryngology, The Johns Hopkins University
School of Medicine, Baltimore, Maryland

AUTHORS

JOSEPH D. BURNS, MD
Department of Neurology, Boston
University School of Medicine, Boston,
Massachusetts

KAISORN L. CHAICHANA, MD
Neurosurgery Resident, Division of
Cerebrovascular Neurosurgery, Department
of Neurosurgery, The Johns Hopkins
University School of Medicine, Baltimore,
Maryland

GEOFFREY P. COLBY, MD, PhD
Resident, Department of Neurosurgery,
The Johns Hopkins University School of
Medicine, Baltimore, Maryland

E. SANDER CONNOLLY Jr, MD
Professor, Department of Neurological
Surgery, Columbia University Medical Center,
New York, New York

ALEXANDER L. COON, MD
Resident, Department of Neurosurgery, The
Johns Hopkins University School of Medicine,
Baltimore, Maryland

PETER DEROSA, BS
Department of Neurological Surgery,
Columbia University Medical Center,
New York, New York

ANDREW F. DUCRUET, MD
Department of Neurological Surgery,
Columbia University Medical Center,
New York, New York

PHILIPPE GAILLOUD, MD
Associate Professor and Director of
Interventional radiology, Division of
Interventional Neuroradiology, The Johns
Hopkins University School of Medicine,
Baltimore, Maryland

DHEERAJ GANDHI, MBBS, MD
Assistant Professor, Division of Interventional Neuroradiology, Department of Radiology; Department of Neurology and Neurosurgery, Johns Hopkins Hospital, The Johns Hopkins University School of Medicine, Baltimore, Maryland

ANAND V. GERMANWALA, MD
Assistant Professor of Neurosurgery, Division of Neurosurgery, University of North Carolina School of Medicine, Chapel Hill, North Carolina

LYDIA GREGG, MA, CMI
Division of Interventional Neuroradiology, The Johns Hopkins University School of Medicine, Baltimore, Maryland

BARTOSZ T. GROBELNY, BA
Department of Neurological Surgery, Columbia University Medical Center, New York, New York

ZACHARY L. HICKMAN, MD
Department of Neurological Surgery, Columbia University Medical Center, New York, New York

STANLEY HOANG, BS
Medical Student, Stanford University, School of Medicine, Palo Alto, California

JUDY HUANG, MD
Associate Professor of Neurosurgery, Department of Neurosurgery, The Johns Hopkins University School of Medicine, Baltimore, Maryland

J. DEDRICK JORDAN, MD, PhD
Instructor, The Johns Hopkins University School of Medicine, Baltimore, Maryland

SUDHIR KATHURIA, MBBS
Division of Interventional Neuroradiology, Department of Radiology, Johns Hopkins Hospital, The Johns Hopkins University School of Medicine, Baltimore, Maryland

IVAN KOTCHETKOV, BA
Department of Neurological Surgery, Columbia University Medical Center, New York, New York

CHRISTOS LAZARIDIS, MD
Assistant Professor, Neurosciences Critical Care, Intensive Care Medicine-EDIC, Vascular Neurology, Medical University of South Carolina, Charleston, South Carolina

ANDRÉ A. LE ROUX, MB, ChB, MD (LMCC) FC Neurosurg(SA)
Cerebrovascular Neurosurgery Fellow, Department of Surgery(Neurosurgery), Faculty of Medicine, University of Toronto, Toronto, Ontario, Canada

SCOTT A. MARSHALL, MD
Division of Neurosciences Critical Care, Departments of Anesthesiology and Critical Care Medicine, Neurology and Neurosurgery, The Johns Hopkins University School of Medicine; Department of Neurology, Uniformed Services University of the Health Sciences, Bethesda, Maryland

STEPHAN A. MAYER, MD, FCCM
Director, Neurologic Intensive Care Unit, New York Presbyterian Hospital/Columbia; Professor, Department of Neurology and Neurosurgery, Columbia University College of Physicians and Surgeons, New York, New York

BEN MCGUINNESS, MBChB, FRANZCR
Division of Interventional Neuroradiology, Department of Radiology, Johns Hopkins Hospital, Baltimore, Maryland

NEERAJ NAVAL, MD
Neurosciences ICU Fellowship Program Director, Neurosciences ICU Associate Director, Oregon Health & Science University (OHSU), Portland, Oregon

PAUL NYQUIST, MD, MPH
Assistant Professor, Departments of Neurology, Anesthesiology/Critical Care Medicine, and Neurosurgery, The Johns Hopkins University School of Medicine, Baltimore, Maryland

MONICA PEARL, MD
Division of Interventional Neuroradiology, The Johns Hopkins University School of Medicine, Baltimore, Maryland

GUSTAVO PRADILLA, MD
Neurosurgery Resident, Division of Cerebrovascular Neurosurgery, Department of Neurosurgery, The Johns Hopkins University School of Medicine, Baltimore, Maryland

RAFAEL J. TAMARGO, MD, FACS
Walter E. Dandy Professor of Neurosurgery,
Director of Cerebrovascular Neurosurgery,
Professor of Neurosurgery and
Otolaryngology, The Johns Hopkins
University School of Medicine, Baltimore,
Maryland

**M. CHRISTOPHER WALLACE, MD, MSc,
FRCSC, FACS**
Professor, Department of
Surgery(Neurosurgery), Faculty of
Medicine, University of Toronto,
Toronto, Ontario, Canada

KATJA E. WARTENBERG, MD, PhD
Department of Neurology, Neurologic
Intensive Care Unit, Martin-Luther University,
Halle-Wittenberg, Leipzig, Germany

EELCO F.M. WIJDICKS, MD, PhD
Department of Neurology, Mayo Clinic,
Rochester, Minnesota

ALAN H. YEE, DO
Department of Neurology, Mayo Clinic,
Rochester, Minnesota

BRAD E. ZACHARIA, MD
Department of Neurological Surgery,
Columbia University Medical Center,
New York, New York

WENDY C. ZIAI, MD, MPH
Division of Neurosciences Critical Care,
Departments of Anesthesiology Critical Care
Medicine, Neurosurgery and Neurology,
The Johns Hopkins University School of
Medicine, Baltimore, Maryland

Contents

INTRODUCTION: THE EPIDEMIOLOGY AND COST OF ANEURYSMAL SUBARACHNOID HEMORRHAGE

> Aneurysmal subarachnoid hemorrhage (aSAH) is a form of hemorrhagic stroke that affects up to 30,000 individuals per year in the United States. The incidence of aSAH has been shown to be associated with numerous nonmodifiable (age, gender, ethnicity, family history, aneurysm location, size) and modifiable (hypertension, body mass index, tobacco and illicit drug use) risk factors. Although early repair of ruptured aneurysms and aggressive postoperative management has improved overall outcomes, it remains a devastating disease, with mortality approaching 50% and less than 60% of survivors returning to functional independence. As treatment modalities change and the percentage of minority and elderly populations increase, it is critical to maintain an up-to-date understanding of the epidemiology of SAH.

> Aneurysmal subarachnoid hemorrhage (aSAH) is a neurosurgical catastrophe. It affects 33,000 patients in the United States annually and has a mortality rate of 50% to 60% at 30 days. Half of the survivors are dependent. Outcome is closely related to the level of consciousness at the time of presentation, global cerebral edema, subarachnoid blood load as seen on CT, and rehemorrhage. Age, hyperglycemia, and medical complications are associated with worse outcomes. The cost impact factor of this condition is high from a financial perspective as well as from a patient perspective. Care givers show increased morbidity when compared with the nonaffected community. Early aggressive treatment of good grade patients seems to provide the best outcome for this serious condition.

SURGICAL AND INTERVENTIONAL RADIOLOGICAL TREATMENT IN ANEURYSMAL SUBARACHNOID HEMORRHAGE

> Aneurysmal subarachnoid hemorrhage (aSAH) is a common and often devastating condition that requires prompt neurosurgical evaluation and intervention. Modern management of aSAH involves a multidisciplinary team of subspecialists, including vascular neurosurgeons, neurocritical care specialists and, frequently, neurointerventional radiologists. This team is responsible for stabilizing the patient on presentation, diagnosing the offending ruptured aneurysm, securing the aneurysm, and managing the patient through a typically prolonged and complicated hospital

course. Surgical intervention has remained a definitive treatment for ruptured cerebral aneurysms since the early 1900s. Over the subsequent decades, many innovations in microsurgical technique, adjuvant maneuvers, and intraoperative and perioperative medical therapies have advanced the care of patients with aSAH. This report focuses on the modern surgical management of patients with aSAH. Following a brief historical perspective on the origin of aneurysm surgery, the topics discussed include the timing of surgical intervention after aSAH, commonly used surgical approaches and craniotomies, fenestration of the lamina terminalis, intraoperative neurophysiological monitoring, intraoperative digital subtraction and fluorescent angiography, temporary clipping, deep hypothermic cardiopulmonary bypass, management of acute hydrocephalus, cerebral revascularization, and novel clip configurations and microsurgical techniques. Many of the topics highlighted in this report represent some of the more debated techniques in vascular neurosurgery. The popularity of such techniques is constantly evolving as new studies are performed and data about their utility become available.

Hydrocephalus After Aneurysmal Subarachnoid Hemorrhage 263

Anand V. Germanwala, Judy Huang, and Rafael J. Tamargo

Hydrocephalus is a common and potentially devastating complication of aneurysmal subarachnoid hemorrhage (SAH). Its incidence is approximately 20% to 30%, and its onset can be acute, within 48 hours after SAH, or rarely chronic, occurring in a delayed fashion weeks and even months after the hemorrhage. Early recognition of its signs and symptoms and accurate interpretation of computed tomography (CT) studies are important for the management of patients with SAH. Clinically, a poor neurologic grade has the highest correlation with an increased incidence of hydrocephalus. Radiographically, the bicaudate index on CT studies has emerged as the best marker of this condition. Although further studies are needed to understand the complex pathophysiology of this condition, hydrocephalus after SAH can be treated effectively using current technology.

Endovascular Treatment of Aneurysmal Subarachnoid Hemorrhage 271

Monica Pearl, Lydia Gregg, and Philippe Gailloud

Aneurysmal subarachnoid hemorrhage is a deadly disease associated with high morbidity and mortality. Surgical clipping has been the gold standard treatment for more than 70 years. Endovascular therapy is now accepted as a valid alternative therapeutic modality. The authors' approach emphasizes collaboration between endovascular and surgical specialists. The array of new endovascular techniques has extended beyond the Guglielmi Detachable Coil to include new stents and flow-diverting devices. The future promises expansion of the number of types of aneurysms that are treatable with endovascular techniques.

Endovascular Management of Cerebral Vasospasm 281

Ben McGuinness and Dheeraj Gandhi

Cerebral vasospasm is a cause of significant morbidity and mortality in patients with subarachnoid hemorrhage (SAH). Most cases of vasospasm can be managed medically. Medical strategies for treatment include hemodynamic augmentation to improve cerebral perfusion pressure and medical therapy to prevent or reduce cerebral vasospasm. In patients with acute neurological deterioration, imaging assessment is essential to triage those patients appropriate for aggressive medical or endovascular therapy. Such imaging assessment can be performed with many radiologic techniques such as transcranial Doppler, computed tomography (CT), magnetic resonance imaging, and single-photon emission CT (SPECT). Advanced CT applications like CT angiography and CT perfusion are gaining popularity and playing an increasingly important role in the decision making. Endovascular techniques for treatment of vasospasm include intra-arterial administration of vasodilators and intracranial angioplasty. This article discusses the use of these endovascular techniques in the management of vasospasm and provides a current review of literature. Sustained efficacy of intra-arterial vasodilators is less well established at this time, and repeated treatments may be necessary. Balloon angioplasty is an effective technique in treating vasospasm and results in durable clinical improvement. It should be used judiciously, however, given a small risk of vessel rupture associated with intracranial angioplasty. The goal of angioplasty should be improvement of vessel caliber to augment flow rather than to achieve a picture-perfect result.

NON-INVASIVE IMAGING IN ANEURYSMAL SUBARACHNOID HEMORRHAGE

Transcranial Doppler ultrasonography (TCD) is a tool employed by the neurosurgeon and neurointensivist in the management of vasospasm in the intensive care unit after aneurysmal subarachnoid hemorrhage. A review of the current indications, monitoring parameters, indices, and relevance of modern TCD technology is provided, as well as algorithms for the use of TCD ultrasonography in the management of patients with subarachnoid hemorrhage. Other current uses of TCD ultrasonography are also discussed in the setting of neurocritical care.

Aneurysmal subarachnoid hemorrhage (aSAH) is a devastating condition, requiring prompt diagnosis and therapeutic intervention as well as close monitoring for the development of complications including vasospasm (VS). Although digital subtraction angiography is still considered the gold standard for the diagnosis of aSAH (and vasospasm), new and less invasive modalities are emerging including ultrasound, CT, CT angiography and CT perfusion, and MR imaging. The current evidence for the use of these newer modalities is described for the diagnosis of aSAH and the management of its sequelae including VS.

THE MEDICAL MANAGEMENT OF ANEURYSMAL SUBARACHNOID HEMORRHAGE AND IT'S SEQUELLA

The prevention and management of medical complications are important for improving outcomes after subarachnoid hemorrhage (SAH). Fever, anemia requiring transfusion, hyperglycemia, hyponatremia, pneumonia, hypertension, and neurogenic cardiopulmonary dysfunction occur frequently after SAH. There is increasing evidence that acute hypoxia and extremes of blood pressure can exacerbate brain injury during the acute phase of bleeding. There are promising strategies to minimize these complications. Randomized controlled trials are needed to evaluate the risks and benefits of these and other medical management strategies after SAH.

Cerebral salt wasting (CSW) is a syndrome of hypovolemic hyponatremia caused by natriuresis and diuresis. The mechanisms underlying CSW have not been precisely delineated, although existing evidence strongly implicates abnormal elevations in circulating natriuretic peptides. The key in diagnosis of CSW lies in distinguishing it from the more common syndrome of inappropriate secretion of antidiuretic hormone. Volume status, but not serum and urine electrolytes and osmolality, is crucial for making this distinction. Volume and sodium repletion are the goals of treatment of patients with CSW, and this can be performed using some combination of isotonic saline, hypertonic saline, and mineralocorticoids.

Vasospasm is a major cause of morbidity and mortality following aneurysmal subarachnoid hemorrhage. This article reviews the risk factors for vasospasm; the various methods for diagnosing vasospasm including the conventional 4-vessel angiography, computed tomographic angiography, and computed tomographic perfusion; the methods to detect vasospasm before clinical onset (including transcranial Doppler ultrasonography); and the recent emergence of multimodality monitoring. A discussion of medical treatment options in the setting of vasospasm is also included; the prophylactic use of "neuroprotectants" such as nimodipine, statins, and magnesium and the role of hemodynamic augmentation in vasospasm amelioration, including the use of inotropic support in addition to traditional triple-H therapy, are discussed.

INFLAMMATION AND VASOSPASM IN SUBARACHNOID HEMORRHAGE

Morbidity and mortality of patients with aneurysmal subarachnoid hemorrhage (aSAH) is significantly related to the development of chronic cerebral vasospasm. Despite extensive clinical and experimental research, the pathophysiology of the events that result in delayed arterial spasm is not fully understood. A review of the published literature on cerebral vasospasm that included but was not limited to all PubMed citations from 1951 to the present was performed. The findings suggest that leukocyte-endothelial cell interactions play a significant role in the pathophysiology of cerebral vasospasm and explain the clinical variability and time course of the disease. Experimental therapeutic targeting of the inflammatory response when timed correctly can prevent vasospasm, and supplementation of endothelial relaxation by nitric oxide-related therapies and other approaches could result in reversal of the arterial narrowing and improved outcomes in patients with aSAH.

Subarachnoid hemorrhage from the rupture of a saccular aneurysm is a devastating neurological disease that has a high morbidity and mortality not only from the initial hemorrhage, but also from the delayed complications, such as cerebral vasospasm. Cerebral vasospasm can lead to delayed ischemic injury 1 to 2 weeks after the initial hemorrhage. Although the pathophysiology of vasospasm has been described for decades, the molecular basis remains poorly understood. With the many advances in the past decade in the development of sensitive molecular biological techniques, imaging, biochemical purification, and protein identification, new insights are beginning to reveal the etiology of vasospasm. These findings will not only help to identify markers of vasospasm and prognostic outcome, but will also yield potential therapeutic targets for the treatment of this disease. This review focuses on the methods available for the identification of biological markers of vasospasm and their limitations, the current understanding as to the utility and prognostic significance of identified biomarkers, the utility of these biomarkers in predicting vasospasm and outcome, and future directions of research in this field.

Neurosurgery Clinics of North America

THE CLINICS ARE NOW AVAILABLE ONLINE!

Access your subscription at:
www.theclinics.com

Preface

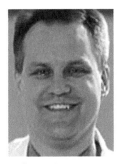

Paul Nyquist, MD, MPH

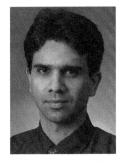

Neeraj Naval, MD

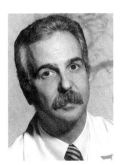

Rafael J. Tamargo, MD

Guest Editors

The incidence of aneurysmal subarachnoid hemorrhage (aSAH) is between 6 and 8 cases per 100,000 persons per annum in the West. It affects some 20,000 to 30,000 Americans each year. In recent decades, the treatment of vasospasm has advanced. Several new clinical trials involving the surgical and endovascular as well as medical management of aSAH have changed the intellectual foundation of the treatment of this disorder. The development of new endovascular techniques has expanded the breadth and effectiveness of the surgical options available to neurosurgeons in caring for these patients. Understanding of the underlying molecular biology of this disorder has given insight into genetic risk factors predisposing to hemorrhage and vasospasm. Inflammation's role in the development of vasospasm is becoming more clearly defined. The proliferation of neurocritical care units and a greater understanding of the issues surrounding the medical management of aSAH have fueled a need for education about the medical treatment of this disorder and its complications.

Centers that ascribe to excellence in the care of patients with subarachnoid hemorrhage must incorporate interdisciplinary approaches. Expert care of these patients requires integration of knowledge from the fields of neurosurgery, neuroradiology, neurocritical care, and stroke neurology. As technology advances and new devices for treatment such as endovascular coiling dramatically change the treatment of these patients, they must be placed in the context of a multidisciplinary approach. As new imaging modalities such as computed tomographic angiography and perfusion computed tomography (CT) are improving, they are allowing for better monitoring of perfusion deficits and increased detection of occult hemorrhages and aneurysms. This growing technological sophistication requires special sensitivity as to how this technology can best be used and integrated into the multi-faceted world of aSAH management to achieve cost-effectiveness and improved outcomes.

There has been a recent explosion of new understanding of the molecular biology of aneurysm development, repair, and its associated clinical sequelae. The role of inflammation and its relation to vasospasm and aSAH is an example of this. This greater understanding of the pathophysiology of vasospasm is leading to new means of detection and treatment of this disorder. It now is recognized that vasospasm is primarily an inflammatory response to the initial hemorrhage. New research approaches involving genomics and proteomics are creating new opportunities in translational research that build on this knowledge. It is hoped that these approaches may yield new techniques for treatment and detection of the delayed clinical effects of aSAH.

This issue of *Neurosurgery Clinics* has been written with the specific intent of updating readers on the advancement of the care of aSAH in a multidisciplinary setting. The goal is to educate the reader about the changing face of the neurosurgical management of this disorder. Special emphasis has been placed on new knowledge about the pathophysiology of the sequelae of aSAH and new imaging and interventional strategies. Chapters have been included on the role of

Neurosurg Clin N Am 21 (2010) xiii–xiv
doi:10.1016/j.nec.2009.10.001
1042-3680/10/$ – see front matter © 2010 Elsevier Inc. All rights reserved.

inflammation on vasospasm, as well as a review on proteomic research and how it has contributed to the understanding of the sequelae of aSAH with the intent of educating the reader about new direction in research. Chapters have been included outlining advances in endovascular and surgical techniques applied to the care of aSAH.

We hope this issue will provide a complete assessment of progress in the neurosurgical management of aSAH that is both timely and up to date. The care of these patients can be quite challenging, and we hope this addition enables the reader to apply current concepts to care for this interesting and challenging group of patients.

We wish to thank all of our colleagues in the field of neurosurgery, interventional neuroradiology and critical care neurology who made this manuscript possible. It is through their academic dedication and hard work that we were able to complete this edition of *Neurosurgery Clinics*. In addition, we would like to thank Ruth Malwitz for her expert editorial skills, administrative efficiency, and good humor. We would also like to thank the publishers at WB Saunders/Elsevier for their support and interest in producing this volume.

Paul Nyquist, MD, MPH
Departments of Neurology
Anesthesiology/Critical Care Medicine
and Neurosurgery
Johns Hopkins School of Medicine
600 North Wolfe Street, Meyer 8-140
Baltimore, MD 21287, USA

Neeraj Naval, MD
Neurosciences ICU
Oregon Health & Science University (OHSU)
3181 SW Sam Jackson Park Road
CR-127
Portland, OR 97239-3098, USA

Rafael J. Tamargo, MD
Department of Neurosurgery
The Johns Hopkins Hospital
600 North Wolfe Street
Meyer Building, Suite 8-181
Baltimore, MD 21287, USA

E-mail addresses:
pnyquis1@jhmi.edu (P. Nyquist)
naval@ohsu.edu (N. Naval)
rtamarg@jhmi.edu (R.J. Tamargo)

Epidemiology of Aneurysmal Subarachnoid Hemorrhage

Brad E. Zacharia, MD*, Zachary L. Hickman, MD,
Bartosz T. Grobelny, BA, Peter DeRosa, BS,
Ivan Kotchetkov, BA, Andrew F. Ducruet, MD,
E. Sander Connolly Jr, MD

KEYWORDS

- Subarachnoid hemorrhage • Aneurysm
- Epidemiology • Stroke

Subarachnoid hemorrhage (SAH) is a devastating stroke subtype, which frequently occurs as the result of a ruptured intracranial aneurysm. Although it accounts for a small percentage of strokes overall, the resultant morbidity and mortality is substantial. This article serves to provide an up-to-date review of the epidemiology of aneurysmal SAH (aSAH), providing a framework for future clinical studies aimed at ameliorating the burden of this neurologic disease.

INCIDENCE

Spontaneous (nontraumatic) SAH most commonly is the result of aneurysmal rupture. Ruptured intracranial aneurysms account for approximately 75% to 80% of spontaneous SAH.[1] Overall, its incidence is between 6 and 8 per 100,000 persons per annum in most Western civilizations.[2,3] There is estimated to be between 16,000 and 30,000 new cases of aSAH in the United States annually.[4,5] Wide variations in aSAH incidence are observed between study populations, with rates reported to be as low as 2.2 per 100,000 persons per annum in China[6] and as high as 33 to 37 per 100,000 persons per annum in Finland[7,8] While the incidence of aSAH has remained relatively constant for the past 4 decades,[3,9] some studies have suggested that the actual incidence of aSAH is significantly higher secondary to misdiagnosis, death before hospital admission, or lack of autopsy in the general population.[10–16] Although developing countries have traditionally had a low burden of disease from aSAH, trends now indicate an increasing prevalence in these countries and a switch from medical problems dominated by infectious diseases to vascular and age-related diseases typically associated with western countries.[17] Overall, however, the epidemiology of aSAH seems to be similar in both developed and developing countries.[17]

PRESENTATION

Sudden onset of worst headache of life often signals a catastrophic event and is associated with high suspicion for aSAH. However, only 25% of individuals with severe, acute, paroxysmal headache actually have aSAH.[18] Other possibilities include benign thunderclap headaches and benign orgasmic cephalgia, both of which do not have subarachnoid blood on computed tomographic (CT) imaging or lumbar puncture. Benign thunderclap headaches may present similarly to SAH, with emesis in approximately 50% of patients, as well as occasional transient focal

Department of Neurological Surgery, Columbia University Medical Center, 630 West 168th Street, P&S Building 5-454, New York, NY 10032, USA
* Corresponding author.
E-mail address: bez2103@columbia.edu

deficits.[19] Benign orgasmic cephalgia is a severe headache with onset just before or at the time of orgasm,[1] and has a strong association with a family history of migraines.[20] Less severe headaches may also mimic major intracranial aneurysm rupture. Sentinel headaches, which are similar in character to the classic aSAH headache, precede 30% to 60% of aSAH and usually resolve within 24 hours. Sentinel headaches might reflect a minor hemorrhage, aneurysmal enlargement, or a hemorrhage confined to the aneurysm wall.[21] Additional signs and symptoms are myriad and may include emesis, syncope, meningismus, and photophobia. The first presentation of such a severe headache should, and often does, prompt a workup for aSAH as this diagnosis carries substantial morbidity and mortality and must be ruled out.

The 2 most frequently used clinical aSAH grading scales by which patients are initially evaluated are the Hunt and Hess[22] and the World Federation of Neurologic Surgeons (WFNS) grading scales, the latter largely using the Glasgow Coma Scale (GCS).[23] Both scales are designed to aid in the prognosis of aSAH patients based on the initial clinical presentation. A study of 235 aneurysmal SAH patients using the Hunt-Hess grading scale found that approximately half of the patients enrolled (105 of 235, 44.7%) presented with less severe grades (I–II).[24] In a study of SAH in neurosurgical units in the United Kingdom and Ireland, the majority of the patients (59.0%) presented with the least severe WFNS grade, Grade I.[25] The next most frequent grade was Grade II. This distribution was confirmed during the International Subarachnoid Aneurysm Trial (ISAT), though this reflected aneurysms that were deemed appropriate for either neurosurgical or endovascular treatment.[26]

RISK FACTORS

Modifiable and nonmodifiable risk factors play an important role in aneurysmal subarachnoid hemorrhage epidemiology. The prevalence of risk factors for aSAH and the ability to address those risk factors may contribute to the wide variation in disease burden of aSAH between regions.[17,27]

Nonmodifiable Risk Factors

Age
The incidence of aSAH increases with age to a peak in the fifth and sixth decades of life.[6] Thereafter, the incidence has been shown to plateau or even decrease slightly with further aging.[6]

Gender
Differences in the incidence of aSAH between genders have also been consistently noted, with aSAH disproportionally affecting women.[28] In a prospective study of aSAH in Texas between 2000 and 2006, women were found to have an age-adjusted risk ratio of 1.74 compared with men.[29] A review of international studies between 1950 and 2005 reported an aSAH incidence in women 1.24 times greater than that observed in men and demonstrated that this difference in incidence began at age 55 and increased thereafter.[30] Studies have also suggested that a relationship exists between hormonal status and development of aSAH. A Japanese study of 124 women, age 30 to 79 years with first occurrence of spontaneous aSAH, found that several factors, including earlier age of menarche (adjusted odds ratio [OR] 3.24), and nulliparity (adjusted OR 4.23), were associated with an increased risk of aSAH. These effects appeared to be additive, and women with both early menarche and null gravidity, had correspondingly increased risk (adjusted OR 6.37).[31]

Ethnicity
Disparities in the incidence of aSAH between ethnic groups has also been recognized in several studies.[32–34] It has been suggested that African Americans in the United States are more likely to suffer from SAH than Caucasians.[35,36] In addition, a study of 27,334 persons presenting with SAH in the United States between 1995 and 1998 found that all minorities had increased risk of aSAH compared with the Caucasian population.[35] These differences were observed in both men and women, with the highest incidence of SAH occurring in Asian/Pacific Islander males. Furthermore, the impact of several other risk factors has been shown to be heterogeneous across different ethnicities.[37]

Family history
In many study populations, across all geographic regions, family history of aSAH has consistently been shown to be one of the strongest predictors of aSAH.[6] Only recently have the genetic underpinnings of this association been explored on a genome-wide basis.[38–41] A review of 10 genome-wide linkage studies of intracranial aneurysms found that only 4 of the identified loci were replicated in different populations[42] In a recent study of a large Caucasian family (n = 35) in the U.S. with familial aggregation of intracranial aneurysms, 250,000 single nucleotide polymorphisms (SNPs) were screened and a possible susceptibility locus was located on chromosome 13q. A similar approach in a large Dutch family with

a high prevalence of intracranial aneurysms found 2 potential susceptibility loci at 1p36 and Xp22.[39] These studies have identified possible target mutations; however, most associations to date have been found in noncoding regions of DNA. More specific loci have also been identified in recent genetic studies, including a SNP in exon 7 of the endothelial nitric oxide synthase gene, G894T, which may be a risk factor for intracranial aneurysm rupture.[38]

Aneurysm location

In a series of 245 consecutive aSAH patients Forget and colleagues[43] demonstrated that the most frequent site of aneurysm rupture was the anterior communicating artery (ACoA, 29.0%). The next most common locations of aneurysm rupture were the posterior communicating artery (PCoA, 19.6%), the basilar artery (14.7%), and the middle cerebral artery (MCA, 11.8%). ISAT provides the largest multicenter series of aSAH patients (n = 2143).[26] Although not a random sample, one can appreciate general trends from this trial. As in the study by Forget and colleagues,[43] the aneurysm location with the highest frequency of rupture was the ACoA. About half of ruptured ACoA aneurysms were midline with the remainder evenly distributed between origins on the right or left side of the ACoA. In addition, ISAT confirmed the high prevalence of ruptured PCoA and MCA aneurysms, but due to the trial's exclusion criteria, there was also a much smaller proportion of posterior circulation aneurysms represented in ISAT than found in natural history studies. Of note, ISAT data also demonstrated differences in laterality of rupture based on aneurysm location.[26] Overall, the ratio of right- to left-sided ruptured anterior circulation aneurysms was 1.24. For MCA and PCoA aneurysms this ratio was 1.40 and 1.55, respectively, whereas for internal carotid artery (ICA) bifurcation aneurysms the laterality was reversed with a ratio of 0.76.

These observations alone, however, are not sufficient to differentiate between whether intracranial aneurysms at specific locations are more prone to rupture or rather if the prevalence of aSAH relative to location reflects the tendency of specific locations in the intracranial circulation to have varying predilections for aneurysm formation. The International Study of Unruptured Intracranial Aneurysms II (ISUIA-II) has helped to shed light on this question. In this study, 4,600 patients with unruptured aneurysms were reported,[44] with ICA aneurysms (excluding the cavernous ICA and PCoA) being the most frequent (29.9%),

followed closely by MCA aneurysms (29.1%). Locations that are most commonly represented amongst ruptured aneurysms, ACoA and PCoA, were third and fourth in incidence, respectively, with 12.3% and 8.5% of the total. Thus, it seems that there is a higher rate of rupture of ACoA and PCoA aneurysms compared with aneurysms of the ICA and MCA, which likely form more frequently. ISUIA also reported a higher rupture rate for a combined group of PCoA and posterior circulation aneurysms, compared with a group that combined ACA, ICA, and MCA aneurysms. It is important to keep in mind that based on the study design, ISUIA data is likely biased toward lower risk lesions, as subjects were those patients who were enrolled after the recommendation of conservative management. Similar results were reported by Juvela and colleagues,[45] in which 181 patients with unruptured aneurysms were prospectively followed in a time when the investigators exclusively recommended conservative management for unruptured aneurysms.

Aneurysm size

Aneurysm size is often felt to be the most significant factor for aneurysm rupture and is generally accepted that the likelihood of aneurysmal rupture increases linearly with the cross-sectional diameter of the aneurysm.[45] However, this does not mean that the natural history of small aneurysms is benign. The International Study of Unruptured Intracranial Aneurysms (ISUIA) reported that in patients with no prior history of SAH, aneurysms less than 10 mm in size carry a very low (0.05%) annual risk of rupture; however, this finding was greeted in the neurosurgical community with much criticism, particularly because the ISUIA inclusion criteria a priori placed patients in a low-risk category.[46] Conversely, Forget and colleagues, found that 210 of 245 (85.7%) consecutive aSAH patients presented with aneurysms smaller than 10 mm. The majority (50.6%) of ruptured aneurysms in their study were 6 to 10 mm in size, and accounted for the largest percentage of ruptured aneurysm in all intracranial locations, except for the superior cerebellar (SCA) and posterior inferior cerebellar (PICA) arteries, For these 2 locations, the majority of ruptured aneurysms were less than 5 mm in size. A study by Langham and colleagues[25] also confirmed that the majority of patients (67.3%) presenting with SAH had aneurysms that were less than 10 mm in size. Findings by Juvela and colleagues[45] further support the assertion that even small aneurysms may pose a significant risk for SAH, with a 1.1% and 2.3% yearly rupture risk for aneurysms 2 to 6 mm and 6 to 9 mm in size, respectively.

Modifiable Risk Factors

Hypertension

Chronically elevated systolic blood pressure (SBP) has been shown to be a strong predictor of intracranial aneurysm rupture. In a recent publication from the Nord-Trøndelag Health (HUNT) study, a large population-based study from in Norway, both mild (SBP 130–139 mm Hg) and severe (SBP >170 mm Hg) chronic elevations of systolic blood pressure were associated with an increased risk of aSAH in the 22-year follow-up period compared with those with SBP of less than 130 mm Hg (hazard ratios of 2.3 and 3.3, respectively).[47] In a Japanese multicenter case control study, a history of hypertension was found to be associated have an increased risk of aSAH, with an OR of 2.65 compared with controls.[48] In 1996, a review of 9 longitudinal and 11 case control studies identified preexisting hypertension as a significant risk factor for the development of SAH, with a relative risk of 2.8 (for longitudinal studies; 95% confidence interval [CI], 2.1–3.6) and an OR of 2.9 (for case control studies; 95% CI 2.4–3.7).[49] Diurnal variations in blood pressure have also been associated with risk of aSAH.[50]

Body mass index

Of note, lower body mass index (BMI) has been reported to be associated with a higher risk of aSAH. A large Finnish population study found a relative risk of 18.3 for lean, hypertensive, smokers compared with matched controls, whereas in the HUNT study, overweight (BMI 25–29.9) and obese (BMI ≥30.0) individuals had a lower risk of developing aSAH during the follow-up period, with hazard ratios of 0.6 and 0.7, respectively, compared with those with a BMI of 18.5 to 24.9.[47]

Tobacco use

Current smoking and a previous history of smoking have both been shown to be important independent risk factors for aSAH.[5,51–56] In the HUNT study, compared with those who had never smoked, former smokers had a hazard ratio of 2.7 (95% CI 1.4–5.1) and current smokers had a hazard ratio of 6.1 (95% CI 3.6–10.4) for development of aSAH.[47] In addition, recent evidence from a study involving 17 hospitals in Cincinnati suggests a gene-environment interaction with smoking. Compared with nonsmokers with no family history of aSAH, current smokers both with and without a positive family history had an increased risk of aSAH (OR 6.4, 95% CI 2.2–4.4; and OR 3.1, 95% CI 3.1–13.2, respectively).[57] Furthermore, differences in susceptibility to the harmful effects of smoking have been noted between ethnicities. Therefore the differences in

incidence of aSAH between ethnic groups may in part be due to the differential effects of smoking.[37] In a study of 120 consecutive SAH patients in Sweden, the relative risk for SAH was approximately 2.5 times greater in smokers compared with the general population, but not elevated in patients who used smokeless tobacco, indicating that nicotine is unlikely to represent the main agent leading to increased SAH risk from tobacco use.[58]

Other risk factors

Recreational cocaine use in within the previous 3 days has been shown to confer an increased risk of SAH (OR 24.97, 95% CI 3.95–∞) in young patients (age 18–49 years).[59] It is possible, however, that undiagnosed, pre-existing vascular malformations may contribute to the increased risk in this population. High daily coffee consumption (>5 cups per day) was also found to be associated with an increased risk of SAH in the Tromso study (OR 3.86, 95% CI 1.01–14.73).[54]

DIAGNOSIS

The evaluation of the patient with symptoms suggestive of SAH begins with confirmation of the presence of subarachnoid blood. This confirmation is primarily accomplished with a noncontrast CT scan, which in the first 12 hours after SAH has a 98% to 100% sensitivity for SAH. This number drops to 93% at 24 hours after SAH, and[60–64] after 6 days decreases further to 57% to 85%.[65,66] In the setting of suggestive symptomatology a negative CT scan should be followed up with a lumbar puncture and analysis of the cerebrospinal fluid for xanthochromia.[67]

The gold standard for evaluation of cerebral aneurysms remains digital subtraction angiography, which demonstrates the source of SAH in approximately 85% of patients. Two less invasive modalities are increasingly being used, magnetic resonance angiography (MRA) and CT angiography. Three-dimensional time of flight MRA has a sensitivity to detect cerebral aneurysms is between 55% and 93%.[68–71] Dichotomizing by size, the sensitivity is 85% to 100% for aneurysms 5 mm or greater, but only 56% for those less than 5 mm in size.[68,70,72,73] CT angiography, however, is the more frequently used noninvasive modality, as it is faster and more readily available. In addition, it has a sensitivity for aneurysms between 77% and 100% and a specificity between 79% and 100%.[74–80]

Nontraumatic Nonaneurysmal Subarachnoid Hemorrhage

One can broadly classify SAH into traumatic and nontraumatic etiologies. Trauma is the most common cause of SAH.[81,82] SAH has been cited as occurring in up to 60% of traumatic brain injury patients,[83] a population with an incidence of approximately 540 per 100,000 in the United States.[84] The pattern of hemorrhage, associated injuries, and clinical history often make this diagnosis readily apparent.

Nontraumatic SAH may also occur in patients not harboring intracranial aneurysms. Perimesencephalic SAH is defined by a relatively distinct radiographic pattern, with hemorrhage centered anterior to the midbrain or pons, with or without extension of blood around the brainstem, into the suprasellar cistern, or into the proximal Sylvian fissures.[85] A negative 4-vessel cerebral angiogram confirms the diagnosis. Nontraumatic SAH has an incidence rate of 0.5 persons per 100,000 in adults.[86] These patients tend to less likely be female, hypertensive, or of older age than aSAH patients.[86] Diffuse, angiographic negative SAH that does not fit the perimesencephalic distribution of blood is thought to be a distinct entity with an incidence rate approximately twice as high as perimesencephalic SAH, and a higher incidence of complications such as hydrocephalus and vasospasm as well as the need for cerebrospinal fluid shunting and frequency of poor outcomes.[87]

Additional possibilities include arteriovenous malformations, vasculitis, tumor, cerebral artery dissection, rupture of a small superficial artery, coagulation disorder, sickle cell disease, rupture of an infundibulum, and pituitary apoplexy.[1] However, no cause can be determined in 14% to 22% of nontraumatic SAH.[1]

TREATMENT

Treatment of SAH requires a multifaceted, collaborative team approach. In addition to acute neurologic concerns aSAH patients are medically ill and require intensive management. Following medical stabilization the primary concern is rebleeding of the ruptured aneurysm, a fact that has resulted in a shift toward early definitive management by either surgical or endovascular means. Of the aforementioned methods of treatment, clipping has long been the mainstay of neurosurgical treatment of aneurysms since it was first performed in 1937. Coiling, on the other hand, is a relatively new development with the Gugliemi detachable coil becoming approved by the Food and Drug Administration in 1995. Since that time, coiling has been gaining popularity, particularly after the publication of the ISAT trial, which revealed a potential benefit of endovascular coiling over clipping for specific ruptured aneurysms.[88]

A longitudinal study by Andaluz and Zuccarello documented these treatment trends using the National Inpatient Sample between 1993 and 2003.[89] These investigators found that while the number of discharges for surgical clip placement has stayed relatively constant over these 10 years, the number of discharges for endovascular treatment has steadily increased. In 1993 both treatments had approximately 12,000 discharges, whereas in 2003 the number of discharges with endovascular treatment (24,638) was approximately double that of surgical clip placement (12,626). The fraction of patients receiving endovascular treatment, however, varies widely between centers. Regardless of center preference, endovascular techniques tend to be the preferred approach for posterior circulation aneurysms, which can be difficult to treat surgically.

There also exists a population of patients with SAH who do not undergo any definitive treatment to secure their aneurysm. An analysis of patients in the United Kingdom and Ireland found that 199 (8.3%) of 2397 patients admitted with SAH over a year did not undergo surgical repair.[25] These patients tended to be older, be of a higher WFNS Grade, have more blood on their CT scans, have larger aneurysms, have more aneurysms in the posterior circulation, have more concurrent medical conditions on admission, and have more frequent prerepair deterioration.

OUTCOME
General Trends and Grading

Over the past 2 decades, mortality following SAH has decreased dramatically.[90] Previous death rates consistently occurred in a range around 50%,[2,8] whereas more recently they have been found in the 10%[91] to 24% range.[89] These reductions likely stem from advances in multiple aspects of SAH management, including improved diagnostic capabilities, aggressive neurocritical care management, and use of modern microsurgical and endovascular instruments and techniques.[26]

The 3 SAH-specific scales most widely used for classifying clinical presentation of SAH patients are the Hunt and Hess (H&H) Scale, the WFNS Scale, and the Fisher Scale.[92] The H&H Scale was designed to gauge surgical risk of admitted SAH patients by evaluating intensity of meningeal inflammatory reaction, severity of neurologic deficit, and level of arousal. Gradation of the scale is 1 to 5, with 1 representing a nearly asymptomatic state and 5 denoting a deep moribund coma.[22] There is evidence that differences between each H&H grade may not correlate with a unique outcome,[93,94] but dichotomizing the scale has demonstrated that a good H&H grade (1 to 3) predicts a better outcome than a high H&H grade (4 and 5). In a series of 230 patients, 19% of good grade H&H patients had an unfavorable outcome compared with 90% of poor grade patients.[95] A later study showed that H&H grades of 4 and 5 had 4.87 times greater odds of unfavorable outcome compared with grades 1 to 3 (95% CI 2.57–9.21; P<.001).[96]

The WFNS Scale, developed in 1988, is also a 5-grade system, but is based on the GCS and is designed to acknowledge the significance of a focal neurologic deficit. Higher grades on the WFNS Scale indicate worse clinical presentation of SAH.[97] The predictive value of this scale has been repeatedly called into question because widely varying outcomes have been observed in patients presenting with the same grade.[98] Some investigations have even failed to predict any difference in outcome among adjacent WFNS grades when assessing patients with Glasgow Outcome Scale (GOS) at 1 month after discharge.[99] In contrast to this, a large study of approximately 3500 SAH cases evaluated patients with the GOS at 3 months following SAH and found that the likelihood ratio of a poor outcome varied linearly with increasing WFNS: WFNS grade 1 = 0.36, WFNS grade 2 = 0.61, WFNS grade 3 = 1.78, WFNS grade 4 = 2.47, and WFNS grade 5 = 5.22.[100]

The Fisher Scale is a radiographically defined score primarily concerned with predicting cerebral vasospasm after SAH. A grade of 1 to 4 is assigned depending on the amount of blood visible on CT imaging and presence of intracerebral or intraventricular clot.[101] Fisher grade 3 is associated with the highest incidence of clinical vasospasm. Although the scale has been used to predict outcome (for scores of 3 or 4, relative risk of poor outcome >4),[102] it is not considered to be comprehensive enough to be used as a primary grading system for SAH.[92]

Several other diagnostic factors on admission have been shown to correlate with outcome following SAH. Specific portions of the GCS can be strong predictors of outcome. In poor grade SAH patients (H&H Grades 4 and 5), an additional point on the GCS motor examination at admission predicted a 1.8-fold increase in the odds of achieving a favorable long-term outcome as defined by a mRS score of 3 or less (95% CI 1.4–2.3). At discharge, an additional point in the eye examination was associated with a 3.1-fold increase in favorable outcome (95% CI 1.8–5.4).[103] In another study, pupillary reactivity at admission predicted a 6.44 increase in the odds of favorable outcome at 12 months (P = .008) in a population of 204 poor grade patients.[104]

The modified Rankin scale (mRS) is an instrument frequently used for outcome assessment following SAH, and the scale is often dichotomized such that scores of 0 to 3 represent a favorable outcome with functional independence, whereas scores of 4 to 6 report a poor outcome with loss of a patient's functional independence.[105] The GOS is a second important measure of outcome composed of 5 points that reflect the following states: death, persistent vegetative state, severe disability, moderate disability, and good recovery.[106]

Rebleeding, Timing of Intervention, and Vasospasm

Rebleeding is the major cause of death in patients who survive the initial hemorrhage but do not undergo surgical intervention.[2,107,108] In untreated SAH, the greatest risk of rebleeding occurs on the first day (4%), with a daily frequency of 1.5% until 13 days. By 2 weeks, the rebleed rate is 15% to 20%, and up to 50% by 6 months.[108] The goal of surgical and endovascular treatment is to prevent this occurrence, and since the 1980s there has been a shift toward early intervention.[90]

Although the timing of intervention is still a source of debate,[109] there are substantial efforts being made to carry out early management protocols[90] on account of broad-based support for their implementation garnered through favorable outcome data.[109–112] In the pursuit of early intervention, there is a widely recognized trade-off between early surgical risk of operative mortality and the benefits it confers in terms of rebleeding prevention. No outcome difference has previously been found between intervention at 0 to 3 days after the original bleed versus 11 to 14 days, but outcomes were definitively worse in the 7- to 10-day interval.[111] Subsequent studies and meta-analyses have argued that the benefits derived from reduction of rebleeding seem to outweigh the risks of early intervention.[109,110,112]

In the current context, the rate of rebleeding is near 7% when pre-hospital events are excluded,[113] although several studies refer to a 10% to 20% incidence of "ultra-early" rebleeds by taking into account events that occur before patients receive neurosurgical attention.[114–117] Overall, rebleed events in the first day are associated with a drastically reduced chance of survival with functional independence at 3 months (mRS score, ≤4; OR 0.08; 95% CI 0.02–0.34).[113]

Ischemic neurologic deterioration secondary to cerebral vasospasm represents another major cause of morbidity after SAH.[118,119] On average, symptomatic vasospasm occurs in 20% to 30%

of patients, but vasospasm can be identified by arteriogram in 30% to 70% of patients with SAH, resulting in observed infarction in 10% to 45% of patients.[119–124] For compounds that attempt to mitigate the effects of vasospasm, class I evidence has been obtained only in demonstrating the beneficial effects of the calcium channel blocker nimodipine. Although this medication does not alter radiographic vasospasm,[125] it does improve the odds of favorable outcome to 1.86:1 ($P<.005$).[126]

Age, Gender, and Race

Patient age is strongly associated with worse outcome following SAH. In a study of 409 patients undergoing craniotomy for SAH, the investigators found that increased age correlated with significantly worse outcome such that a patient older than 63 years was at a 30-times greater risk for a poor outcome (GOS scores 1–3) than a patient aged 43 to 52 years.[102] Less drastically, a study of 98 patients treated for SAH demonstrated that those who were 65 years or older fared significantly worse than younger patients on mRS outcome measures (hazard ratio 6.6; 95% CI 1.8–24.1; $P<.001$).[127] Despite a higher mortality rate for elderly SAH patients, Stachniak and colleagues[128] determined that quality of life (QOL) scores appeared acceptable for elderly survivors of SAH, suggesting that surgery need not be ruled out as an option for this population.

Mortality rates for female SAH patients have been reported to be higher than those for males.[129–131] In an analysis of national death certificate data of SAH (n = 27,334) from 1995 to 1998, women had a higher death rate compared with men following SAH (4.9% versus 3.1%; Rate Ratio = 1.58; 95% CI 1.54–1.62).[129] Although there exists a significant difference in mortality among men and women, gender has not been found to predict severity of presentation, outcome, or survival following SAH.[132,133] In a trial for high-dose intravenous nicardipine, after adjustment for age, no difference was observed between women and men in terms of favorable outcomes at 3 months as measured by the GOS (69.7% for women versus 73.4% for men, P = .243; n = 565 women and 320 men).[133] Thus, some investigators conclude that higher death rates in women may simply be the result of higher SAH incidence among females.[134]

Although there exist variations in incidence and presentation of SAH among racial groups, the same cannot be concluded about differences in outcome, as several studies have shown no relation between outcome and race.[29,94,128,135–137] In a 1970 study of SAH patients (n = 319) selected from a 20% systematic sample of hospital veterans, there were no racial differences in terms of survival after SAH.[137] A retrospective case series from a single-center study of patients (1971–1976) similarly reports that race was not associated with adverse events in surgery.[136] Although these 2 studies were conducted before the establishment of current guidelines for early treatment of SAH, subsequent and more recent work corroborates their conclusions.

In an analysis of 107 patients prospectively identified from 2000 to 2006 in the Brain Attack Surveillance in Corpus Christi Project, no ethnic difference in outcome or discharge was found between whites and Mexican Americans.[29] Likewise, a prospective/retrospective case series of patients undergoing craniotomy for clipping of ruptured aneurysms (n = 219, recruited from 1989 to 1994), demonstrated no racial difference in QOL score after clipping for SAH.[128] Lastly, a retrospective study of prospectively collected data for a randomized-control trial of tirilazad in SAH patients (1991–1997) found no difference in 3-month outcome as measured by GOS.[94] A retrospective case series of cranial surgery among Medicare beneficiaries, however, demonstrated that black SAH patients had a longer length of hospital stay than the average SAH patient (12.2 days versus average 9.6 days, P = .001).[138] Interpretation of these results is inherently limited as only 5.7% of the study subjects were diagnosed with SAH (2526 SAH cases of 44,078 enrolled patients), while the stated results are for all cranial surgeries. The preponderance of studies that report a lack of association between race and outcome, coupled with the consistency of that observation before and after the shift to early treatment guidelines, would suggest that outcome following SAH is largely unaffected by race.

Other Prognostic Indicators

Hospitals with a high volume of SAH admissions generate better treatment outcomes for SAH than do low-volume hospitals.[89,139–144] In a large-sample study that examined 16,399 hospitalizations for SAH from 18 states in the US, patients who were treated in hospitals that see a low volume of SAH had 1.4 times the odds of dying in the hospital (95% CI 1.2–1.6) as patients admitted to high-volume hospitals.[142] Larger hospital size seems to be associated with lower mortality rates especially in patients who undergo aneurysm clipping ($P<.01$).[89] In New York state hospitals, those treatment centers that performed more than 30 craniotomies per year reported a 43% (95% CI 29%–57%) lower mortality rate for SAH patients compared with hospitals performing less surgery.[144] Furthermore, country or continent has no bearing on outcome after SAH,[145] and outcome is unaffected by weekend versus weekday admission.[146]

SUMMARY

aSAH is a form of hemorrhagic stroke that affects up to 30,000 individuals per year in the United States. The incidence of aSAH has been shown to be associated with numerous nonmodifiable (age, gender, ethnicity, family history, aneurysm location and size) and modifiable (hypertension, BMI, tobacco and illicit drug use) risk factors. Although early repair of ruptured aneurysms and aggressive postoperative management has improved overall outcomes, it remains a devastating disease, with mortality approaching 50% and less than 60% of survivors returning to functional independence. As treatment modalities change and the percentage of minority and elderly populations increase it is critical to maintain an up-to-date understanding of subarachnoid hemorrhage epidemiology.

REFERENCES

1. Greenberg M. Handbook of neurosurgery. 6th edition. New York: Thieme; 2006.
2. Broderick J, Brott T, Tomsick T, et al. Intracerebral hemorrhage more than twice as common as subarachnoid hemorrhage. J Neurosurg 1993;78: 188.
3. Linn FH, Rinkel GJ, Algra A, et al. Incidence of subarachnoid hemorrhage: role of region, year, and rate of computed tomography: a meta-analysis. Stroke 1996;27:625.
4. Bederson JB, Connolly ES Jr, Batjer HH, et al. Guidelines for the management of aneurysmal subarachnoid hemorrhage: a statement for healthcare professionals from a special writing group of the Stroke Council, American Heart Association. Stroke 2009;40:994.
5. Kissela BM, Sauerbeck L, Woo D, et al. Subarachnoid hemorrhage: a preventable disease with a heritable component. Stroke 2002;33:1321.
6. Ingall T, Asplund K, Mahonen M, et al. A multinational comparison of subarachnoid hemorrhage epidemiology in the WHO MONICA stroke study. Stroke 2000;31:1054.
7. Knekt P, Reunanen A, Aho K, et al. Risk factors for subarachnoid hemorrhage in a longitudinal population study. J Clin Epidemiol 1991;44:933.
8. Sarti C, Tuomilehto J, Salomaa V, et al. Epidemiology of subarachnoid hemorrhage in Finland from 1983 to 1985. Stroke 1991;22:848.
9. Harmsen P, Tsipogianni A, Wilhelmsen L. Stroke incidence rates were unchanged, while fatality rates declined, during 1971–1987 in Goteborg, Sweden. Stroke 1992;23:1410.
10. Fridriksson S, Hillman J, Landtblom AM, et al. Education of referring doctors about sudden onset headache in subarachnoid hemorrhage. A prospective study. Acta Neurol Scand 2001;103:238.
11. Inagawa T, Takechi A, Yahara K, et al. Primary intracerebral and aneurysmal subarachnoid hemorrhage in Izumo City, Japan. Part I: incidence and seasonal and diurnal variations. J Neurosurg 2000;93:958.
12. Kowalski RG, Claassen J, Kreiter KT, et al. Initial misdiagnosis and outcome after subarachnoid hemorrhage. JAMA 2004;291:866.
13. Mayer PL, Awad IA, Todor R, et al. Misdiagnosis of symptomatic cerebral aneurysm. Prevalence and correlation with outcome at four institutions. Stroke 1996;27:1558.
14. Mori K, Kasuga C, Nakao Y, et al. Intracranial pseudoaneurysm due to rupture of a saccular aneurysm mimicking a large partially thrombosed aneurysm ("ghost aneurysm"): radiological findings and therapeutic implications in two cases. Neurosurg Rev 2004;27:289.
15. Polmear A. Sentinel headaches in aneurysmal subarachnoid haemorrhage: what is the true incidence? A systematic review. Cephalalgia 2003; 23:935.
16. Vannemreddy P, Nanda A, Kelley R, et al. Delayed diagnosis of intracranial aneurysms: confounding factors in clinical presentation and the influence of misdiagnosis on outcome. South Med J 2001; 94:1108.
17. Sridharan SE, Unnikrishnan JP, Sukumaran S, et al. Incidence, types, risk factors, and outcome of stroke in a developing country. The Trivandrum Stroke Registry. Stroke 2009;40:1212–8.
18. Linn FH, Wijdicks EF, van Gijn J, et al. Prospective study of sentinel headache in aneurysmal subarachnoid haemorrhage. Lancet 1994;344:590.
19. Linn FH, Rinkel GJ, Algra A, et al. Headache characteristics in subarachnoid haemorrhage and benign thunderclap headache. J Neurol Neurosurg Psychiatr 1998;65:791.
20. Lance JW. Headaches related to sexual activity. J Neurol Neurosurg Psychiatr 1976;39:1226.
21. Verweij R, Wijdicks E, van Gijn J. Warning headache in aneurysmal subarachnoid hemorrhage. A case-control study. Arch Neurol 1988;45:1019.
22. Hunt W, Hess R. Surgical risk as related to time of intervention in the repair of intracranial aneurysms. J Neurosurg 1968;28:14.

23. Report of World Federation of Neurological Surgeons Committee on a Universal Subarachnoid Hemorrhage Grading Scale. J Neurosurg 1988;68: 985.

24. Mack W, Ducruet A, Hickman Z, et al. Doppler ultrasonography screening of poor-grade subarachnoid hemorrhage patients increases the diagnosis of deep venous thrombosis. Neurol Res 2008;30:889.

25. Langham J, Reeves BC, Lindsay KW, et al. Variation in outcome after subarachnoid hemorrhage: a study of neurosurgical units in UK and Ireland. Stroke 2009;40:111.

26. Molyneux A, Kerr R, Stratton I, et al. International Subarachnoid Aneurysm Trial (ISAT) of neurosurgical clipping versus endovascular coiling in 2143 patients with ruptured intracranial aneurysms: a randomised trial. Lancet 2002;360:1267.

27. Feigin VL, Lawes CM, Bennett DA, et al. Worldwide stroke incidence and early case fatality reported in 56 population-based studies: a systematic review. Lancet Neurol 2009;8:355.

28. King JT Jr. Epidemiology of aneurysmal subarachnoid hemorrhage. Neuroimaging Clin N Am 1997;7: 659.

29. Eden SV, Meurer WJ, Sanchez BN, et al. Gender and ethnic differences in subarachnoid hemorrhage. Neurology 2008;71:731.

30. de Rooij NK, Linn FH, van der Plas JA, et al. Incidence of subarachnoid haemorrhage: a systematic review with emphasis on region, age, gender and time trends. J Neurol Neurosurg Psychiatr 2007; 78:1365.

31. Okamoto K, Horisawa R, Kawamura T, et al. Menstrual and reproductive factors for subarachnoid hemorrhage risk in women: a case-control study in Nagoya, Japan. Stroke 2001;32:2841.

32. Chong JY, Sacco RL. Epidemiology of stroke in young adults: race/ethnic differences. J Thromb Thrombolysis 2005;20:77.

33. Sacco RL, Boden-Albala B, Gan R, et al. Stroke incidence among white, black, and Hispanic residents of an urban community: the Northern Manhattan Stroke Study. Am J Epidemiol 1998; 147:259.

34. Smeeton NC, Heuschmann PU, Rudd AG, et al. Incidence of hemorrhagic stroke in black Caribbean, black African, and white populations: the South London stroke register, 1995–2004. Stroke 2007;38:3133.

35. Ayala C, Greenlund KJ, Croft JB, et al. Racial/ethnic disparities in mortality by stroke subtype in the United States, 1995–1998. Am J Epidemiol 2001;154:1057.

36. Gillum RF. Stroke mortality in blacks. Disturbing trends. Stroke 1999;30:1711.

37. Krishna V, Kim DH. Ethnic differences in risk factors for subarachnoid hemorrhage. J Neurosurg 2007; 107:522.

38. Ozum U, Bolat N, Gul E, et al. Endothelial nitric oxide synthase gene [G894T] polymorphism as a possible risk factor in aneurysmal subarachnoid haemorrhage. Acta Neurochir (Wien) 2008;150:57.

39. Ruigrok YM, Wijmenga C, Rinkel GJ, et al. Genomewide linkage in a large Dutch family with intracranial aneurysms: replication of 2 loci for intracranial aneurysms to chromosome 1p36.11-p36.13 and Xp22.2-p22.32. Stroke 2008;39:1096.

40. Santiago-Sim T, Depalma SR, Ju KL, et al. Genomewide linkage in a large Caucasian family maps a new locus for intracranial aneurysms to chromosome 13q. Stroke 2009;40:S57.

41. Zhang J, Claterbuck RE. Molecular genetics of human intracranial aneurysms. Int J Stroke 2008; 3:272.

42. Ruigrok YM, Rinkel GJ. Genetics of intracranial aneurysms. Stroke 2008;39:1049.

43. Forget TR Jr, Benitez R, Veznedaroglu E, et al. A review of size and location of ruptured intracranial aneurysms. Neurosurgery 2001;49:1322.

44. Wiebers DO. Unruptured intracranial aneurysms: natural history, clinical outcome, and risks of surgical and endovascular treatment. Lancet 2003;362:103.

45. Juvela S, Porras M, Poussa K. Natural history of unruptured intracranial aneurysms: probability of and risk factors for aneurysm rupture. J Neurosurg 2000;93:379.

46. Unruptured intracranial aneurysms—risk of rupture and risks of surgical intervention. The international study of unruptured intracranial aneurysms investigators. N Engl J Med 1998;339:1725.

47. Sandvei MS, Romundstad PR, Muller TB, et al. Risk factors for aneurysmal subarachnoid hemorrhage in a prospective population study. The HUNT study in Norway. Stroke 2009;40:1958–62.

48. Kubota M, Yamaura A, Ono J. Prevalence of risk factors for aneurysmal subarachnoid haemorrhage: results of a Japanese multicentre case control study for stroke. Br J Neurosurg 2001;15: 474.

49. Teunissen LL, Rinkel GJ, Algra A, et al. Risk factors for subarachnoid hemorrhage: a systematic review. Stroke 1996;27:544.

50. Fogelholm RR, Turjanmaa VM, Nuutila MT, et al. Diurnal blood pressure variations and onset of subarachnoid haemorrhage: a population-based study. J Hypertens 1995;13:495.

51. Clarke M. Systematic review of reviews of risk factors for intracranial aneurysms. Neuroradiology 2008;50:653.

52. Feigin V, Parag V, Lawes CM, et al. Smoking and elevated blood pressure are the most important

risk factors for subarachnoid hemorrhage in the Asia-Pacific region: an overview of 26 cohorts involving 306,620 participants. Stroke 2005;36: 1360.

53. Feigin VL, Rinkel GJ, Lawes CM, et al. Risk factors for subarachnoid hemorrhage: an updated systematic review of epidemiological studies. Stroke 2005; 36:2773.

54. Isaksen J, Egge A, Waterloo K, et al. Risk factors for aneurysmal subarachnoid haemorrhage: the Tromso study. J Neurol Neurosurg Psychiatr 2002; 73:185.

55. Kleinpeter G, Lehr S. Is hypertension a major risk factor in aneurysmal subarachnoid hemorrhage? Wien Klin Wochenschr 2002;114:307.

56. Okamoto K, Horisawa R, Ohno Y. The relationships of gender, cigarette smoking, and hypertension with the risk of aneurysmal subarachnoid hemorrhage: a case-control study in Nagoya, Japan. Ann Epidemiol 2005;15:744.

57. Woo D, Khoury J, Haverbusch MM, et al. Smoking and family history and risk of aneurysmal subarachnoid hemorrhage. Neurology 2009;72:69.

58. Koskinen LO, Blomstedt PC. Smoking and non-smoking tobacco as risk factors in subarachnoid haemorrhage. Acta Neurol Scand 2006;114:33.

59. Broderick JP, Viscoli CM, Brott T, et al. Major risk factors for aneurysmal subarachnoid hemorrhage in the young are modifiable. Stroke 2003;34: 1375.

60. Morgenstern L, Luna-Gonzales H, Huber J, et al. Worst headache and subarachnoid hemorrhage: prospective, modern computed tomography and spinal fluid analysis. Ann Emerg Med 1998;32:297.

61. Sames T, Storrow A, Finkelstein J, et al. Sensitivity of new-generation computed tomography in subarachnoid hemorrhage. Acad Emerg Med 1996;3:16.

62. Sidman R, Connolly E, Lemke T. Subarachnoid hemorrhage diagnosis: lumbar puncture is still needed when the computed tomography scan is normal. Acad Emerg Med 1996;3:827.

63. Tomasello F, d'Avela D, de Divitiis O. Does lamina terminalis fenestration reduce the incidence of chronic hydrocephalus after subarachnoid hemorrhage? Neurosurgery 1999;45:827.

64. van der Wee N, Rinkel GJ, Hasan D, et al. Detection of subarachnoid haemorrhage on early CT: is lumbar puncture still needed after a negative scan? J Neurol Neurosurg Psychiatr 1995;58:357.

65. Edlow J. Diagnosis of subarachnoid hemorrhage. Neurocrit Care 2005;2:99.

66. van Gijn J, van Dongen K. The time course of aneurysmal haemorrhage on computed tomograms. Neuroradiology 1982;23:153.

67. Cruickshank A, Auld P, Beetham R, et al. Revised national guidelines for analysis of cerebrospinal fluid for bilirubin in suspected subarachnoid haemorrhage. Ann Clin Biochem 2008;45:238.

68. Anzalone N, Triulzi F, Scotti G. Acute subarachnoid haemorrhage: 3D time-of-flight MR angiography versus intra-arterial digital angiography. Neuroradiology 1995;37:257.

69. Horikoshi T, Fukamachi A, Nishi H, et al. Detection of intracranial aneurysms by three-dimensional time-of-flight magnetic resonance angiography. Neuroradiology 1994;36:203.

70. Huston J, Nichols D, Luetmer P, et al. Blinded prospective evaluation of sensitivity of MR angiography to known intracranial aneurysms: importance of aneurysm size. AJNR Am J Neuroradiol 1994;15: 1607.

71. Schuierer G, Huk W, Laub G. Magnetic resonance angiography of intracranial aneurysms: comparison with intra-arterial digital subtraction angiography. Neuroradiology 1992;35:50.

72. Atlas S. Magnetic resonance imaging of intracranial aneurysms. Neuroimaging Clin N Am 1997;7: 709.

73. Wilcock D, Jaspan T, Holland I, et al. Comparison of magnetic resonance angiography with conventional angiography in the detection of intracranial aneurysms in patients presenting with subarachnoid haemorrhage. Clin Radiol 1996;51:330.

74. Alberico RA, Patel M, Casey S, et al. Evaluation of the circle of Willis with three-dimensional CT angiography in patients with suspected intracranial aneurysms. AJNR Am J Neuroradiol 1995;16:1571.

75. Hope JK, Wilson JL, Thomson FJ. Three-dimensional CT angiography in the detection and characterization of intracranial berry aneurysms. AJNR Am J Neuroradiol 1996;17:439.

76. Korogi Y, Takahashi M, Katada K, et al. Intracranial aneurysms: detection with three-dimensional CT angiography with volume rendering-comparison with conventional angiographic and surgical findings. Radiology 1999;211:497.

77. Liang EY, Chan M, Hsiang JH, et al. Detection and assessment of intracranial aneurysms: value of CT angiography with shaded-surface display. Am J Roentgenol 1995;165:1497.

78. Ogawa T, Okudera T, Noguchi K, et al. Cerebral aneurysms: evaluation with three-dimensional CT angiography. AJNR Am J Neuroradiol 1996;17: 447.

79. Vieco P, Shuman W, Alsofrom G, et al. Detection of circle of Willis aneurysms in patients with acute subarachnoid hemorrhage: a comparison of CT angiography and digital subtraction angiography. Am J Roentgenol 1995;165:425.

80. Wilms G, Guffens M, Gryspeerdt S, et al. Spiral CT of intracranial aneurysms: correlation with digital subtraction and magnetic resonance angiography. Neuroradiology 1996;38:S20.

81. Greene K, Marciano F, Johnson B, et al. Impact of traumatic subarachnoid hemorrhage on outcome in nonpenetrating head injury. Part I: a proposed computerized tomography grading scale. J Neurosurg 1995;83:445.

82. Taneda M, Kataoka K, Akai F, et al. Traumatic subarachnoid hemorrhage as a predictable indicator of delayed ischemic symptoms. J Neurosurg 1996;84:762.

83. Morris G, Bullock R, Marshall S, et al. Failure of the competitive N-methyl-D-aspartate antagonist Selfotel (CGS 19755) in the treatment of severe head injury: results of two phase III clinical trials. J Neurosurg 1999;91:737.

84. Rutland-Brown W, Langlois JA, Thomas KE, et al. Incidence of traumatic brain injury in the United States, 2003. J Head Trauma Rehabil 2006;21:544.

85. Schwartz TH, Solomon RA. Perimesencephalic nonaneurysmal subarachnoid hemorrhage: review of the literature. Neurosurgery 1996;39:433.

86. Flaherty M, Haverbusch M, Kissela B, et al. Perimesencephalic subarachnoid hemorrhage: incidence, risk factors, and outcome. J Stroke Cerebrovasc Dis 2005;14:267.

87. Hui F, Tumialán L, Tanaka T, et al. Clinical differences between angiographically negative, diffuse subarachnoid hemorrhage and perimesencephalic subarachnoid hemorrhage. Neurocrit Care 2009;11(1):64–70.

88. Molyneux AJ, Kerr RS, Yu LM, et al. International subarachnoid aneurysm trial (ISAT) of neurosurgical clipping versus endovascular coiling in 2143 patients with ruptured intracranial aneurysms: a randomised comparison of effects on survival, dependency, seizures, rebleeding, subgroups, and aneurysm occlusion. Lancet 2005;366:809.

89. Andaluz N, Zuccarello M. Recent trends in the treatment of cerebral aneurysms: analysis of a nationwide inpatient database. J Neurosurg 2008;108:1163.

90. Komotar RJ, Schmidt JM, Starke RM, et al. Resuscitation and critical care of poor-grade subarachnoid hemorrhage. Neurosurgery 2009;64:397.

91. Molyneux AJ, Kerr RS, Birks J, et al. Risk of recurrent subarachnoid haemorrhage, death, or dependence and standardised mortality ratios after clipping or coiling of an intracranial aneurysm in the International Subarachnoid Aneurysm Trial (ISAT): long-term follow-up. Lancet Neurol 2009;8:427–33.

92. Rosen DS, Macdonald RL. Subarachnoid hemorrhage grading scales: a systematic review. Neurocrit Care 2005;2:110.

93. Oshiro EM, Walter KA, Piantadosi S, et al. A new subarachnoid hemorrhage grading system based on the Glasgow Coma Scale: a comparison with the Hunt and Hess and World Federation of Neurological Surgeons Scales in a clinical series. Neurosurgery 1997;41:140.

94. Rosen D, Novakovic R, Goldenberg FD, et al. Racial differences in demographics, acute complications, and outcomes in patients with subarachnoid hemorrhage: a large patient series. J Neurosurg 2005;103:18.

95. Proust F, Hannequin D, Langlois O, et al. Causes of morbidity and mortality after ruptured aneurysm surgery in a series of 230 patients. The importance of control angiography. Stroke 1995;26:1553.

96. Ogilvy CS, Cheung AC, Mitha AP, et al. Outcomes for surgical and endovascular management of intracranial aneurysms using a comprehensive grading system. Neurosurgery 2006;59:1037.

97. Teasdale GM, Drake CG, Hunt W, et al. A universal subarachnoid hemorrhage scale: report of a committee of the World Federation of Neurosurgical Societies. J Neurol Neurosurg Psychiatr 1988;51:1457.

98. Takagi K, Tamura A, Nakagomi T, et al. How should a subarachnoid hemorrhage grading scale be determined? A combinatorial approach based solely on the Glasgow Coma Scale. J Neurosurg 1999;90:680.

99. Lagares A, Gomez PA, Lobato RD, et al. Prognostic factors on hospital admission after spontaneous subarachnoid haemorrhage. Acta Neurochir (Wien) 2001;143:665.

100. Rosen DS, Macdonald RL. Grading of subarachnoid hemorrhage: modification of the World Federation of Neurosurgical Societies scale on the basis of data for a large series of patients. Neurosurgery 2004;54:566.

101. Fisher CM, Kistler JP, Davis JM. Relation of cerebral vasospasm to subarachnoid hemorrhage visualized by computerized tomographic scanning. Neurosurgery 1980;6:1.

102. Ogilvy CS, Carter BS. A proposed comprehensive grading system to predict outcome for surgical management of intracranial aneurysms. Neurosurgery 1998;42:959.

103. Starke RM, Komotar RJ, Otten ML, et al. Predicting long-term outcome in poor grade aneurysmal subarachnoid haemorrhage patients utilising the Glasgow Coma Scale. J Clin Neurosci 2009;16:26.

104. Mack WJ, Hickman ZL, Ducruet AF, et al. Pupillary reactivity upon hospital admission predicts long-term outcome in poor grade aneurysmal subarachnoid hemorrhage patients. Neurocrit Care 2008;8:374.

105. Rankin J. Cerebral vascular accidents in patients over the age of 60. III. Diagnosis and treatment. Scott Med J 1957;2:254.

106. Jennett B, Bond M. Assessment of outcome after severe brain damage. Lancet 1975;1:480.

107. Kassell NF, Torner JC. Aneurysmal rebleeding: a preliminary report from the Cooperative Aneurysm Study. Neurosurgery 1983;13:479.

108. Winn HR, Richardson AE, Jane JA. The long-term prognosis in untreated cerebral aneurysms: I. The incidence of late hemorrhage in cerebral aneurysm: a 10-year evaluation of 364 patients. Ann Neurol 1977;1:358.

109. van der Jagt M, Hasan D, Dippel DW, et al. Impact of early surgery after aneurysmal subarachnoid haemorrhage. Acta Neurol Scand 2009;119:100.

110. de Gans K, Nieuwkamp DJ, Rinkel GJ, et al. Timing of aneurysm surgery in subarachnoid hemorrhage: a systematic review of the literature. Neurosurgery 2002;50:336.

111. Kassell NF, Torner JC, Jane JA, et al. The International Cooperative Study on the timing of aneurysm surgery. Part 2: surgical results. J Neurosurg 1990; 73:37.

112. Milhorat TH, Krautheim M. Results of early and delayed operations for ruptured intracranial aneurysms in two series of 100 consecutive patients. Surg Neurol 1986;26:123.

113. Naidech AM, Janjua N, Kreiter KT, et al. Predictors and impact of aneurysm rebleeding after subarachnoid hemorrhage. Arch Neurol 2005;62: 410.

114. Fujii Y, Takeuchi S, Sasaki O, et al. Ultra-early rebleeding in spontaneous subarachnoid hemorrhage. J Neurosurg 1996;84:35.

115. Hillman J, Fridriksson S, Nilsson O, et al. Immediate administration of tranexamic acid and reduced incidence of early rebleeding after aneurysmal subarachnoid hemorrhage: a prospective randomized study. J Neurosurg 2002;97:771.

116. Ohkuma H, Tsurutani H, Suzuki S. Incidence and significance of early aneurysmal rebleeding before neurosurgical or neurological management. Stroke 2001;32:1176.

117. Sorteberg W, Slettebo H, Eide PK, et al. Surgical treatment of aneurysmal subarachnoid haemorrhage in the presence of 24-h endovascular availability: management and results. Br J Neurosurg 2008;22:53.

118. Bendok BR, Getch CC, Malisch TW, et al. Treatment of aneurysmal subarachnoid hemorrhage. Semin Neurol 1998;18:521.

119. Starke RM, Kim GH, Komotar RJ, et al. Endothelial nitric oxide synthase gene single-nucleotide polymorphism predicts cerebral vasospasm after aneurysmal subarachnoid hemorrhage. J Cereb Blood Flow Metab 2008;28:1204.

120. Kassell NF, Sasaki T, Colohan AR, et al. Cerebral vasospasm following aneurysmal subarachnoid hemorrhage. Stroke 1985;16:562.

121. Lanzino G, Kassell NF, Dorsch NW, et al. Double-blind, randomized, vehicle-controlled study of high-dose tirilazad mesylate in women with aneurysmal subarachnoid hemorrhage. Part I. A cooperative study in Europe, Australia, New Zealand, and South Africa. J Neurosurg 1999;90:1011.

122. Song MK, Kim MK, Kim TS, et al. Endothelial nitric oxide gene T-786C polymorphism and subarachnoid hemorrhage in Korean population. J Korean Med Sci 2006;21:922.

123. Vajkoczy P, Meyer B, Weidauer S, et al. Clazosentan (AXV-034343), a selective endothelin A receptor antagonist, in the prevention of cerebral vasospasm following severe aneurysmal subarachnoid hemorrhage: results of a randomized, double-blind, placebo-controlled, multicenter phase IIa study. J Neurosurg 2005;103:9.

124. Wurm G, Tomancok B, Nussbaumer K, et al. Reduction of ischemic sequelae following spontaneous subarachnoid hemorrhage: a double-blind, randomized comparison of enoxaparin versus placebo. Clin Neurol Neurosurg 2004; 106:97.

125. Allen GS, Ahn HS, Preziosi TJ, et al. Cerebral arterial spasm—a controlled trial of nimodipine in patients with subarachnoid hemorrhage. N Engl J Med 1983;308:619.

126. Barker FG 2nd, Ogilvy CS. Efficacy of prophylactic nimodipine for delayed ischemic deficit after subarachnoid hemorrhage: a metaanalysis. J Neurosurg 1996;84:405.

127. Mocco J, Ransom ER, Komotar RJ, et al. Preoperative prediction of long-term outcome in poor-grade aneurysmal subarachnoid hemorrhage. Neurosurgery 2006;59:529.

128. Stachniak JB, Layon AJ, Day AL, et al. Craniotomy for intracranial aneurysm and subarachnoid hemorrhage. Is course, cost, or outcome affected by age? Stroke 1996;27:276.

129. Ayala C, Croft JB, Greenlund KJ, et al. Sex differences in US mortality rates for stroke and stroke subtypes by race/ethnicity and age, 1995–1998. Stroke 2002;33:1197.

130. Johnston SC, Selvin S, Gress DR. The burden, trends, and demographics of mortality from subarachnoid hemorrhage. Neurology 1998;50:1413.

131. Truelsen T, Bonita R, Duncan J, et al. Changes in subarachnoid hemorrhage mortality, incidence, and case fatality in New Zealand between 1981–1983 and 1991–1993. Stroke 1998;29:2298.

132. Ingall TJ, Whisnant JP, Wiebers DO, et al. Has there been a decline in subarachnoid hemorrhage mortality? Stroke 1989;20:718.

133. Kongable GL, Lanzino G, Germanson TP, et al. Gender-related differences in aneurysmal subarachnoid hemorrhage. J Neurosurg 1996; 84:43.

134. Kaptain GJ, Lanzino G, Kassell NF. Subarachnoid haemorrhage: epidemiology, risk factors, and treatment options. Drugs Aging 2000;17:183.

135. Eden SV, Heisler M, Green C, et al. Racial and ethnic disparities in the treatment of cerebrovascular diseases: importance to the practicing neurosurgeon. Neurocrit Care 2008;9:55.

136. Kaufman DM, Portenoy RK, Lesser ML, et al. The influence of race and other factors on the outcome of intracranial surgery for cerebral artery aneurysms. N Y State J Med 1984;84:549.

137. Keller AZ. Hypertension, age and residence in the survival with subarachnoid hemorrhage. Am J Epidemiol 1970;91:139.

138. Buczko W. Cranial surgery among Medicare beneficiaries. J Trauma 2005;58:40.

139. Bardach NS, Zhao S, Gress DR, et al. Association between subarachnoid hemorrhage outcomes and number of cases treated at California hospitals. Stroke 2002;33:1851.

140. Berman MF, Solomon RA, Mayer SA, et al. Impact of hospital-related factors on outcome after treatment of cerebral aneurysms. Stroke 2003;34:2200.

141. Cowan JA Jr, Dimick JB, Wainess RM, et al. Outcomes after cerebral aneurysm clip occlusion in the United States: the need for evidence-based hospital referral. J Neurosurg 2003;99:947.

142. Cross DT 3rd, Tirschwell DL, Clark MA, et al. Mortality rates after subarachnoid hemorrhage: variations according to hospital case volume in 18 states. J Neurosurg 2003;99:810.

143. Dudley RA, Johansen KL, Brand R, et al. Selective referral to high-volume hospitals: estimating potentially avoidable deaths. JAMA 2000;283:1159.

144. Solomon RA, Mayer SA, Tarmey JJ. Relationship between the volume of craniotomies for cerebral aneurysm performed at New York state hospitals and in-hospital mortality. Stroke 1996;27:13.

145. Lipsman N, Tolentino J, Macdonald RL. Effect of country or continent of treatment on outcome after aneurysmal subarachnoid hemorrhage. J Neurosurg 2009;111:67–74.

146. Crowley RW, Yeoh HK, Stukenborg GJ, et al. Influence of weekend versus weekday hospital admission on mortality following subarachnoid hemorrhage. J Neurosurg 2009;111:60–6.

Outcome and Cost of Aneurysmal Subarachnoid Hemorrhage

André A. le Roux, MB, ChB, MD (LMCC), FCNeurosurg(SA), M. Christopher Wallace, MD, MSc, FRCSC*

KEYWORDS
• Aneurysmal subarachnoid hemorrhage • Outcome
• Risk factors • Cost

Aneurysmal subarachnoid hemorrhage (aSAH) is a neurosurgical disaster. Few conditions in neurosurgery consume so many resources, with such a relatively poor outcome, as does aSAH. Of the patients who present with aSAH, 75% to 85% will have a ruptured intracranial aneurysm. Aneurysmal subarachnoid hemorrhage is reported to be responsible for 2% to 5% of all stroke cases. It affects between 21,000 and 33,000 people in the United States per year[1,2] and 5000 patients per year in the United Kingdom.[3] The incidence of aSAH is most commonly quoted as 6 to 9 per 100,000 person-years in most communities.[4–7] It is well recognized that subarachnoid hemorrhage is more common in Finland and Japan, with an incidence of 20 per 100,000 person-years.[5] China reports a 2 per 100,000 annual incidence with South and Central America reporting low incidences.[8] Overall, women are affected 1.6 times more commonly than men[9] and black patients show a 2.1 increased risk over whites.[10,11] In a review of the incidence over the past 45 years, a 0.6% decrease has been noted.[7]

OUTCOME AND ASSOCIATED RISK FACTORS

The natural history of aSAH shows that the mortality rate in the Cooperative Study on Intracranial Aneurysms is 50% at 29 days.[12] The mortality rate has been seen to decrease over the past couple of decades.[13–15] Recent case fatality rates vary from 33% to 45%.[16,17] The exact reasons for this is not clear but may be related to better primary health care, improved blood pressure control, and a decreasing trend in cigarette smoking. There is also a variation in mortality rates among various regions and countries.[13–15] Aneurysmal subarachnoid hemorrhage patients show a 25% mortality rate within 24 hours of the initial hemorrhage, 10% to 15% acute mortality before reaching hospital, and 10% mortality within 24 hours of hospitalization. One-month mortality is estimated at 50% to 60%. Of those who survive, up to two-thirds will have a significantly reduced quality of life with 50% of these patients remaining dependent.[18] Between 25% and 30% of the morbidity and mortality of aSAH is attributed to secondary ischemia, most commonly caused by vasospasm.[19]

The major cause of poor outcome (major morbidity and death) in aSAH patients is related to neurologic injury caused by the hemorrhage itself. This is often determined by the initial hemorrhage and the neurologic sequelae that follow. The direct causes of death and major morbidity as documented by The International Cooperative Study on the Timing of Aneurysm Surgery[20,21] were: (1) cerebral infarction secondary to vasospasm—33.5%, (2) direct effect of hemorrhage—25.5%, (3) rehemorrhage before treatment—17.3%, (4) treatment complications—8.9%, (5) intracerebral hematoma—4.5%, and (6) hydrocephalus—3.0%. The strongest predictors of death and

Department of Surgery, Division of Neurosurgery, Toronto Western Hospital, University Health Network, WW 4-450, 399 Bathurst Street, Toronto, Ontario M5T 2S8, Canada
* Corresponding author.
E-mail address: chris.wallace@uhn.on.ca

Neurosurg Clin N Am 21 (2010) 235–246
doi:10.1016/j.nec.2009.10.014
1042-3680/10/$ – see front matter © 2010 Elsevier Inc. All rights reserved.

poor outcome include an increasing patient age, poor World Federation of Neurological Surgeons (WFNS) grade (decreased level of consciousness) upon initial presentation, and a large volume of blood on initial CT scan.

Grade

Patients with poor WFNS (4–5), Hunt and Hess (4–5), grade do poorly.[22] If no treatment is offered, the mortality rate approaches 100%.[23] Ross and colleagues[24] report on treating poor-grade aSAH patients with late surgery and early coiling. Their data suggest no added benefit by early coiling of poor-grade patients.[24] With active treatment, good outcome has been reported in 50% of Grade 4 patients and 20% of Grade 5 patients.[25] Patients older than 80 years do poorly. Poor-grade patients more often have associated hydrocephalus with an incidence estimated to be 50%.[23] Management of these patients includes placement of an external ventricular drain (EVD) and following 24 hours of observation, 47% of this subgroup will have had made no improvement. In their series,[23] these patients were treated conservatively with a mortality rate of 100% (mean of 2.6 days after presentation). Interestingly, men seem to do worse than woman, with the outcome discrepancy independent of age. Other clinical series[26,27] show some improvement in 40% to 80% of cases following EVD placement.

Global Cerebral Edema

Global cerebral edema, as seen on CT scan, is associated with poorer outcome. Claassen and colleagues[27] found that the admission CT scan showed edema in 6% to 8%[20,27] and that edema developed later in 12%. Global cerebral edema is clinically suggested by an altered level of consciousness and or poor WFNS grade upon presentation. When reviewing mortality at 3 months, the global edema subgroup had a 48% to 50% mortality rate as compared with those without at 18%. Kreiter and colleagues[28] also found poorer cognitive outcome in patients with global brain edema.

Rehemorrhage

The most treatable cause of poor outcome is rehemorrhage.[29] Rehemorrhage poses the greatest threat to life during the initial stages of aSAH and is associated with a mortality rate of 50% to 70%. Rehemorrhage is the highest on day 1 post ictus[30] (4%), then decreasing to 2% per day for the following 4 weeks. After 3 months, the rehemorrhage rate is at 3% per year.[31] In patients managed conservatively, a mortality of 20% to 30% is

reported at 30 days.[32,33] Some studies report the incidence of ultra-early bleeding at 15%.[34,35] Ultra-early rehemorrhage occurs within 24 hours of the initial ictus, with most hemorrhages occurring between 0 and 12 hours.[36] Some reports indicate 87% of events occurring within the first 6 hours,[37,38] specifically the first 2 hours.[35] Risk factors for ultra-early bleeding is poorer grade at time of presentation, high initial blood pressure, and extended period between ictus and presentation to hospital.

Rehemorrhage rates for poor-grade patients are higher (20%) than good-grade patients (5%). The rehemorrhage rate in coiled patients was higher but the mortality rate in any rehemorrhaged patient is exceedingly high. Sluzewski and colleagues[39] reported a 1.27% incidence of late rehemorrhage following coiling. Late rehemorrhage had less of an effect on patient outcome than early rehemorrhage. The rehemorrhage events occurred between 8 and 40 months in this review. Factors associated with early rehemorrhage included small aneurysm size and an associated intracerebral hematoma on the initial CT scan. Risk factors for late rehemorrhage include large aneurysm size and incomplete occlusion/obliteration of the aneurysm.

Age

Age affects associated clinical outcomes as well as the initial risk of aSAH. Data from the Framingham study showed an increased incidence in aSAH as the population grows older.[40] The International Cooperative Study of the Timing of Aneurysm Surgery[20,21] found a linear association between advancing age and worse outcome. Aging patients have a higher probability of dying or sustaining permanent neurologic damage or dying from vasospasm than younger patients. The complication rate increased from 28% in the sub-40-year group to 46% in the patients older than 70 years. Discharge glasgow outcome scores at 3 months are worse for older patients. In Lanzino and colleagues'[41] series, patients aged 40 years or younger made a good recovery 73% of the time, with the same degree of recovery found in only 25% of patients aged 70 years or older. Mortality rates are also worse for older patients (35% in the >70-year group) as compared with younger patients (12% in the <40-year group) with the same clinical presentation.

Lanzino and colleagues[41] extensively analyzed the effect of age on aSAH. They found that older patients were more likely to present with a lower level of consciousness, have a poorer WFNS score, have a thicker subarachnoid blood load, and were more likely to have associated intraventricular blood. These patients were more likely to have hydrocephalus and showed an increased re-hemorrhage rate (4.5% in the sub-40-year group to 16.4% in the above 70-year group). The thicker SAH blood load and increased intraventricular hemorrhage is in part explained by the increased subarachnoid spaces and ventricular size secondary to atrophy of the aging brain.

In older patients, increased systolic blood pressure is more common and is associated with a poorer WFNS grade. Advancing age was also associated with increased comorbidities, including hypertension, diabetes, pulmonary dysfunction, cardiac disease, and cerebrovascular disease. Older patients were also found not to have larger aneurysms. Despite having a larger subarachnoid blood load, older patients showed less angiographic vasospasm.[41–44] This might be related to decreasing vascular compliance and a more rigid vascular vessel wall secondary to hypertension and increasing age.

The exact age at which poor outcome seems to be more common is hard to predict. In most studies,[40,41] the relationship between advancing age and poor outcome is a linear one. Statistical series suggests that better outcomes are to be anticipated in patients younger than 60 years of age. The aging brain seems to be less able to cope with the secondary effects of an aSAH. The reasons are a combination of factors,[45–47] ranging from structural changes, biochemical, and reduced plasticity.

Hyperglycemia

Hyperglycemia and its predictive role in outcome has been investigated.[48] It is well known that following aSAH, plasma glucose levels are elevated.[49–51] This may reflect a stress response. Studies have found plasma glucose levels, taken less than 72 hours following the ictus, to be elevated and to correlate with the severity of the bleed and clinical condition of the patient. Juvela and colleagues,[48] testing admission plasma glucose levels, found that hyperglycemia predicted a poor outcome. Lanzino and colleagues[51] suggested that hyperglycemia does not increase the risk for vasospasm (radiographic and/or symptomatic) or cerebral infarction. Finding hyperglycemia (day 3–7 post aSAH) in a patient with vasospasm was associated with a poorer outcome.[51] The harmful effects of hyperglycemia during episodes of cerebral ischemia have also been reported.[49–51]

Medical Complications

Solenski and colleagues[52] reported on the medical complications associated with aSAH and the associated impact on outcome. Their work found

that extracranial causes directly contributed to death in 23% of cases, increasing the significance of extracranial causes on par with vasospasm and rehemorrhage as a cause of poor outcome and death. Management of these patients needs a multidisciplinary approach.

Gruber and colleagues[53] reviewed aSAH patient admissions to a neuro critical care unit over a 5-year period. Neurologic failure (Hunt and Hess grades 4 and 5) occurred in 36.8% of patients with an associated mortality rate of 40.4%. Of these patients, 51.7% had isolated neurologic failure and 48.3% showed at least one additional organ system failure. Isolated central nervous system (CNS) failure carried a17.4% mortality but the addition of an extracerebral organ failure increased mortality to 65.1%. Eighty-one percent of patients admitted developed some degree of organ dysfunction, 26% developing organ failure. Single-organ failure was the commonest (16%) followed by two organ system failure (4.9%) and 3 or more system failure in 4.1%. Mortality rates increased from 30.7% (single-system failure) to 91% for two and 100% for 3 or more organ failure.

Le Roux and colleagues[54] found that medical conditions complicated and negatively affected the outcome of subarachnoid patients. Pneumonia and sepsis were common culprits. Close to half (41.8%) of patient deaths, excluding prehospital deaths, are associated some degree of extracranial organ dysfunction. The development of the systemic inflammatory response syndrome (SIRS) heralds a negative turning point in disease progression. SIRS may be the common initiating pathway to patient demise. The detailed pathophysiology of this process is beyond the scope of this article and the reader is referred to the references listed.[55–60] Suffice to say that Gruber and colleagues[53] found 29% of patients admitted to ICU to develop SIRS and 10.3% develop septic shock. The associated mortality rates were 40.3% for SIRS and 80.0% for septic shock against the backdrop of aSAH.

The association of poor outcome and fever has been reviewed. Oliveira-Filho and colleagues[60] found that patients with vasospasm had an increased risk of developing fever. They concluded that the risk of a poor outcome increased with the duration of a fever, independent from vasospasm, disease severity, and infections per se.

Alcohol Consumption

Alcohol consumption has been implicated in the outcome of aSAH. Juvela and colleagues[61–63] reported on this association and found that patients with a history of heavy alcohol intake were more likely to have a poor outcome. In their series,[62] 12% to 13% of aSAH could be attributed to heavy alcohol intake. Heavy drinking more often preceded episodes of aSAH and most patients who presented following alcohol intake, did so in the "hungover" phase. Patients with heavy alcohol intake were more likely to present in a poorer grade following an ictus and were more likely to die following rehemorrhage or a delayed ischemic event. They were also more prone to additional medical problems. In this regard, a history of heavy alcohol intake probably represents a marker of a specific lifestyle, associated with increased incidence of cigarette smoking, poor nutritional practices with increased body mass index, hypertension, dyslipidemias, and limited physical exercise.

Cocaine

Conway and Tamargo[64] reviewed patients who presented with aSAH following cocaine use. Conflicting reports in the literature[65] initially suggested a worse outcome in this subset of patients.[66,67] Their analysis suggested that there is an increased incidence of vasospasm (63% vs 30% in control group) following aSAH but that outcome is not statistically any different. Consensus has not yet been reached with other authors reporting poorer results.[68] If aSAH was related to cocaine usage, the patient population tended to be younger (average 36 years) and a disproportionate number of anterior circulation aneurysms (97% vs 84% in the control group) were present. Most patients in this subset practiced polypharmacy (81% of cocaine users) and had other comorbid factors associated, including HIV, bacterial infections, and viral hepatitis.

Statins

Statin users were reported to show a better outcome following aSAH.[69] This was attributable to reduced vasospasm and improved cerebral hemodynamics. Parra and colleagues[70] could not demonstrate this benefit. Tseng and colleagues[3] in a follow-up to their initial[69] article indicated benefit by reduced incidence of vasospasm or need to treat vasospasm and improved psychological outcome. The Statins for Aneurysmal Subarachnoid Hemorrhage (STASH) trial, assessing statin therapy on long-term outcome, is ongoing.

Aneurysm Size and Location

Some authors have suggested a larger SAH volume with the rupture of small aneurysms.[71,72] As SAH blood load is associated with vasospasm, this may lead to poorer outcome. Although Taylor and colleagues[72] found smaller aneurysms to produce larger bleeds, outcome was not affected by size. Salary and colleagues[73] found no relationship between aneurysm size and SAH blood load or outcome.

The effect on outcome of location of the aneurysm has been investigated. Kassell and colleagues[20,21] found that patients with aneurysms located on the internal carotid artery or middle cerebral artery had an overall better outcome as compared with patients with lesions of the anterior cerebral artery and/or vertebrobasilar system. Säveland and Brandt[74] concurred with this. Anterior circulation aneurysms tend to fare better than posterior circulation lesions.[75]

Gender

Gender differences do not seem to affect the outcome of aSAH.[76] Females predominate in most series (ruptured and unruptured, clinical or autopsy-based[20,76–82]). Women tend to be older at presentation (51.4 years vs 47.3 years for males) and more often have multiple aneurysms (32.4% vs 17.6% for males). In children and adolescents, males predominate. The sex ratio remains 1:1 up to the third decade and then gradually changes to a female predominance. Female patients tended to have more aneurysms on the internal carotid artery (36.8% vs 18.0% in males), whereas men had more on the anterior cerebral artery system (46.1% vs 26.6% in females).[76] Vasospasm was encountered equally in both sexes.

WFNS Grades 1 and 2

Predicting outcome in patients with a good WFNS grade (Grades 1 and 2) is more complicated. Historically, Grade 1 patients made a good outcome 72% of the time and Grade 2 in 52% (3-month outcome).[23,83,84] When applying the National Institutes of Health Stroke Scale (NIHSS)[84] to admission clinical findings, different outcome data are obtained. The NIHSS allows for a more detailed neurologic assessment. When evaluating the various aspects of the NIHSS, four clinical aspects are found to have statistical significance. These include (1) worst motor (arm) score, (2) dysphasia, (3) visual field deficits, and (4) level of consciousness. The presence of a positive sign (any one of the four clinical aspects) would imply a poorer outcome. Patients classified as WFNS

Grade 1 with positive findings of the NIHSS showed a good outcome in 48% (vs 72%). The same was found for Grade 2 WFNS with positive NIHSS findings with good outcome found in 41% (vs 52%). The addition of these additional clinical factors thus improves the predictive value, but the practically of this has been doubted by some.

Biomarkers

Various biochemical markers have been tested to try to predict outcome following aSAH. No biomarker has yet been shown to provide a prediction method with enough sensitivity and specificity to accurately estimate clinical outcomes. Some of these tested methods have shown promise. These methods include serum S-100 plasma protein levels[85] (associated and indicative of brain damage following SAH), plasma endothelin levels[86] (associated with vasospasm and delayed cerebral ischemia), free fatty acid concentration in cerebrospinal fluid[87] (may play a role in evolution of and hence prediction of vasospasm), and genetic markers such as apolipoprotein E genotype.[88] Genetic testing may aid in the future outcome prediction of patients with aSAH.

OUTCOME AND RECOVERY

Patients who have had an aSAH tend to show higher unemployment rates than controls. They showed more emotional distress and reduced social independence up to 5 years following the event.[89] This outcome is more commonly found in patients who require inpatient rehabilitation.[90,91] Higher than normal rates of mood disturbance, anxiety, depression, and neglect of social contact were found in some patients who had made a good neurologic recovery.[92,93] Researchers found a decrease in general well-being with patients having difficulties with interpersonal relationships, low energy levels, and a feeling of being unwell. Ogden and colleagues[94] reported that 1 year following the ictus up to 59% of patients with good outcomes were still not back to their pre-event employment, and 86% experienced ongoing fatigue. Patients also suffered from lack of motivation, loss of drive, and emotional strain. Investigation showed that patients who suffered an aSAH tended to have experienced a more stressful year before the event. These events may explain, in part, the reduced quality of life experienced by some despite a good neurologic outcome. Another explanation for this phenomenon was that of an organic brain syndrome. McKenna and colleagues[95] did a prospective comparison between patients who suffered an aSAH and those who had a myocardial infarction.

They found that about half of each group had a decreased sense of well-being/reduced quality-of-life experience. This may reflect a posttraumatic stress disorder.[95] Powell and colleagues[89] reviewed patients who made a good neurologic recovery. Some 60% showed features of clinical significant posttraumatic stress symptoms at 3 months and 30% at 9 months following the ictus. They were also more prone to increased mood disturbance, dependence, and decreased social functioning. Mood status of patients at 9 months after the event was related to physical and mental health status before the ictus.

Often, the neuropsychological outcome of patients is measured in isolation. The disease impact on the partners and family members is immense.[96] A large proportion of carers found the discharge phase more stressful than the initial acute event. Hop and colleagues[97] showed that partners of patients discharged with a Rankin Score (RS) of 0, were unaffected as compared with the general population. Emotional problems were more common though. The main areas of change in quality of life for family members/partners of patients with RS of 1 to 5, was in "emotional behavior," "social interactions," "work," and "recreation and pastime." Interestingly, the partners sometimes showed a larger degree of reduction than the patients themselves. This report clearly shows the huge impact of aSAH on the lives of patients and their partners.

Pritchard and colleagues[98] found 54% of patients felt depressed following discharge and 33% experienced increased anxiety. Up to 19% of patients attended medical services because of psychosocial reasons. Half of the carers felt that they were negatively affected and 40% felt they were able to cope better with the acute event than when the patient was at home post discharge. Up to 33% reported financial issues and a quarter needed to medicate themselves for stress and anxiety. Mezue and colleagues[99] reviewed the impact of caretaking on family members. They found that 53.8% felt social and personal (emotional) stress with close to half (46.4%) being completely overwhelmed. Their study showed that patients who have a poor outcome induce more stress to the caretaker. Most of the carers are not trained to cope with the various aspects of taking care of a chronically ill patient. This in itself induces huge amounts of stress and anxiety.

THE COST OF CARE

The economic impact of an aneurysmal subarachnoid hemorrhage is devastating. This is true for both the patient and the health care system. The cost implications to any disease process can be either direct or indirect. Not only is there a direct dollar value to a specific illness or pathologic process, but the chronic care cost is often concealed in various forms, including that of rehabilitation, ongoing medical care, medication and follow-up investigations, and long-term and possible repeated surgical procedures because of complications. Components of indirect cost, among others, include the fiscal amounts related to the loss of income of the patient and the ripple effect this has on the community at large. These amounts (dollar value) and costs (socioeconomic) are harder to calculate or predict.

Direct cost can be attributed to acute and chronic care. Acute care costs include the ambulance transport, emergency room, diagnostic and treatment (medication, surgical, and endovascular) cost, staff cost, facility cost, and initial in-hospital rehabilitation cost. Chronic care cost entails the financial aspects of a rehabilitation facility or chronic care or nursing home. For patients who are sent home for outpatient rehabilitation, the costs include those for home visitation, physiotherapy, occupational therapy, and speech therapy.

Long-term cost depends largely on the survival duration and the degree of disability. Affected patients who are young will incur greater cost than those who are elderly, as the life expectancy is longer. This is also true for patients with greater degrees of impairment. Young patients with a minor degree of disability may not add greatly to the dollar value of chronic care costs, but the decrease in actual earning power will, at least on a fiscal basis, be cumulative over the years. The social impact (neuropsychological cost) of the latter group will be higher than those who are significantly cognitively obtunded.

Indirect costs are influenced by the educational status, work status, number of dependents, and location of the patient and secondary complications that occurred during the primary event may contribute. The degree of impact largely depends on the degree of residual disability. Patients with a high level of dependency will incur higher costs. Certain cost factors cannot be calculated. The loss of the ability to work may be calculated by actuarial manner but the emotional cost to the patient and immediate family is far greater than what can be calculated in fiscal terms.

Hospitalization

When reviewing treatment costs in the initial stages (first 12 months), most of the cost is made up of hospitalization. This creates a large window of opportunity as any treatment or intervention that would shorten hospital, and specifically ICU, stay, will have a huge beneficial cost impact. Ross and colleagues[100] found that 85% of the cost during the first year was made up of hospital admission and radiological and treatment costs. Of this amount, two thirds is devoted to hospitalization and the rest to imaging and therapeutic costs. This latter group is subdivided with 45% of cost going to radiological studies, with angiography consuming 52% of this budget. From the rest of the radiological/treatment budget, 42% is consumed by surgery or coiling. Medications only comprised 3% of the treatment budget.

Regardless of what mode of treatment is used to secure an aneurysm, the presence of complications will increase costs. The development of vasospasm will not only incur costs in extending the duration of ICU stay, hospital stay, and treatment costs per se, with the potential poor outcome escalating rehabilitation and chronic care costs. The same could be said for any complication.

The adoption of newer treatment strategies has also brought along increased cost. The pharmaceutical industry invests heavily into research and development and hence has to recoup their investment via product costs. The evolution of endovascular treatment systems has shown this clearly. The initial introduction of coils has been compounded by the addition of newer types of coils, balloons, and now, stents. All these products are aimed at achieving a better outcome, but this implies increased cost. There are also specific associated complications with these newer devices, this in itself escalating the cost in the acute phase.

As one would expect, the cost of the whole experience will differ from country to country and continent to continent. Costs, although high, seem to be more contained within a national health system/state-funded system than a private sector system.

Coiling Versus Clipping

Direct cost comparison of surgical clipping versus coiling has been done by various authors, each proclaiming their method is better or just as cost effective as that or their competitor. Proponents of endovascular coiling state that their method is less invasive with better outcome at 1 year. Bairstow and colleagues[101] indicated that although endovascular treatment was associated with higher upfront costs, specifically related to consumables (coils, balloons, and stents), the shorter hospital stay associated with better outcome and a sooner return to work period made this treatment option cost equal to neurosurgical clipping of aneurysms. Follow-up costs and specifically imaging costs are higher in the endovascular group. Retreatment costs are also higher as incomplete coiling will necessitate repeat treatment. Wolstenholme and colleagues[102] found that the endovascular-treated group had a lower cost of treatment when compared with the surgical-clipping group for the acute event and follow-up to 1 year. However, by 2 years, repeated imaging studies, more frequent follow-up, and repeat endovascular treatments eroded this financial advantage and a close to equal costing between the two treatment methods remained. Other studies have also come to similar conclusions.[100,101,103,104]

Javadpour and colleagues[103] did a cost analysis of patients treated for aSAH, in the largest cohort of North American contributor to International Subarachnoid Aneurysm Trial (ISAT).[72] They found no difference in hospital stay between the two groups and also concurred with other authors about the increased imaging cost in the endovascular group. The total cost between the two groups was once again similar. Assessing return to work, the ISAT data were reviewed. More patients in the endovascular treatment group had returned to work by 12-month follow-up. This advantage was not present by the 24-month follow-up. When reviewing total cost following discharge, close to 60% of costs were related to transportation and rehabilitation. Reviews from developing countries indicate a wide array of cost differences. Some of these countries do not have access to regular neurosurgical services, let alone endovascular facilities. Yentur and colleagues[105] from Turkey reported a beneficial cost outcome in the surgical clipping group. They related this to the increased cost associated with importing endovascular consumables. These products are not manufactured locally, resulting in an exaggerated expense in importing products. This translates into increased cost to the endovascular group that is not regained by the reported shorter hospital stay.

Community Impact

When reviewing the community economic impact of aSAH, Pritchard and colleagues[98] reported that 11% of patients lost their employment following the management of a ruptured aneurysm. In excess of 50% were off work for 6 months and 22% off more than 1 year. Family members and caretakers of patients involved in looking after them post event were also heavily affected. Eighty six percent were off work at least 2 weeks with 15% off a quarter of the year (17 weeks) or more.

They attributed this to inadequate medical support to the patient, necessitating them to be involved. The lost or diminished productivity is significant.

Screening for New Aneurysms

In patients with a history of a previous treated aneurysm, screening for new aneurysms has been found not to be cost effective, despite an increased risk of a repeat event. The risk of new aneurysm formation and rupture is higher than in the general population. The risk of repeat aSAH following successful surgical clipping is 3% in 10 years.[106] This is more than 20 times the risk in the general population.[106,107] The case fatality rate seen in rehemorrhage following a previous aSAH is 40%.[108] Wermer and colleagues,[108] as part of the Aneurysm Screening after Treatment for Ruptured Aneurysms (ASTRA) study group, reviewed this topic in detail. They documented a 16% incidence of newly diagnosed aneurysms in patients with a previously surgically clipped aneurysm. Of these, 81.4% were aneurysms at new locations and 18.6% were at the previous clip site. Upon reviewing the old imaging, 68% of the "new lesions" were actually present (retrospective diagnosis) previously and only 32% were "de novo" lesions. Of patients with a known second aneurysm that was treated, enlargement of the second lesion took place in 25%. Treatment was offered to 23% of patients and the others were followed. In reviewing the data, they concluded that screening of these patients was not cost effective.

Clinical Grade

In assessing factors that may predict cost outcome following aSAH, Elliot and colleagues[109] found that clinical grade at time of presentation best predicts not only the length of stay but also the predicted total hospital cost involved. Wiebers and colleagues[110] postulated that the treatment of ruptured aneurysms is 150% more expensive than treating unruptured aneurysms.

Regionalization of Cerebrovascular Services

Regionalization of cerebrovascular services has shown to improve outcome.[16] Solomon and colleagues[111] found that units that do more than 30 surgical clippings per year have a 43% reduced mortality compared with lower case-load units. This was echoed by Berman and colleagues[112] and Luft and colleagues.[113] The health facility's availability to provide endovascular services improves outcome as well. From a neurosurgical perspective, cost evaluation brings into discussion the issue of neurosurgical subspecialization.[114] It is well recognized that if a specific practitioner devotes a larger percentage of time to a specific disease process, his or her proficiency in treating this disorder increases ("practice-makes-perfect"). This will have a cost-saving effect on the whole.

Bardach and colleagues[115] found that an increased patient load did lead to a better patient outcome when comparing low-volume (<20 cases per year) to high-volume (>20 cases per year) treatment facilities. The improved outcome was also associated with an increased cost but better outcome. When the treating facility was treating more than 50 cases per year, costs were reduced and the outcome was improved. Transfer of sick patients is a difficult situation. Not only does the risk of adverse outcome increase during transport, but the costs associated with this specific case increases. Bardach and colleagues[115] did however find this transfer cost effective, more so if the accepting facility offered endovascular coiling services. Of note is that high-volume centers tend to treat patients more rapidly. This time gain eliminates the time lost in the transfer process. The presence of neurosurgical residents was associated with increased cost of treatment.[112] Berman and colleagues[112] found that treatment volume impacted more so on the outcome of surgical outcomes than the outcome of endovascular coiling.

SUMMARY

Despite the huge advances made in neurosurgical management of aSAH over recent decades, there has not been a proportional improvement in outcome of this condition. Although more people may survive, our ability to impact on the primary pathology has been minimal. It remains a high-cost investment (both fiscal and medical) disease with poor return for the efforts of the treating multidisciplinary team.

REFERENCES

1. Lytle RA, Diringer M, Dacey RG. Complications of subarachnoid haemorrhage: cerebral vasospasm. Contemp Neurosurg 2004;26(5):1–8.
2. Suarez JI, Tarr RW, Selman WR. Aneurysmal subarachnoid hemorrhage. N Engl J Med 2006; 354:387–96.
3. Tseng M-Y, Hutchinson PJ, Czosnyka M, et al. Effects of acute pravastatin treatment on intensity of rescue therapy, length of inpatient stay, and 6-month outcome in patients after aneurysmal subarachnoid hemorrhage. Stroke 2007;38: 1545–50.
4. van Gijn J, Kerr RS, Rinkel GJE. Subarachnoid haemorrhage. Lancet 2007;369:306–18.
5. Linn FHH, Rinkel GJE, Algra A, et al. Incidence of subarachnoid haemorrhage: role of region, year, and rate of computed tomography: a meta-analysis. Stroke 1996;27:625–9.
6. Da Costa LB, Gunnarsson T, Wallace MC. Unruptured intracranial aneurysms: natural history and management decisions. Neurosurg Focus 2004;17(5):E6.
7. de Rooij NK, Linn FHH, van der Plas JA, et al. Incidence of subarachnoid haemorrhage: a systematic review with emphasis on region, age, gender and time trends. J Neurol Neurosurg Psychiatr 2007; 78:1365–72.
8. Ingall T, Asplund K, Mahonen M, et al. A multinational comparison of subarachnoid hemorrhage epidemiology in the WHO MONICA stroke study. Stroke 2000;31:1054–61.
9. Lindsay KW, Teasdale GM, Knill-Jones RP. Observer variability in assessing the clinical features of subarachnoid hemorrhage. J Neurosurg 1983;58: 57–62.
10. Sacco RL, Mayer SA. Epidemiology of intracerebral hemorrhage. In: Armok Feldmann E, editor. Intracerebral hemorrhage. New York: Futura Publishing; 1994. p. 3–23.
11. Broderick JP, Brott T, Tomsick T, et al. The risk of subarachnoid and intracerebral hemorrhages in blacks as compared with whites. N Engl J Med 1992;326:733–6.
12. Locksley HB, Sahs AL, Sandler R. Report on the cooperative study of intracranial aneurysms and subarachnoid hemorrhage. J Neurosurg 1966; 24(6):1034–56.
13. Harmsen P, Tsipogianni A, Wilhelmsen L. Stroke incidence rates were unchanged, while fatality rates declined, during 1971–1987 in Göteborg, Sweden. Stroke 1992;23:1410–5.
14. Ingall TJ, Whisnant JP, Wiebers DO, et al. Has there been a decline in subarachnoid hemorrhage mortality? Stroke 1989;20:718–24.
15. Stegmayr B, Eriksson M, Asplund K. Declining mortality from subarachnoid hemorrhage: changes in incidence and case fatality from 1985 through 2000. Stroke 2004;35:2059–63.
16. Cross DT 3rd, Tirschwell DL, Clark MA, et al. Mortality rates after subarachnoid hemorrhage: variations according to hospital case volume in 18 states. J Neurosurg 2003;99:810–7.
17. Broderick JP, Brott TG, Duldner JE, et al. Initial and recurrent bleeding are the major causes of death following subarachnoid hemorrhage. Stroke 1994; 25:1342–7.
18. Al-Shahi R, White PM, Davenport RJ, et al. Subarachnoid haemorrhage. BMJ 2006;333:235–40.
19. Feigin VL, Rinkel GJE, Algra A, et al. Calcium antagonists in patients with aneurysmal

subarachnoid hemorrhage, a systematic review. Neurology 1998;50:876–83.

20. Kassell NF, Torner JC, Haley EC Jr, et al. The international cooperative study on the timing of aneurysm surgery. Part 1: overall management results. J Neurosurg 1990;73:18–36.

21. Kassell NF, Torner JC, Jane JA, et al. The international co-operative study on the timing of aneurysm surgery. Part 2: surgical results. J Neurosurg 1990; 73:37–47.

22. Cesarini KG. Improved survival after subarachnoid haemorrhage: review of case management during a twelve year period. J Neurosurg 1999;90:664–72.

23. Leira EC, Davis PH, Martin CO, et al. Improving prediction of outcome in "good grade" subarachnoid hemorrhage. Neurosurgery 2007;61:470–4.

24. Ross J, O'Sullivan MG, Grant IS, et al. Impact of early endovascular aneurysmal occlusion on outcome of patients in poor grade after subarachnoid haemorrhage: a prospective, consecutive study. J Clin Neurosci 2002;9(6):648–65.

25. Wijdicks EFM, Kallmes DF, Manno EM, et al. Subarachnoid hemorrhage: neurointensive care and aneurysm repair. Mayo Clin Proc 2005;80(4): 550–9.

26. Rajshekhar V, Harbaugh RE. Results of routine ventriculostomy with external ventricular drainage for acute hydrocephalus following subarachnoid haemorrhage. Acta Neurochir (Wien) 1992;115: 8–14.

27. Claassen J, Carhuapoma JR, Kreiter KT, et al. Global cerebral edema after subarachnoid hemorrhage: frequency, predictors, and impact on outcome. Stroke 2002;33:1225–32.

28. Kreiter KT, Copeland D, Bernardini GL, et al. Predictors of cognitive dysfunction after subarachnoid hemorrhage. Stroke 2002;33:200–9.

29. Benderson JB, Connolly ES Jr, Batjer HH, et al. Guidelines for the management of aneurysmal subarachnoid hemorrhage: a statement for healthcare professionals from a special writing group of the stroke council, American Heart Association. Stroke 2009;40:994–1025.

30. Kassell NF, Torner JC. Aneurysmal rebleeding: a preliminary report from the cooperative aneurysm study. Neurosurgery 1983;13:479–81.

31. Winn HR, Richardson AE, Jane JA. The long-term prognosis in untreated cerebral aneurysms, I: the incidence of late hemorrhage in cerebral aneurysm: a 10-year evaluation of 364 patients. Ann Neurol 1977;1:358–70.

32. Richardson AE, Jane JA, Yashon D. Prognostic factors in the untreated course of posterior communicating aneurysms. Arch Neurol 1966;14:172–6.

33. Henderson WG, Torner JC, Nibbelink DW. Intracranial aneurysms and subarachnoid hemorrhage: report on a randomized treatment study, IV-B: regulated bed rest: statistical evaluation. Stroke 1977;8:579–89.

34. Hillman J, Fridriksson S, Nilsson O, et al. Immediate administration of tranexamic acid and reduced incidence of early rebleeding after aneurysmal subarachnoid hemorrhage: a prospective randomized study. J Neurosurg 2002;97:771–8.

35. Ohkuma H, Tsurutani H, Suzuki S. Incidence and significance of early aneurysmal rebleeding before neurosurgical or neurological management. Stroke 2001;32:1176–80.

36. Laidlaw JD, Siu KH. Poor-grade aneurysmal subarachnoid hemorrhage: outcome after treatment with urgent surgery. Neurosurgery 2003;53: 1275–80.

37. Laidlaw JD, Siu KH. Ultra-early surgery for aneurysmal subarachnoid hemorrhage: outcomes for a consecutive series of 391 patients not selected by grade or age. J Neurosurg 2002;97:250–8.

38. Fujii Y, Takeuchi S, Sasaki O, et al. Ultra-early rebleeding in spontaneous subarachnoid hemorrhage. J Neurosurg 1996;84:35–42.

39. Sluzewski M, van Rooij WJ, Beute GN. Late rebleeding of ruptured intracranial aneurysms treated with detachable coils. AJNR Am J Neuroradiol 2005;26:2542–9.

40. Sacco RL, Wolf PA, Bharucha NE, et al. Subarachnoid and intracerebral hemorrhage: natural history, prognosis, and pre-cursive factors in the Framingham Study. Neurology 1984;34:847–54.

41. Lanzino G, Kassell NF, Germanson TP, et al. Age and outcome after aneurysmal subarachnoid hemorrhage: why do older patients fare worse? J Neurosurg 1996;85:410–8.

42. Artiola I, Fortuny L, Adams CBT, et al. Surgical mortality in an aneurysm population: effects of age, blood pressure and preoperative neurological stage. J Neurol Neurosurg Psychiatr 1980;43:879–82.

43. Inagawa T. Cerebral vasospasm in elderly patients treated by early operation for ruptured intracranial aneurysms. Acta Neurochir 1992;115:79–85.

44. Inagawa T. Cerebral vasospasm in elderly patients with ruptured intracranial aneurysms. Surg Neurol 1991;36:91–8.

45. Mehlhorn RJ. Oxidants and antioxidants in aging. In: Timiras PS, editor. Physiological basis of aging and geriatrics. 2nd edition. Boca Raton (FL): CRC Press; 1994. p. 61–73.

46. Strehler BL. Time, cells, and aging. 2nd edition. New York: Academic Press; 1977. p. 292–4.

47. Timiras PS. Aging of the nervous system: structural and biochemical changes. In: Timiras PS, editor. Physiological basis of aging and geriatrics. 2nd edition. Boca Raton (FL): CRC Press; 1994. p. 89–102.

48. Juvela S, Shronen J, Kuhmonen J. Hyperglycemia, excess weight, and history of hypertension as risk

factors for poor outcome and cerebral infarction after aneurysmal subarachnoid hemorrhage. J Neurosurg 2005;102:998–1003.

49. Alberti O, Becker R, Benes L, et al. Initial hyperglycemia as indicator of severity of the ictus in poor-grade patients with spontaneous subarachnoid hemorrhage. Clin Neurol Neurosurg 2000;102:78–83.

50. Dorhout Mees SMD, van Dijk GW, Algra A, et al. Glucose levels and outcome after subarachnoid hemorrhage. Neurology 2003;61:1132–3.

51. Lanzino G, Kassell NF, Germanson T, et al. Plasma glucose levels and outcome after aneurysmal subarachnoid hemorrhage. J Neurosurg 1993;79: 885–91, 19.

52. Solenski N, Haley C, Kassell NF, et al. Medical complications of aneurysmal subarachnoid hemorrhage: a report of the multicenter, cooperative aneurysm study. Crit Care Med 1995;23:1007–17.

53. Gruber A, Reinprecht A, Illievich UM. Extracerebral organ dysfunction and neurologic outcome after aneurysmal subarachnoid hemorrhage. Crit Care Med 1999;27(3):505–14.

54. Le Roux PD, Elliott JP, Newell D, et al. Predicting outcome in poor grade patients with subarachnoid hemorrhage: a review of 159 aggressively managed cases. J Neurosurg 1996;85:39–49.

55. Smith RR, Clower BR, Homma Y, et al. The constrictive angiopathy of subarachnoid hemorrhage: an immunopathological approach. In: Wilkins RH, editor. Vasospasm. New York: Raven Press; 1988. p. 247–52.

56. Mathiesen T, Andersson B, Loftenius A, et al. Increased interleukin-6 levels in cerebrospinal fluid following subarachnoid hemorrhage. J Neurosurg 1993;78:562–7.

57. Ostergaard JR, Kristensen BO, Svehag SE. Immune complexes and complement activation following rupture of intracranial saccular aneurysms. J Neurosurg 1987;66:891–7.

58. Weir B, Disney L, Grace M, et al. Daily trends in white cell count and temperature after subarachnoid hemorrhage from aneurysm. Neurosurgery 1989;25:161–5.

59. Tremblay L, Valenza F, Ribeiro SP, et al. Injurious ventilatory strategies increase cytokines and c-FOS mRNA expression in an isolated rat lung model. J Clin Invest 1997;99:944–52.

60. Oliveira–Filho J, Ezzeddine MA, Segal AZ, et al. Fever in subarachnoid hemorrhage: relationship to vasospasm and outcome. Neurology 2001;56:1299–304.

61. Juvela S. Alcohol consumption as a risk factor for poor outcome after aneurysmal subarachnoid haemorrhage. BMJ 1992;304:1663–7.

62. Juvela S, Hillbom M, Numminen H, et al. Cigarette smoking and alcohol consumption as risk factors for aneurysmal subarachnoid hemorrhage. Stroke 1993;24:639–46.

63. Juvela S, Porras M, Poussa K. Natural history of unruptured intracranial aneurysms: probability of and risk factors for aneurysm rupture. J Neurosurg 2000;93:379–87.

64. Conway JE, Tamargo RJ. Cocaine use is an independent risk factor for cerebral vasospasm after aneurysmal subarachnoid hemorrhage. Stroke 2001;32:2338–43.

65. Nanda A, Vannemreddy PS, Polin RS, et al. Intracranial aneurysms and cocaine abuse: analysis of prognostic indicators. Neurosurgery 2000;46: 1063–7.

66. Oyesiku NM, Colohan AR, Barrow DL, et al. Cocaine-induced aneurysmal rupture: an emergent factor in the natural history of intra-cranial aneurysms? Neurosurgery 1993;32:518–25.

67. Simpson RK Jr, Fischer DK, Narayan RK, et al. Intravenous cocaine abuse and subarachnoid haemorrhage: effect on outcome. Br J Neurosurg 1990; 4:27–30.

68. Howington JU, Kutz SC, Wilding G, et al. Cocaine use as a predictor of outcome in aneurysmal subarachnoid hemorrhage. J Neurosurg 2003;99: 271–5.

69. Tseng M-Y, Czosnyka M, Richards H, et al. Effects of acute treatment with pravastatin on cerebral vasospasm, autoregulation, and delayed ischemic deficits after aneurysmal subarachnoid hemorrhage: a phase II randomized placebo-controlled trial. Stroke 2005;36:1627–32.

70. Parra A, Kreiter KT, Williams S, et al. Effect of prior statin use on functional outcome and delayed vasospasm after acute aneurysmal subarachnoid hemorrhage: a matched controlled cohort study. Neurosurgery 2005;56:476–84.

71. Russell SM, Lin K, Hahn SA, et al. Smaller cerebral aneurysms producing more extensive subarachnoid hemorrhage following rupture: a radiological investigation and discussion of theoretical determinants. J Neurosurg 2003;99:248–53.

72. Taylor CL, Steele D, Kopitnik TA Jr, et al. Outcome after subarachnoid hemorrhage from a very small aneurysm: a case-control series. J Neurosurg 2004;100:623–5.

73. Salary M, Quigley MR, Wilberger JE Jr. Relation among aneurysm size, amount of subarachnoid blood, clinical outcome. J Neurosurg 2007;107: 13–7.

74. Säveland H, Brandt L. Which are the major determinants for outcome in aneurysmal subarachnoid hemorrhage? A prospective total management study from a strictly unselected series. Acta Neurol Scand 1994;90:245–50.

75. Schievink WI, Wijdicks EFM, Piepgras DG, et al. The poor prognosis of ruptured intracranial aneurysms of the posterior circulation. Neurosurgery 1995;82:791–5.

76. Kongable GL, Lanzino G, Germanson TP, et al. Gender related differences in aneurysmal subarachnoid hemorrhage. J Neurosurg 1996;84: 43–8.

77. Haberman S, Capildeo R, Rose FC. Sex differences in the incidence of cerebrovascular disease. J Epidemiol Community Health 1981; 35:45–50.

78. Simpson RK, Contant CF, Fischer DK, et al. Epidemiological characteristics of subarachnoid hemorrhage in an urban population. J Clin Epidemiol 1991;44:641–8.

79. Sekhar LN, Heros RC. Origin, growth, and rupture of saccular aneurysms: a review. Neurosurgery 1981;8:248–60.

80. Inagawa T, Hirano A. Autopsy study of unruptured incidental intracranial aneurysms. Surg Neurol 1990;34:361–5.

81. Inagawa T, Hirano A. Ruptured intracranial aneurysms: an autopsy study of 133 patients. Surg Neurol 1990;33:117–23.

82. Rosenørn J, Eskesen V, Schmidt K. Clinical features and outcome in females and males with ruptured intracranial ular aneurysms. Br J Neurosurg 1993;7:287–90.

83. Cavanagh SJ, Gordon VL. Grading scales used in the management of aneurysmal subarachnoid hemorrhage: a critical review. J Neurosci Nurs 2002;34:288–95.

84. Drake CG. Report of the World Federation of Neurological Surgeons Committee on a universal subarachnoid haemorrhage grading scale. J Neurosurg 1988;68:985–8.

85. Weismann M, Missler U, Hagenström H, et al. S-100 protein plasma levels after aneurysmal subarachnoid haemorrhage. Acta Neurochir 1997; 139(12):1155–60.

86. Juvela S. Plasma endothelin concentrations after aneurysmal subarachnoid hemorrhage. J Neurosurg 2000;92:390–400.

87. Pilitsis JG, Coplin WM, O'Regan MH, et al. Free fatty acids in human cerebrospinal fluid following subarachnoid hemorrhage and their potential role in vasospasm: a preliminary observation. J Neurosurg 2002;97:272–9.

88. Leung CHS, Poon WS, Yu LM. Apolipoprotein E genotype and outcome in aneurysmal subarachnoid hemorrhage. Stroke 2002;33:548–52.

89. Powell J, Kitchen N, Heslin J, et al. Psychosocial outcomes at three and nine months after good neurological recovery from aneurismal subarachnoid haemorrhage: predictors and prognosis. J Neurol Neurosurg Psychiatr 2002;72:772–81.

90. Dombovy ML, Drew-Cates J, Serdans R. Recovery and rehabilitation following subarachnoid haemorrhage. Part I. Outcome after inpatient rehabilitation. Brain Inj 1998;12:443–54.

91. Dombovy ML, Drew-Cates J, Serdans R. Recovery and rehabilitation following subarachnoid haemorrhage. Part II. Long-term follow-up. Brain Inj 1998; 12:887–94.

92. Freckmann N, Stegen G, Valdueza JM. Long-term follow-up and quality of life after aneurysmal subarachnoid haemorrhage. Aktuelle Neurol 1994;21:84–8.

93. Beristain X, Gaviria M, Dujony M, et al. Evaluation of outcome after intracranial aneurysm surgery: the neuropsychiatric approach. Surg Neurol 1996;45: 422–9.

94. Ogden JA, Mee E, Henning M. A prospective study of psychosocial adaptation following subarachnoid haemorrhage. Neuropsychol Rehabil 1994;4:7–30.

95. McKenna P, Willison JR, Lowe D, et al. Cognitive outcome and quality of life one year after subarachnoid haemorrhage. Neurosurgery 1989;24:361–7.

96. Ross YB, Dijkgraaf MG, Albrecht KW, et al. Direct costs of modern treatment of aneurysmal subarachnoid hemorrhage in the first year after diagnosis. Stroke 2002;33:1595–9.

97. Hop JW, Rinkel GJE, Algra A, et al. Quality of life in patients and partners after aneurysmal subarachnoid haemorrhage. Stroke 1998;29:798–804.

98. Pritchard C, Foulkes L, Lang DA, et al. Psychosocial outcomes for patients and carers after aneurismal subarachnoid haemorrhage. Br J Neurosurg 2001;15(6):456–63.

99. Mezue W, Mathew B, Draper P, et al. The impact of care on carers of patients treated for aneurysmal subarachnoid haemorrhage. Br J Neurosurg 2004; 18(2):135–7. Available at: http://www.informaworld.com/smpp/title~content=t713407147~db=all~tab=issueslist~branches=18-v18.

100. Ross YB, Dijkgraaff MG, Albrecht KW, et al. Direct costs of modern treatment of aneurysmal subarachnoid hemorrhage in the first year after diagnosis. Stroke 2002;33:1595–9.

101. Bairstow P, Dodgson A, Linto J, et al. Comparison of cost and outcome of endovascular and neurosurgical procedures in the treatment of ruptured intracranial aneurysms. Australas Radiol 2002;46:249–51.

102. Wolstenholme J, Rivero-Arias O, Gray A, et al. Treatment pathways, resource use, and costs of endovascular coiling versus surgical clipping after aSAH. Stroke 2008;39:111–9.

103. Javadpour M, Jain H, Wallace MC, et al. Analysis of cost related to clinical and angiographic outcomes of aneurysm patients enrolled in the international subarachnoid aneurysm trial in a North American setting. Neurosurgery 2005;56:886–93.

104. Niskanen M, Koivisto T, Ronkainen A, et al. Resource use after subarachnoid hemorrhage: comparison between endovascular and surgical treatment. Neurosurgery May 2004;54(5):1081–8.

105. Yentur E, Gurbuz S, Tanriverdi T, et al. Clipping and coiling of intracerebral aneurysms—a cost analysis from a developing country. Neurosurg Q 2004;14:127–32.

106. Tsutsumi K, Ueki K, Usui M, et al. Risk of recurrent subarachnoid hemorrhage after complete obliteration of cerebral aneurysms. Stroke 1998;29:2511–3.

107. Wermer MJH, Greebe P, Algra A, et al. Incidence of recurrent subarachnoid hemorrhage after clipping for ruptured intracranial aneurysms. Stroke 2005; 36:2394–9.

108. Wermer MJH, Rinkel GJE, Greebe P, et al. Late recurrence of subarachnoid hemorrhage after treatment for ruptured aneurysms: patient characteristics and outcomes. Neurosurgery 2005;56: 197–204.

109. Elliott JP, Le Roux PD, Ransom G, et al. Predicting length of hospital stay and cost by aneurysm grade on admission. J Neurosurg 1996;85:388–91.

110. Wiebers DO, Torner JC, Meissner I. Impact of unruptured intracranial aneurysms on public health in the United States. Stroke 1992;23: 1416–9.

111. Solomon RA, Mayer SA, Tarmey JJ. Relationship between the volume of craniotomies for cerebral aneurysm performed at New York state hospital and in-hospital mortality. Stroke 1996;27:13–7.

112. Berman MF, Johnston SC, Solomon RA, et al. Impact on hospital related factors on outcome following treatment of cerebral aneurysms. Stroke 2003;34:2200–7.

113. Luft HS, Hunt SS, Maerki SC. The volume-outcome relationship: practice makes perfect or selective referral patterns? Health Serv Res 1987;22:157–82.

114. Ashkan K, Guy N, Norris J. Sub-specialisation in neurosurgery: perspective from a small specialty. Ann R Coll Surg Engl 2003;85:149–53.

115. Bardach NS, Olson SJ, Elkins JS, et al. Regionalization of treatment for subarachnoid hemorrhage—a cost utility analysis. Circulation 2004; 109:2207–12.

Surgical Management of Aneurysmal Subarachnoid Hemorrhage

Geoffrey P. Colby, MD, PhD, Alexander L. Coon, MD,
Rafael J. Tamargo, MD*

KEYWORDS

- Aneurysmal subarachnoid hemorrhage
- Surgical management
- Vascular neurosurgery • Neurocritical care

Aneurysmal subarachnoid hemorrhage (aSAH) comprises approximately 2% to 5% of all strokes in the United States, affecting about 30,000 people annually,[1] and the worldwide incidence is approximately 10.5 cases per 1000,000 individuals.[2] Despite advances in diagnostic tools, perioperative management, and definitive surgical or endovascular interventions, aSAH remains a devastating condition. Following aSAH, at least 12% of patients die before receiving medical attention,[3] 46% die within 30 days,[4] and many survivors have significant morbidity and require long term assistance.[1] Cognitive dysfunction is common among aSAH survivors, with up to 50% showing deficits and unable to return to work.[5–7] Because aSAH occurs at a relatively young age and has such a poor prognosis, it is estimated that the loss of productive years from SAH is a significant portion of years lost from ischemic stroke.[8] Outcomes following aSAH are primarily determined by the severity of the initial bleed, early rebleeding, and delayed cerebral ischemia secondary to vasospasm.

Intracranial aneurysm formation and subsequent rupture is a complex multifactorial process that is not well understood. Epidemiology of aSAH is dependent on age, sex, race, and location. Aneurysmal SAH can occur in any age group, but is most common in the fourth to sixth decades.

Women have 1.6 times greater risk than men of aSAH[9] and African Americans have 2.1 times the risk of whites.[10] Incidence of aSAH varies greatly among different countries, with Japan (23 to 32 per 100,000) and Finland (22.5 per 100,000) having the highest statistics.[1] Modifiable risk factors include smoking, hypertension, heavy alcohol intake, and use of sympathomimetic agents (eg, cocaine).[1,11] Nonmodifiable risk factors include a family history of SAH and autosomal-dominant polycystic kidney disease, as well as various uncharacterized genetic susceptibility loci.[12,13] Familial intracranial aneurysms tend to rupture at earlier ages than sporadic aneurysms.[12]

Aneurysmal SAH is a life-threatening condition that requires prompt medical and surgical attention. This article reviews the surgical management of aSAH, describing frequently used craniotomies and certain additional techniques and surgical maneuvers that are currently debated in the literature.

HISTORICAL PERSPECTIVE

Early treatment of cerebral aneurysms involved ligation of the proximal parent artery, a technique named Hunterian ligation after John Hunter (1728–1793), who popularized the technique in peripheral arteries in the mid 1700s.[14] Victor

Department of Neurosurgery, The Johns Hopkins University School of Medicine, 600 North Wolfe Street, Meyer 8-181, Baltimore, MD 21287, USA
* Corresponding author.
E-mail address: rtamarg@jhmi.edu

Neurosurg Clin N Am 21 (2010) 247–261
doi:10.1016/j.nec.2009.10.003

Horsley (1857–1916) was the first person to apply this technique to the cerebral circulation when he performed internal carotid artery (ICA) ligation for a giant intracranial aneurysm in 1885.[14,15] Norman Dott (1897–1973) subsequently performed the first planned intracranial surgery for treatment of a ruptured cerebral aneurysm in 1931, in which he wrapped the aneurysm with muscle for hemostasis.[16] Dott learned the technique of using muscle pledgets while training under Harvey Cushing (1869–1939), who is thought to be the first surgeon to pack and wrap an unruptured intracranial aneurysm.[15] Dott also pioneered the technique of aneurysm suture ligation in 1933, although this technically challenging maneuver was eventually supplanted by aneurysm clips.[14]

Cushing introduced hemostatic silver vessel clips to neurosurgery in 1911, first using these clips in tumor surgeries to achieve hemostasis on vessels not accessible to suture ligation.[15] Walter Dandy (1886–1946) used a modified Cushing V-shaped silver clip in 1937 to perform the first clipping of an ICA aneurysm.[17] Over the subsequent decades, aneurysm clips underwent many design modifications, particularly with respect to the size and shape of clips suitable for microsurgery and to the materials required for compatibility with magnetic resonance imaging (eg, titanium).[17] In the late 1970s, clipping of ruptured aneurysms was shown to be better than the alternatives of bed rest and carotid artery ligation,[18] and neurosurgical practices shifted toward using clips for routine treatment.

TIMING OF SURGICAL INTERVENTION

Practice regarding the timing of surgery following aneurysm rupture has been historically controversial and has gone through changes over the years.[19] From the 1950s to the mid 1970s, most surgeons advocated delaying surgical intervention for aneurysm clipping at least 1 week until the patient was medically stable. Early surgery was presumed to be more technically demanding due to brain swelling, thought to worsen vasospasm, and was associated with high operative morbidity and worse outcomes.[19–21] While delayed surgical intervention led to excellent operative results, overall patient outcomes remained poor because of high rates of rebleeding and significant vasospasm-related morbidity and mortality in patients waiting for surgery.[22] Rebleeding is a major concern following aSAH, as mortality from such an event reaches 70%.[1] The risk of rebleeding following aSAH without intervention is up to 40% within 30 days,[23] with the rate greatest within the first 24 hours (4%) versus a daily rate of 1% to

2% for the subsequent 4 weeks.[24] Certain studies have demonstrated higher rebleed rates (15%) within the first day, especially within 2 to 12 hours.[25,26] Following the 30-day peak period, the risk of rebleed settles out at about 3% per year.[27]

Interest in early surgery increased in the late 1970s as surgical techniques improved, operations became safer, and as medical management failed to significantly reduce rates of vasospasm and rebleeding before surgery.[19] Following favorable initial results from early surgery, primarily from Japanese groups, the International Cooperative Study on the Timing of Aneurysm Surgery sought to better characterize the relationship between outcomes for early (0–3 days) versus late (11–14 days) surgery after aSAH.[22] This study showed that the overall patient outcome of early surgery was equivalent to that of late surgery. Of note, patients in the late surgery group had better surgical outcomes at 6 months than the early surgery group, most likely secondary to natural selection of survivors. However, up to 30% of patients with aSAH do not survive to have surgery at the later time points, and waiting 2 weeks for surgery was associated with a 30% risk of focal ischemic deficit and 12% risk of rebleeding. Thus, the additional risks associated with delayed surgery negated the better surgical outcomes seen in this group, and early surgery became a feasible option. Additional impetus for early surgery is that these patients, having a secured aneurysm, would greatly benefit from any future advances in vasospasm management. It is now common practice that patients are operated on within 48 hrs of presentation if an aneurysm is present.

COMMON SURGICAL APPROACHES

Surgery for intracranial aneurysms relies on 2 main principles: gaining access to the aneurysm through a craniotomy and subsequently securing the aneurysm. The basic principles of turning a craniotomy and the microsurgical principles used for the management of acute aSAH (eg, opening of the arachnoid, drainage of cerebral cisterns, use of microinstruments, use of the operating microscope, and brain retraction) have been thoroughly reviewed in numerous articles and textbooks. This section reviews common craniotomies used in most operative cases for acute aSAH. The surgical approach to any given aneurysm depends on a variety of factors, including aneurysm location, morphology, orientation, and neck anatomy. There are 3 main surgical approaches, with possible extensions, required to treat the majority of anterior and posterior circulation aneurysms.[28] Each of these approaches is described briefly below.

Frontosphenotemporal (Pterional) Craniotomy, and the Orbitozygomatic and Subtemporal Extensions

The frontosphenotemporal or pterional craniotomy[29] (**Fig. 1**) is the workhorse of vascular neurosurgery and can be used for most anterior circulation aneurysms and upper posterior circulation aneurysms. For this approach, the head is placed in a radiolucent skull immobilizer, rotated (up to 60 degrees depending on surgical target), and the neck is extended (approximately 30 degrees) so that the malar eminence is the highest point. The scalp is incised from the root of the zygomatic arch, to the linea temporalis, and anteriorly to the midline just short of the patient's hairline. The scalp and temporalis muscles are elevated using a subfascial dissection to preserve the frontalis branch of the facial nerve.[30]

In the authors' practice, the craniotomy is performed using 5 burr holes: keyhole, above the zygomatic root, approximately 1 cm above the temporal squamosa (in line with zygomatic root), intersection of coronal suture with linea temporalis, and frontal bone above frontal sinus and orbit.

The burr holes are connected with a Gigli saw (allows for maximum beveling and superior aesthetic results) except for the segment between the keyhole and zygomatic root, which is drilled. Additional squamosal temporal bone is removed with a rongeur to expose the floor of the middle cranial fossa. The greater and lesser wings of the sphenoid are then drilled until the dural flap covering the orbitomeningeal artery is exposed. The dura is opened with a semicircular incision and reflected anterior.

To improve access to the basilar apex and upper clivus regions, the orbitozygomatic and subtemporal extensions (see **Fig. 1**) can be performed following a traditional pterional craniotomy. Since Jane and colleagues[31] first described the supraorbital craniotomy, it has evolved considerably through many adjustments.[32–36] The traditional orbitozygomatic craniotomy as described by Zabramski and colleagues[37] and the modified orbitozygomatic craniotomies as described by Lemole and colleagues[38] are commonly used today. For the traditional orbitozygomatic craniotomy, the temporal fascia is elevated to expose the zygoma and superior orbital rim, and the periorbita is detached from the orbital roof with the use of an Adson elevator. The orbital and zygomatic osteotomies are then performed using a series of 6 bone cuts involving the orbital roof, lateral orbit,

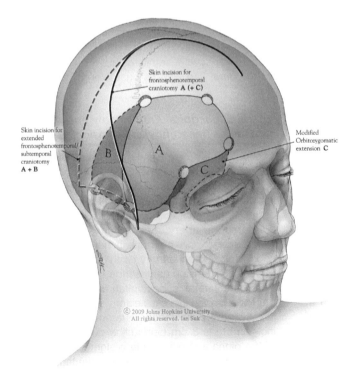

Fig. 1. Frontosphenotemporal craniotomy (A) with subtemporal (B) or modified orbitozygomatic (C) extensions. The skin incision for the frontosphenotemporal craniotomy with or without the modified orbitozygomatic extension (*solid line*) is curvilinear and extends from the root of the zygoma to the hairline in the midline. The frontosphenotemporal craniotomy (A) is centered on the sphenoid wing and keyhole. For the modified orbitozygomatic extension (C), the orbital rim and frontal process of the zygomatic bone are removed. For the frontosphenotemporal craniotomy with subtemporal extension, the skin incision extends posteriorly from the root of the zygoma to the region of the mastoid (*dashed line*) and then arcs superiorly to the hairline in the midline. The craniotomy for the subtemporal extension (C) includes removal of more temporal and parietal bone. (*Courtesy* of Johns Hopkins University, Baltimore, MD.)

maxillary root, and zygomatic root as previously described.[37] Subtemporal and supraorbital modifications of the traditional orbitozygomatic craniotomy can be performed to better tailor the craniotomy to treat lesions in the temporal fossa or the anterior/middle cranial fossae, respectively.[38] In general, the authors favor the modified orbitozygomatic craniotomy over the full version of this extension.

The subtemporal craniotomy was popularized by Charles Drake in 1961[39] as an approach to the basilar apex. In brief, the subtemporal approach is performed through a horseshoe-shaped incision starting at the zygoma in front of the ear, extending superiorly and posteriorly along the linea temporalis, and then inferior behind the mastoid. The craniotomy flap is turned using burr holes at the corners of the intended boney exposure and by drilling a trough across the base of the bone flap. Once the bone flap is removed, the inferior edge of the craniotomy is drilled flush with the floor of the middle cranial fossa, and a horseshoe-shaped dural flap is reflected inferiorly. The limitations of this approach include a narrow surgical corridor, the need for significant brain retraction, and difficult access to the contralateral P1 segment and nearby perforators. In the setting of aSAH, a swollen temporal lobe can be problematic when this approach is used.

Most neurosurgeons today use the subtemporal craniotomy as an extension of the frontosphenotemporal craniotomy. The "half and half" approach, originally mentioned by Drake in 1978[40] and popularized by Batjer and Samson,[41] combines the pterional craniotomy with a subtemporal craniotomy. This combined approach essentially eliminates the disadvantages of a pure subtemporal approach, and it provides good access to the basilar bifurcation, the superior cerebellar artery takeoff, and the P1 segment.

As with all surgical procedures, cosmetically superior reconstruction following craniotomy for aSAH is paramount to prevent disfigurement and negative psychosocial effects on the patient and the family. Patients undergoing pterional craniotomies for aneurysm clipping commonly have depression of the frontozygomatic fossa 6 to 12 months after surgery secondary to atrophy of the temporalis muscle. Such cosmetic defects can be avoided by careful dissection to maintain the neurovascular supply to the temporalis muscle[42] and by a simple use of a frontozygomatic fossa titanium cranioplasty.[43] Raza and colleagues[43] described the use of a frontozygomatic titanium cranioplasty in 194 patients who underwent a pterional craniotomy with average follow-up of 9.5

months. In this series, 93% of patients had excellent cosmetic outcomes with virtually no evidence of surgery, and the remaining 7% had only slight depression of the temporalis fossa. This method and other such techniques should be used when possible to achieve outstanding cosmesis in aSAH patients.

Anterior Parasagittal Craniotomy

The anterior parasagittal craniotomy (**Fig. 2**) is used for interhemispheric approaches to distal anterior cerebral artery aneurysms as described by Tamargo and colleagues.[44] For this approach, a radiolucent skull immobilizer is placed and then the head is distracted, flexed, and rotated to the contralateral side. Many variations in positioning have been described, with some surgeons preferring more lateral head position to facilitate gravity retraction and increased exposure of the interhemispheric fissure.

The scalp is incised in a bicoronal fashion and the flap is reflected anteriorly. Following identification of the coronal and sagittal sutures, a pentagonal craniotomy is planned with 5 burr holes so that the craniotomy straddles the midline and extends 4 to 5 cm in front and 2 to 3 cm behind the coronal suture. The anterior-posterior position of the craniotomy in relation to the coronal suture can be modified depending on the location of the aneurysm. Two burr holes are placed ipsilateral to the lesion, 2 burr holes directly over the sagittal sinus, and a single burr hole is placed on the contralateral side. The burr holes are connected with a Gigli saw. A semicircular incision is made for the dural flap with its base along the sagittal sinus.

Lateral Suboccipital Craniectomy and the Far-Lateral Transcondylar Extension

Although there are many different described approaches to aneurysms of the posterior circulation, most aneurysms of the vertebral trunk, the mid and lower basilar trunk, and their associated branches (superior cerebellar artery, anterior inferior cerebellar artery, and posterior inferior cerebellar artery) can be approached by a lateral suboccipital craniectomy with or without the far-lateral extension as described (**Fig. 3**).[28]

For the lateral suboccipital craniectomy, the patient is placed in a skull clamp and is positioned in either the park-bench or lateral position. The incision starts 3 cm behind the posterior margin of the pinna and extends in a sigmoid fashion to the spinous process of C2. After reflection of the suboccipital musculature, the asterion is identified (landmark for junction of transverse and sigmoid

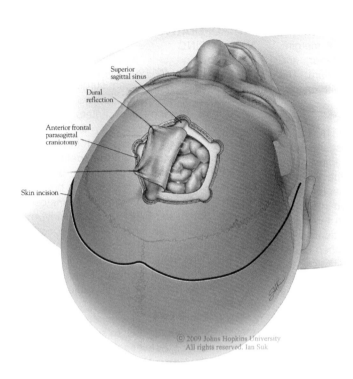

Superior
sagittal sinus

Dural
reflection

Anterior frontal
parasagittal
craniotomy

Skin incision

Fig. 2. Anterior parasagittal craniotomy. A bicoronal skin incision is made (*solid line*). The pentagonal craniotomy straddles the midline. The anterior-posterior position of the craniotomy in relation to the coronal suture is tailored to the location of the aneurysm. A semicircular dural incision is made with its base along the superior sagittal sinus and is reflected toward the midline. (*Courtesy of* Johns Hopkins University, Baltimore, MD.)

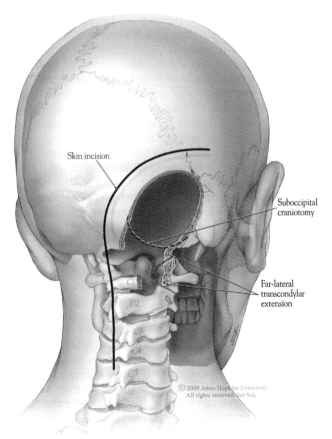

Skin incision

Suboccipital
craniotomy

C1
C2

Far-lateral
transcondylar
extension

Fig. 3. Lateral suboccipital craniectomy and the far-lateral transcondylar extension. A "hockey stick" skin incision (*solid line*) is made with the lateral arm beginning superior and posterior to the ear, descending medial, and ending midline in the upper to mid cervical level. The suboccipital craniectomy extends from the asterion to just above the foramen magnum (*dashed line*). For the far-lateral extension, the lip of the foramen magnum, the C1 arch, and the posteromedial third of the atlanto-occipital joint are removed. (*Courtesy of* Johns Hopkins University, Baltimore, MD.)

sinuses). A craniectomy is then performed that extends from the asterion (supralateral margin), to just above the foramen magnum (inferior), and medially to expose the lateral cerebellum. The dura is opened in a lambdoid incision with respect to the sigmoid and transverse sinuses.

For the far-lateral extension, a "hockey stick" incision is performed with the lateral arm beginning superior and posterior to the ear, descending to the superior nuchal line, crossing medial to the midline, and then descending to the spinous process of C2 or C3. A musculocutaneous flap is then elevated to expose the foramen magnum, the mastoid, and C1 from the arch to the transverse process. The vertebral artery is identified at the point where it enters the dura and then traced to the sulcus arteriosus. The main additions of the far-lateral are removal of the C1 arch, the lip of the foramen magnum, and the posteromedial third of the atlanto-occipital joint. Following completion of the craniectomy, the dura is opened from the transverse sigmoid junction to the arch of C1 and reflected laterally.

FENESTRATION OF THE LAMINA TERMINALIS

Aneurysmal SAH can cause fibrosis of the arachnoid granulations and leptomeninges,[45,46] leading to altered cerebrospinal fluid (CSF) dynamics and persistent hydrocephalus that requires CSF diversion. Shunt-dependent hydrocephalus occurs in > 20% of patients with aSAH,[47] representing a significant complication. Microsurgical fenestration of the lamina terminalis during aneurysm surgery was proposed in the mid to late 1990s as a means of facilitating CSF dynamics and reducing the incidence of shunt-dependent hydrocephalus in patients with aSAH[48,49]; however, subsequent studies have been inconclusive regarding the benefit of this technique. Komotar and colleagues,[47] in a retrospective study of 582 patients with aSAH, demonstrated greater than 80% reduction in shunt-dependent hydrocephalus if the lamina terminalis was fenestrated at the time of surgery. However, a more recent retrospective analysis of 369 patients[50] and a literature review comparing results from 11 different studies[51] failed to find a significant association between lamina terminalis fenestration and decreased shunt dependency. This latest review, in particular, is limited by unmatched cohorts, and all studies of this technique are limited by lack of prospective, randomized data. Pending more definitive studies, this technique is generally favorable and continues to be used by the senior author of this article.

INTRAOPERATIVE ELECTROPHYSIOLOGICAL MONITORING

Intraoperative neurophysiological monitoring during intracranial aneurysm surgery has become standard practice at the authors' institution as well as other major medical centers. Intraoperative neurophysiological monitoring is an important adjunct to meticulous surgical inspection and intraoperative angiography to detect cerebral ischemia from temporary clipping, unintentional parent vessel or perforator occlusion, brain manipulation, and retraction injury. Somatosensory evoked potentials (SSEPs), particularly median and posterior tibial nerve SSEPs, are commonly monitored during anterior circulation procedures, whereas dual monitoring with SSEPs and brainstem auditory evoked responses (BAERs) are preferred for posterior circulation aneurysm surgeries.[52,53]

The rationale for employing electrophysiological monitoring during aneurysm surgery is the significant correlation between alterations in electrical signals and regional cerebral blood flow (rCBF), with transient electrophysiological changes generally corresponding to good outcomes[52] and permanent changes corresponding to postoperative deficits.[54,55] However, SSEP false-negative rates can reach up to 25% in some studies, and patients with unchanged SSEPs can still have new postoperative motor and other neurologic deficits.[53,56] Motor deficits with the false-negative SSEP results are commonly attributed to subcortical (internal capsule or brainstem) strokes.[57–59] Monitoring of motor evoked potentials (MEPs) has been evaluated for efficacy in detecting impending motor deficits. Studies by Neuloh and Schramm,[56] using transcranial electrical stimulation, and Horiuchi and colleagues,[60] using direct cortical stimulation, have demonstrated that MEP deterioration is a more sensitive and reliable predictor of postoperative motor paresis than SSEPs. This technique is promising, but further evaluation in a controlled trial is needed to assess if monitoring with MEPs can reduce morbidity from aneurysm surgery in patients with aSAH.

Electroencephalography (EEG) is also commonly used during surgery for intracranial aneurysm clipping. Prior to temporary clip application, the neuroanesthesia team titrates the brain-protective anesthetic regimen to achieve burst suppression on EEG. Burst suppression helps to decrease metabolic demand so that the cerebral tissue can better tolerate induced ischemia, such as during temporary clipping. EEG is less commonly used to detect ischemia during such surgeries because the airspaces between the dura and arachnoid as a result of the craniotomy and brain relaxation can interfere with scalp EEG recordings.[53,61] Intraoperative multilobar EEG using subdural electrodes are more sensitive than scalp EEG for detecting ischemic events during aneurysm surgery,[62] but these are not currently in widespread use.

DIGITAL SUBTRACTION INTRAOPERATIVE ANGIOGRAPHY

Egas Moniz (1874–1955) developed cerebral angiography in 1927,[17] but it was not until 1933 when the first angiogram to demonstrate an intracranial aneurysm was performed by Norman Dott.[16] The technology to perform intraoperative angiography was available by the 1960s,[63] however, its routine use did not occur until the 1990s. The interest for intraoperative evaluation of aneurysm clip placement stemmed from reports of routine postoperative angiography that demonstrated unexpected rates of residual aneurysms and major vessel compromise.[64–66] In such studies, the incidence of residual aneurysms and incidence of parent or branch vessel occlusion were as high as 12% and 19%, respectively, for a possible combined 31% total incidence of unexpected findings. Incompletely treated aneurysms are dangerous as they are prone to regrowth with a 20% to 80% risk of rehemorrhage and 10% to 30% risk of mass effect over 10 to 20 years.[64,67–69] These reports, combined with improvements in portable digital subtraction (DS) angiography equipment and practitioner expertise led to more widespread use of intraoperative angiography and subsequent studies evaluating its efficacy.

Various groups have evaluated and demonstrated the efficacy of intraoperative angiography during surgery for aneurysm clipping as an adjunct to methodical surgical technique and clip inspection.[70–72] In a series of 337 aneurysms by Chiang and colleagues,[71] findings on intraoperative angiography led to clip repositioning in 37 (11%) of aneurysm cases, with 22 (6.5%) being related to residual aneurysm, 10 (3%) parent vessel occlusion, and 5 (1.5%) a combination of residual aneurysm and vessel occlusion. Intraoperative angiography is particularly useful in large (>10 mm) and giant (>25 mm) aneurysms, as these lesions are more likely to be unsatisfactorily clipped and require revision than smaller aneurysms.[70–72] It is also particularly useful in peri-clinoidal, basilar apex, and anterior communicating region aneurysms. Complications from intraoperative angiography include vessel occlusion, embolic events, and dissection. Chiang and colleagues[71] reported an overall complication rate of 2.6%, with stroke in 1 of 303 (0.3%) operations, whereas Tang and colleagues[72] reported 2 strokes in 517 aneurysms treated (0.4% stroke risk). The false-negative rate of intraoperative angiography ranges from 5% to 8%,[70–73] but this number is limited by the lack of routine postoperative angiography in such cases. In general, intraoperative angiography is an important tool to evaluate for aneurysm residuals and vessel occlusion, and it is used routinely at the authors' institution. Drawbacks are that, it is not available in all centers, it is an invasive technique, and it does not provide immediate feedback.

INTRAOPERATIVE FLUORESCENT ANGIOGRAPHY

Intraoperative fluorescent angiography has been a recent addition to the neurosurgical armamentarium to assess intraoperative blood flow dynamics, aneurysm sac obliteration, and vessel patency. Angiography using fluorescein sodium has been used by some groups[74,75] in the treatment of cerebral aneurysms; however, the near-infrared dye indocyanine green (ICG) has emerged as the preferred agent for microsurgical use[76–82] secondary to superior contrast of vessels during primary and subsequent dye applications.[81]

ICG has been evaluated in several studies of aneurysm clipping,[76–80,82] and integration of ICG near-infrared video technology into the surgical microscope[79] has greatly facilitated its application. ICG use is noninvasive, safe, simple, and provides the surgeon with rapid feedback after clip application. ICG provides high resolution imaging of vessel anatomy, arterial and venous blood flow, and incomplete aneurysm clipping. Raabe and colleagues[78] demonstrated that ICG angiography correlated with intraoperative or postoperative DS angiography in 90% of cases, and it provided significant information in 9% of cases, many of which led to clip repositioning. This technique is also unique in that it can visualize perforating arteries with good resolution.[78,80]

ICG videoangiography is not without limitations and is not suited for all applications. Only vessels within the microscope field can be visualized with ICG. Blood clots (subarachnoid, intramural, or intraluminal), vessel wall calcification, atherosclerotic plaque, and arachnoid scarring can all obscure visualization.[78,82] For the aforementioned reasons, ICG angiography is not currently a replacement for intraoperative DS angiography, but rather a complement to it.

TEMPORARY CLIPPING

Temporary arterial occlusion, or induced reversible arrest of local arterial flow, is an important adjunct technique used in the management of cerebral aneurysms. This technique was developed in the 1940s by Norman Dott,[21] and has been a vital tool for cerebrovascular neurosurgeons since that time. Temporary arterial arrest can be useful to decrease the risk of rupture during dissection of cerebral aneurysms ranging from those that are seemingly mundane to those that are complex and giant. The technique softens the aneurysm neck and sac, facilitates microdissection of aneurysms that are adherent to efferent vessels or perforating arteries, and allows for evacuation of calcified larger aneurysms before definitive clip placement. In the event of an intraoperative rupture, targeted temporary clip placement halts flow to the involved vessel and provides the neurosurgeon with critical minutes to enact a definitive treatment plan. Temporary arterial occlusion on vascular territories at greatest risk for infarction following temporary clipping are those with significant numbers of perforating arteries, such as the distal basilar artery and the proximal middle cerebral artery.[83]

The goal of temporary clip placement is to limit the duration of occlusion so that iatrogenic ischemia is not converted to permanent infarction. Prior to temporary clipping, intravenous brain-protection anesthesia titrated to EEG burst suppression is initiated to increase tolerance of brain tissue to temporary ischemia by decreasing cellular metabolic demand. Hypertension is also commonly induced to increase collateral perfusion.

Although temporary clipping of parent vessels is routinely used in the operating room, reported "safe limit" times of occlusion are variable, mostly secondary to the wide variety of patient, technical, and anesthetic factors involved. Various studies have tried to determine the occlusion time tolerable before infarction occurs; however, the acceptable occlusion time depends on the location of the aneurysm, the presence of nearby perforating arteries, the degree of collateral flow, and the anesthetic regime used to achieve brain protection. Samson and colleagues,[83] in a study of 100 patients undergoing temporary arterial occlusion under normothermic, normotensive conditions with etomidate-mediated burst suppression, demonstrated that temporary ischemia converted to fixed infarction within 15 to 20 minutes of temporary clip time. In this study, none of 49 (0%) patients with temporary clip time less than 14 minutes developed an infarction

linked to the temporary clipping, whereas 5 of 27 (19%) patients with temporary clip times between 14 and 21 minutes developed an infarction. Furthermore, patients over 61 years of age and those with poorer preoperative neurologic condition (Hunt and Hess Grade III to IV) developed permanent infarction after shorter periods of arterial occlusion. Ogilvy and colleagues,[84] using mild hypothermia, hypertension, and mannitol for brain protection also found that the risk of stroke increased after approximately 15 to 20 minutes, with a stroke rate of 1 in 67 (1.5%) in patients with temporary clipping duration less than 20 minutes and stroke rate of 12 in 65 (18%) for longer clip durations. Tolerable temporary ischemia varies depending on the vascular territory. For example, Lavine and colleagues[85] demonstrated that infarction was more common after only 10 minutes of occlusion time for middle cerebral artery aneurysms despite the use of brain-protection anesthesia, as the middle cerebral artery (MCA) territory is particularly sensitive to ischemia.

One modification of the temporary clipping technique is the use of intermittent reperfusion, or short periods of temporary occlusion separated by reperfusion periods. Although intermittent reperfusion is beneficial in decreasing ischemia in rat[86–88] and rabbit[89] stroke models, few clinical studies have addressed this question. Samson and colleagues[83] did not show any benefit to the use of intermittent reperfusion.

DEEP HYPOTHERMIC CARDIOPULMONARY BYPASS

Some aneurysms cannot be safely clipped while fully arterialized. Such aneurysms are typically large, deep in location, have atherosclerotic walls, are partially thrombosed, are intimately associated with critical perforators, or incorporate branch vessels in the wall and the dome. Perforating arteries and the cerebral territories they perfuse do not tolerate temporary clipping well. As such, special circumstances arise when temporary clipping is not sufficient, and reduced blood flow (or complete circulatory arrest) in combination with deep hypothermia for brain protection is necessary to decrease pressure in the aneurysm dome for proper dissection and clipping.

Circulatory arrest, or no-flow deep hypothermic circulatory arrest, was first introduced in the 1960s and subsequently underwent many modifications, including adaptation to the neurosurgical arena. The specifics of this complex technique are described elsewhere.[90] Several series have been published regarding hypothermic circulatory arrest for aneurysm treatment.[91–94] Mack and colleagues[94] published a 15-year, single institution experience with deep hypothermic circulatory arrest for complex aneurysms in 66 patients, 15 (23%) of whom presented as SAH. In this series, aneurysms were clipped in 57 (86%) patients and unclipped in 9 (14%) patients. Unclipped aneurysms were treated by Hunterian ligation (n = 3), trapping (n = 4), or left untreated (n = 2). The surgical mortality was 11% based on 7 perioperative deaths, with 2 of the deaths resulting from complication of the cardiopulmonary bypass. Patient age and duration of cardiac arrest were independent predictors of early clinical outcome ($P<.05$), with patients younger than 60 years and circulatory arrest times less than 30 minutes associated with better outcomes. This group found that the volume of cases requiring hypothermic circulatory arrest decreased over the study period, likely secondary to the increase of endovascular capability and early diagnosis of aneurysms before they reach large sizes necessitating bypass procedures.

During the development and refinement of cardiac arrest protocols over the past several decades, concern for adverse neurologic sequelae as a result of complete circulatory arrest gave rise to the alternative method of low-flow deep hypothermic cardiopulmonary bypass (DHCPB), in which cerebral and body circulation is maintained at a reduced rate. Several early studies, primarily in animals, provided evidence for superior neurologic outcomes using low-flow DHCPB versus cardiac arrest.[95–97] This result was confirmed by Newburger and colleagues[98] in a study of perioperative neurologic effects of no-flow versus low-flow DHCPB open cardiac surgery in 171 infants. Cardiac arrest was associated with higher risk of seizure, longer EEG-based recovery time, and greater release of brain isoenzyme and creatine kinase within 6 hours after surgery compared with low-flow DHCPB. Bellinger and colleagues[99] studied developmental and neurologic function at 1-year follow-up for 155 of the 171 original patients. Compared with the low-flow DHCPB group, patients in the cardiac arrest group scored significantly lower on the Psychomotor Development Index of the Bayley Scales of Infant Development and had nonstatistically significant trends toward poorer results on other tests of development. Furthermore, worse test results and increased risk of neurologic abnormalities correlated with duration of circulatory arrest. Low-flow DHCPB is used extensively in cardiac and general vascular surgery; however, only few reports exist of its use in neurovascular procedures[100,101] despite data indicating superior outcomes versus cardiac arrest. At the authors' institution, the use of low-flow DHCPB is

favored for the reasons mentioned. Temporary clipping is used as an adjunct maneuver to achieve local flow arrest as needed during aneurysm dissection and clipping.

All neurosurgical procedures involving either low-flow DHCPB or no-flow hypothermic circulatory arrest require pharmacologic- and temperature-mediated brain protection. Mild (33°C) or deep (15°C) hypothermia and pharmacologic agents such as etomidate, propofol, and isoflurane are used to decrease cerebral oxygen consumption and protect the brain from ischemia. When using deep hypothermia, the surgeon must be aware of its many side effects,[90] especially the common side effect of coagulopathy secondary to platelet dysfunction and slowing of the coagulation cascade.[102] Hemostasis is of critical importance during the craniotomy and dissection not only because of the hypothermic coagulopathy but also because heparin is given prior to cannulation and initiation of bypass. A seemingly small ooze can quickly result in significant bleeding if not given due attention. Once hypothermia is induced and the bypass is setup, blood flow can be titrated down as needed, including turning the pump off for total circulatory arrest. Of note, small vessels can appear as arachnoid bands when devoid of blood, so the aneurysm should be dissected as much as possible before cardiac arrest to limit potential damage to these vessels.

Due to the complexity and significant risk of low-flow DHCPB and circulatory arrest procedures, they should only be done at major centers with advanced neurosurgical and cardiothoracic capabilities.

MANAGEMENT OF ACUTE HYDROCEPHALUS

Acute hydrocephalus (ventriculomegaly within 72 hours) is a common manifestation of aSAH that occurs in 20% to 30% of patients, particularly in patients with poor clinical grade and high Fisher Scale scores.[1] In a retrospective study of 433 patients with aSAH, Heuer and colleagues[103] demonstrated increased intracranial pressure (ICP) in approximately 50% of patients with good clinical grade (Hunt and Hess Grades I–III) and more than 60% of patients with poor clinical grade (Hunt and Hess Grades IV–V). Progressive decline in mental status, slow pupillary responses to light, and upward gaze palsy are known presenting signs of acute hydrocephalus,[11] and the diagnosis can be confirmed by computed tomography scan. Patients with acute hydrocephalus following aSAH should receive medical ICP management and be promptly evaluated for external CSF diversion. Elevated ICP following aSAH is associated with poor patient outcome, with higher ICPs leading to worse outcomes.[103] Many centers, including the authors', prefer ventricular drainage, especially when the hydrocephalus is obstructive secondary to intraventricular clot. Other groups prefer lumbar drainage, citing that this technique is more effective than ventricular drainage in washing blood from the basal cisterns,[104,105] and that it may have the added benefit of decreasing vasospasm.[104]

It is generally accepted that timely ventricular drainage for acute hydrocephalus following aSAH in poor clinical grade patients (Hunt and Hess Grades IV–V) is beneficial,[106–109] but is more controversial in good grade patients, particularly Hunt and Hess Grade III.[110] Controversy stems from the belief that CSF drainage before securing a ruptured aneurysm lowers the ICP and, as a result, increases transmural pressure across the aneurysm wall and increases the rebleed risk.[111] Some studies demonstrate an increased rebleed rate with CSF drainage before aneurysm repair,[112–114] whereas other studies demonstrate similar frequency of rebleeding in patients with and without CSF drainage.[105,106,115,116] This topic was recently discussed at a Symposium on the Controversies in the Management of Cerebral Aneurysms,[110] where the audience members preferred noninvasive management for good grade patients.

CEREBRAL REVASCULARIZATION

Some aneurysms are difficult to clip without significant surgical risk of stroke. These aneurysms are often giant or complex, fusiform aneurysms that incorporate the parent artery or other arterial branches into the aneurysm neck and base. Atherosclerosis, calcification, and previous coil embolization[117] can also make aneurysm clipping difficult, if not dangerous. Surgical options for such lesions include parent vessel ligation or aneurysm trapping. However, these maneuvers risk cerebral ischemia and stroke, and extracranial-intracranial (EC-IC) bypass may be necessary to restore distal blood flow. EC-IC bypass procedures were first conceptualized in the early 1950s, but did not become a surgical reality until 1967 when introduced by Yasargil and Donaghy.[118,119] This technique has subsequently been refined by different groups over the decades,[120–123] and many strategies for bypass following parent artery occlusion are currently available for the treatment of aneurysms in the anterior and posterior circulations. Detailed descriptions of these techniques are well described in the literature and in textbooks and are outside the scope of this article. In brief, arterial bypasses have been categorized into 4 main types.[124] Type I is a saphenous vein interposition graft for carotid artery replacement. Type II is a saphenous vein bypass graft from the extracranial carotid artery to the middle or posterior cerebral artery. Type III is a superficial temporal or occipital artery bypass to an intracranial artery. Type IV is the anastomosis of one intracranial artery to an adjacent intracranial artery, or the primary reanastomosis of an artery following aneurysm excision. Important to note is that patients that undergo bypass procedures are commonly on postoperative aspirin, and this might complicate subsequent interventions on sick patients with aSAH.

NOVEL CLIP CONFIGURATIONS AND TECHNIQUES

The neurosurgical literature has numerous technical notes describing novel approaches and maneuvers for treating complex cerebral aneurysms and intraoperative complications, such as aneurysm rupture. Two such reports are described here as examples.

Surgical management of complex multilobed aneurysms, such as those that frequently occur at the MCA bifurcation, presents a challenge to the operator. Many techniques are available to treat these lesions: temporary arterial occlusion, reconstruction with multiple clips in series, coagulation of the aneurysm fundus, wrapping, and in the case of giant aneurysms, hypothermia and circulatory bypass. Novel clip configurations, using combinations of fenestrated and nonfenestrated aneurysm clips, are also effective for obliteration of complex aneurysms and reconstruction of the pertinent normal vascular anatomy.[125,126] Clatterbuck and colleagues[126] reported a series of 15 morphologically complex MCA aneurysms treated successfully with a novel orthogonal interlocking tandem clip arrangement. For this technique, a straight clip is applied to obliterate a portion of the fundus, and then a fenestrated clip is applied to obliterate the residual fundus. The advantage is that the blades of the initial straight clip are incorporated into the fenestration of the second clip, with the angle between the 2 clips 90° or more. This technique can help reduce incidence of aneurysm remnants, while maintaining patency of critical associated normal vasculature.

Intraoperative aneurysm rupture is a known serious complication of surgical intervention for SAH. One type of rupture that can be tricky to manage is partial avulsion of the aneurysm neck.

Lanzino and Spetzler[127] describe the simple, yet effective, technique of clip wrapping to manage this problem. In their case of a woman with SAH from a ruptured anterior communicating artery aneurysm, the aneurysm neck was partially avulsed from the anterior communicating artery during clip placement. The avulsed region was then wrapped, and simultaneously tamponaded, with cotton. The clip was then re-applied to the aneurysm neck so that the clip partially covered the cotton and secured it in place over the avulsion. Novel techniques such as this add to the list of tricks available to the neurosurgeon when dealing with difficult intraoperative situations.

SUMMARY

Aneurysmal SAH is a neurosurgical emergency with significant morbidity and mortality. Successful management of patients with aSAH involves a multidisciplinary team including neurosurgeons, critical care specialists, and in many cases interventional radiologists. Surgical clipping remains a definitive treatment for ruptured cerebral aneurysms, and many techniques have improved over the years to better approach, dissect, and secure both simple and complex aneurysms following aSAH. This report highlights some of these techniques and adjuvant therapies; however, these techniques are constantly evolving and being scrutinized. Future studies, particularly randomized prospective trials, are required to further advance the field and improve outcomes following aSAH.

REFERENCES

1. Bederson JB, Connolly ES Jr, Batjer HH, et al. Guidelines for the management of aneurysmal subarachnoid hemorrhage: a statement for healthcare professionals from a special writing group of the Stroke Council, American Heart Association. Stroke 2009;40:994.
2. Suarez JI, Tarr RW, Selman WR. Aneurysmal subarachnoid hemorrhage. N Engl J Med 2006; 354:387.
3. Schievink WI, Wijdicks EF, Parisi JE, et al. Sudden death from aneurysmal subarachnoid hemorrhage. Neurology 1995;45:871.
4. Broderick JP, Brott T, Tomsick T, et al. Intracerebral hemorrhage more than twice as common as subarachnoid hemorrhage. J Neurosurg 1993;78: 188.
5. Bonita R, Thomson S. Subarachnoid hemorrhage: epidemiology, diagnosis, management, and outcome. Stroke 1985;16:591.
6. Hutter BO, Kreitschmann-Andermahr I, Mayfrank L, et al. Functional outcome after aneurysmal subarachnoid hemorrhage. Acta Neurochir Suppl 1999;72:157.
7. Kreiter KT, Copeland D, Bernardini GL, et al. Predictors of cognitive dysfunction after subarachnoid hemorrhage. Stroke 2002;33:200.
8. Johnston SC, Selvin S, Gress DR. The burden, trends, and demographics of mortality from subarachnoid hemorrhage. Neurology 1998;50:1413.
9. Linn FH, Rinkel GJ, Algra A, et al. Incidence of subarachnoid hemorrhage: role of region, year, and rate of computed tomography: a meta-analysis. Stroke 1996;27:625.
10. Broderick JP, Brott T, Tomsick T, et al. The risk of subarachnoid and intracerebral hemorrhages in blacks as compared with whites. N Engl J Med 1992;326:733.
11. van Gijn J, Rinkel GJ. Subarachnoid haemorrhage: diagnosis, causes and management. Brain 2001; 124:249.
12. Nahed BV, Bydon M, Ozturk AK, et al. Genetics of intracranial aneurysms. Neurosurgery 2007;60: 213.
13. Ruigrok YM, Rinkel GJ. Genetics of intracranial aneurysms. Stroke 2008;39:1049.
14. Polevaya NV, Kalani MY, Steinberg GK, et al. The transition from Hunterian ligation to intracranial aneurysm clips: a historical perspective. Neurosurg Focus 2006;20:E3.
15. Cohen-Gadol AA, Spencer DD, Harvey W. Cushing and cerebrovascular surgery: part I, Aneurysms. J Neurosurg 2004;101:547.
16. Todd NV, Howie JE, Miller JD. Norman Dott's contribution to aneurysm surgery. J Neurol Neurosurg Psychiatr 1990;53:455.
17. Louw DF, Wilson WT, Sutherland GR. A brief history of aneurysm clips. Neurosurg Focus 2001;11:1.
18. Jane JA, Winn HR, Richardson AE. The natural history of intracranial aneurysms: rebleeding rates during the acute and long term period and implication for surgical management. Clin Neurosurg 1977;24:176.
19. Stein SC. Brief history of surgical timing: surgery for ruptured intracranial aneurysms. Neurosurg Focus 2001;11:E3.
20. Norlen G, Olivecrona H. The treatment of aneurysms of the circle of Willis. J Neurosurg 1953;10:404.
21. Dott NM. Intracranial aneurysmal formations. Clin Neurosurg 1969;16:1.
22. Kassell NF, Torner JC, Jane JA, et al. The International Cooperative Study on the timing of aneurysm surgery. Part 2: surgical results. J Neurosurg 1990; 73:37.
23. Hijdra A, Vermeulen M, van Gijn J, et al. Rerupture of intracranial aneurysms: a clinicoanatomic study. J Neurosurg 1987;67:29.

24. Kassell NF, Torner JC. Aneurysmal rebleeding: a preliminary report from the Cooperative Aneurysm Study. Neurosurgery 1983;13:479.

25. Ohkuma H, Tsurutani H, Suzuki S. Incidence and significance of early aneurysmal rebleeding before neurosurgical or neurological management. Stroke 2001;32:1176.

26. Hillman J, Fridriksson S, Nilsson O, et al. Immediate administration of tranexamic acid and reduced incidence of early rebleeding after aneurysmal subarachnoid hemorrhage: a prospective randomized study. J Neurosurg 2002;97:771.

27. Winn HR, Richardson AE, Jane JA. The long-term prognosis in untreated cerebral aneurysms: I. The incidence of late hemorrhage in cerebral aneurysm: a 10-year evaluation of 364 patients. Ann Neurol 1977;1:358.

28. Clatterbuck RE, Tamargo RJ. Surgical positioning and exposures for cranial procedures. In: Winn HR, Youmans JR, editors. Youmans neurological surgery. 5th edition. Philadelphia: WB Saunders; 2004. p. 624–9.

29. Yasargil MG, Antic J, Laciga R, et al. Microsurgical pterional approach to aneurysms of the basilar bifurcation. Surg Neurol 1976;6:83.

30. Yasargil MG, Reichman MV, Kubik S. Preservation of the frontotemporal branch of the facial nerve using the interfascial temporalis flap for pterional craniotomy. Technical article. J Neurosurg 1987;67:463.

31. Jane JA, Park TS, Pobereskin LH, et al. The supraorbital approach: technical note. Neurosurgery 1982;11:537.

32. Pellerin P, Lesoin F, Dhellemmes P, et al. Usefulness of the orbitofrontomalar approach associated with bone reconstruction for frontotemporosphenoid meningiomas. Neurosurgery 1984;15:715.

33. Al-Mefty O. Supraorbital-pterional approach to skull base lesions. Neurosurgery 1987;21:474.

34. Hakuba A, Liu S, Nishimura S. The orbitozygomatic infratemporal approach: a new surgical technique. Surg Neurol 1986;26:271.

35. Al-Mefty O, Anand VK. Zygomatic approach to skull-base lesions. J Neurosurg 1990;73:668.

36. Seckin H, Avci E, Uluc K, et al. The work horse of skull base surgery: orbitozygomatic approach. Technique, modifications, and applications. Neurosurg Focus 2008;25:E4.

37. Zabramski JM, Kiris T, Sankhla SK, et al. Orbitozygomatic craniotomy. Technical note. J Neurosurg 1998;89:336.

38. Lemole GM Jr, Henn JS, Zabramski JM, et al. Modifications to the orbitozygomatic approach. Technical note. J Neurosurg 2003;99:924.

39. Drake CG. Bleeding aneurysms of the basilar artery. Direct surgical management in four cases. J Neurosurg 1961;18:230.

40. Drake CG. Microsurgical evaluation of the pterional approach to aneurysms of the distal basilar circulation [comment]. Neurosurgery 1978;3:140–1.

41. Batjer HH, Samson DS. Causes of morbidity and mortality from surgery of aneurysms of the distal basilar artery. Neurosurgery 1989;25:904.

42. Kadri PA, Al-Mefty O. The anatomical basis for surgical preservation of temporal muscle. J Neurosurg 2004;100:517.

43. Raza SM, Thai QA, Pradilla G, et al. Frontozygomatic titanium cranioplasty in frontosphenotemporal ("pterional") craniotomy. Neurosurgery 2008;62:262.

44. Tamargo RJ, Haroun RI, Rigamonti D, et al. Artery aneurysms. In: Winn HR, Youmans JR, editors. Youmans neurological surgery. 5th edition. Philadelphia: WB Saunders; 2004. p. 1938–44.

45. Torvik A, Bhatia R, Murthy VS. Transitory block of the arachnoid granulations following subarachnoid haemorrhage. A postmortem study. Acta Neurochir (Wien) 1978;41:137.

46. Kosteljanetz M. CSF dynamics in patients with subarachnoid and/or intraventricular hemorrhage. J Neurosurg 1984;60:940.

47. Komotar RJ, Olivi A, Rigamonti D, et al. Microsurgical fenestration of the lamina terminalis reduces the incidence of shunt-dependent hydrocephalus after aneurysmal subarachnoid hemorrhage. Neurosurgery 2002;51:1403.

48. Sindou M. Favourable influence of opening the lamina terminalis and Lilliequist's membrane on the outcome of ruptured intracranial aneurysms. A study of 197 consecutive cases. Acta Neurochir (Wien) 1994;127:15.

49. Tomasello F, d'Avella D, de Divitiis O. Does lamina terminalis fenestration reduce the incidence of chronic hydrocephalus after subarachnoid hemorrhage? Neurosurgery 1999;45:827.

50. Komotar RJ, Hahn DK, Kim GH, et al. The impact of microsurgical fenestration of the lamina terminalis on shunt-dependent hydrocephalus and vasospasm after aneurysmal subarachnoid hemorrhage. Neurosurgery 2008;62:123.

51. Komotar RJ, Hahn DK, Kim GH, et al. Efficacy of lamina terminalis fenestration in reducing shunt-dependent hydrocephalus following aneurysmal subarachnoid hemorrhage: a systematic review. J Neurosurg 2009;111:147–54.

52. Lopez JR, Chang SD, Steinberg GK. The use of electrophysiological monitoring in the intraoperative management of intracranial aneurysms. J Neurol Neurosurg Psychiatr 1999;66:189.

53. Lopez JR. The use of evoked potentials in intraoperative neurophysiologic monitoring. Phys Med Rehabil Clin N Am 2004;15:63.

54. Friedman WA, Kaplan BL, Day AL, et al. Evoked potential monitoring during aneurysm operation:

observations after fifty cases. Neurosurgery 1987; 20:678.

55. Friedman WA, Chadwick GM, Verhoeven FJ, et al. Monitoring of somatosensory evoked potentials during surgery for middle cerebral artery aneurysms. Neurosurgery 1991;29:83.

56. Neuloh G, Schramm J. Monitoring of motor evoked potentials compared with somatosensory evoked potentials and microvascular Doppler ultrasonography in cerebral aneurysm surgery. J Neurosurg 2004;100: 389.

57. Little JR, Lesser RP, Luders H. Electrophysiological monitoring during basilar aneurysm operation. Neurosurgery 1987;20:421.

58. Krieger D, Adams HP, Albert F, et al. Pure motor hemiparesis with stable somatosensory evoked potential monitoring during aneurysm surgery: case report. Neurosurgery 1992;31:145.

59. Holland NR. Subcortical strokes from intracranial aneurysm surgery: implications for intraoperative neuromonitoring. J Clin Neurophysiol 1998;15:439.

60. Horiuchi K, Suzuki K, Sasaki T, et al. Intraoperative monitoring of blood flow insufficiency during surgery of middle cerebral artery aneurysms. J Neurosurg 2005;103:275.

61. Emerson RG, Turner CA. Monitoring during supratentorial surgery. J Clin Neurophysiol 1993; 10:404.

62. Dehdashti AR, Pralong E, Debatisse D, et al. Multilobar electrocorticography monitoring during intracranial aneurysm surgery. Neurocrit Care 2006;4:215.

63. Loop JW, Foltz EL. Applications of angiography during intracranial operation. Acta Radiol Diagn (Stockh) 1966;5:363.

64. Lin T, Fox AJ, Drake CG. Regrowth of aneurysm sacs from residual neck following aneurysm clipping. J Neurosurg 1989;70:556.

65. Macdonald RL, Wallace MC, Kestle JR. Role of angiography following aneurysm surgery. J Neurosurg 1993;79:826.

66. Le Roux PD, Elliott JP, Eskridge JM, et al. Risks and benefits of diagnostic angiography after aneurysm surgery: a retrospective analysis of 597 studies. Neurosurgery 1998;42:1248.

67. Drake CG, Vanderlinden RG. The late consequences of incomplete surgical treatment of cerebral aneurysms. J Neurosurg 1967;27:226.

68. Feuerberg I, Lindquist C, Lindqvist M, et al. Natural history of postoperative aneurysm rests. J Neurosurg 1987;66:30.

69. Giannotta SL, Litofsky NS. Reoperative management of intracranial aneurysms. J Neurosurg 1995;83:387.

70. Alexander TD, Macdonald RL, Weir B, et al. Intraoperative angiography in cerebral aneurysm surgery: a prospective study of 100 craniotomies. Neurosurgery 1996;39:10.

71. Chiang VL, Gailloud P, Murphy KJ, et al. Routine intraoperative angiography during aneurysm surgery. J Neurosurg 2002;96:988.

72. Tang G, Cawley CM, Dion JE, et al. Intraoperative angiography during aneurysm surgery: a prospective evaluation of efficacy. J Neurosurg 2002;96: 993.

73. Derdeyn CP, Moran CJ, Cross DT, et al. Intraoperative digital subtraction angiography: a review of 112 consecutive examinations. AJNR Am J Neuroradiol 1995;16:307.

74. Wrobel CJ, Meltzer H, Lamond R, et al. Intraoperative assessment of aneurysm clip placement by intravenous fluorescein angiography. Neurosurgery 1994;35:970.

75. Suzuki K, Kodama N, Sasaki T, et al. Confirmation of blood flow in perforating arteries using fluorescein cerebral angiography during aneurysm surgery. J Neurosurg 2007;107:68.

76. Imizu S, Kato Y, Sangli A, et al. Assessment of incomplete clipping of aneurysms intraoperatively by a near-infrared indocyanine green-video angiography (NiICG-Va) integrated microscope. Minim Invasive Neurosurg 2008;51:199.

77. Raabe A, Beck J, Gerlach R, et al. Near-infrared indocyanine green video angiography: a new method for intraoperative assessment of vascular flow. Neurosurgery 2003;52:132.

78. Raabe A, Beck J, Seifert V. Technique and image quality of intraoperative indocyanine green angiography during aneurysm surgery using surgical microscope integrated near-infrared video technology. Zentralbl Neurochir 2005;66:1.

79. Raabe A, Nakaji P, Beck J, et al. Prospective evaluation of surgical microscope-integrated intraoperative near-infrared indocyanine green videoangiography during aneurysm surgery. J Neurosurg 2005;103:982.

80. de Oliveira JG, Beck J, Seifert V, et al. Assessment of flow in perforating arteries during intracranial aneurysm surgery using intraoperative near-infrared indocyanine green videoangiography. Neurosurgery 2007;61:63.

81. Raabe A, Spetzler RF. Fluorescence angiography. J Neurosurg 2008;108:429.

82. Dashti R, Laakso A, Niemela M, et al. Microscope-integrated near-infrared indocyanine green videoangiography during surgery of intracranial aneurysms: the Helsinki experience. Surg Neurol 2009;71:543.

83. Samson D, Batjer HH, Bowman G, et al. A clinical study of the parameters and effects of temporary arterial occlusion in the management of intracranial aneurysms. Neurosurgery 1994;34:22.

84. Ogilvy CS, Carter BS, Kaplan S, et al. Temporary vessel occlusion for aneurysm surgery: risk factors for stroke in patients protected by induced hypothermia and hypertension and intravenous mannitol administration. J Neurosurg 1996;84:785.

85. Lavine SD, Masri LS, Levy ML, et al. Temporary occlusion of the middle cerebral artery in intracranial aneurysm surgery: time limitation and advantage of brain protection. J Neurosurg 1997;87:817.

86. Goldman MS, Anderson RE, Meyer FB. Effects of intermittent reperfusion during temporal focal ischemia. J Neurosurg 1992;77:911.

87. Kurokawa Y, Tranmer BI. Interrupted arterial occlusion reduces ischemic damage in a focal cerebral ischemia model of rats. Neurosurgery 1995;37:750.

88. David CA, Prado R, Dietrich WD. Cerebral protection by intermittent reperfusion during temporary focal ischemia in the rat. J Neurosurg 1996;85:923.

89. Steinberg GK, Panahian N, Sun GH, et al. Cerebral damage caused by interrupted, repeated arterial occlusion versus uninterrupted occlusion in a focal ischemic model. J Neurosurg 1994;81:554.

90. Connolly ES, Solomon RA. Techniques for deep hypothermic circulatory arrest. In: Winn HR, Youmans JR, editors. Youmans neurological surgery. 5th edition. Philadelphia: WB Saunders; 2004. p. 1528–39.

91. Spetzler RF, Hadley MN, Rigamonti D, et al. Aneurysms of the basilar artery treated with circulatory arrest, hypothermia, and barbiturate cerebral protection. J Neurosurg 1988;68:868.

92. Lawton MT, Raudzens PA, Zabramski JM, et al. Hypothermic circulatory arrest in neurovascular surgery: evolving indications and predictors of patient outcome. Neurosurgery 1998;43:10.

93. Sullivan BJ, Sekhar LN, Duong DH, et al. Profound hypothermia and circulatory arrest with skull base approaches for treatment of complex posterior circulation aneurysms. Acta Neurochir (Wien) 1999;141:1.

94. Mack WJ, Ducruet AF, Angevine PD, et al. Deep hypothermic circulatory arrest for complex cerebral aneurysms: lessons learned. Neurosurgery 2007; 60:815.

95. Rebeyka IM, Coles JG, Wilson GJ, et al. The effect of low-flow cardiopulmonary bypass on cerebral function: an experimental and clinical study. Ann Thorac Surg 1987;43:391.

96. Wilson GJ, Rebeyka IM, Coles JG, et al. Loss of the somatosensory evoked response as an indicator of reversible cerebral ischemia during hypothermic, low-flow cardiopulmonary bypass. Ann Thorac Surg 1988;45:206.

97. Swain JA, McDonald TJ Jr, Griffith PK, et al. Low-flow hypothermic cardiopulmonary bypass protects the brain. J Thorac Cardiovasc Surg 1991;102:76.

98. Newburger JW, Jonas RA, Wernovsky G, et al. A comparison of the perioperative neurologic effects of hypothermic circulatory arrest versus low-flow cardiopulmonary bypass in infant heart surgery. N Engl J Med 1993;329:1057.

99. Bellinger DC, Jonas RA, Rappaport LA, et al. Developmental and neurologic status of children after heart surgery with hypothermic circulatory arrest or low-flow cardiopulmonary bypass. N Engl J Med 1995;332:549.

100. Bendok BR, Getch CC, Frederiksen J, et al. Resection of a large arteriovenous fistula of the brain using low-flow deep hypothermic cardiopulmonary bypass: technical case report. Neurosurgery 1999; 44:888.

101. Dufour H, Levrier O, Bruder N, et al. Resection of a giant intracranial dural arteriovenous fistula with the use of low-flow deep hypothermic cardiopulmonary bypass after partial embolization: technical case report. Neurosurgery 2001;48:1381.

102. Patt A, McCroskey BL, Moore EE. Hypothermia-induced coagulopathies in trauma. Surg Clin North Am 1988;68:775.

103. Heuer GG, Smith MJ, Elliott JP, et al. Relationship between intracranial pressure and other clinical variables in patients with aneurysmal subarachnoid hemorrhage. J Neurosurg 2004;101:408.

104. Klimo P Jr, Kestle JR, MacDonald JD, et al. Marked reduction of cerebral vasospasm with lumbar drainage of cerebrospinal fluid after subarachnoid hemorrhage. J Neurosurg 2004;100:215.

105. Ruijs AC, Dirven CM, Algra A, et al. The risk of rebleeding after external lumbar drainage in patients with untreated ruptured cerebral aneurysms. Acta Neurochir (Wien) 2005;147:1157.

106. Kusske JA, Turner PT, Ojemann GA, et al. Ventriculostomy for the treatment of acute hydrocephalus following subarachnoid hemorrhage. J Neurosurg 1973;38:591.

107. Steinke D, Weir B, Disney L. Hydrocephalus following aneurysmal subarachnoid haemorrhage. Neurol Res 1987;9:3.

108. Hasan D, Vermeulen M, Wijdicks EF, et al. Management problems in acute hydrocephalus after subarachnoid hemorrhage. Stroke 1989;20:747.

109. Rajshekhar V, Harbaugh RE. Results of routine ventriculostomy with external ventricular drainage for acute hydrocephalus following subarachnoid haemorrhage. Acta Neurochir (Wien) 1992;115:8.

110. Komotar RJ, Zacharia BE, Mocco J, et al. Controversies in the surgical treatment of ruptured intracranial aneurysms: the First Annual J. Lawrence Pool Memorial Research Symposium—controversies in the management of cerebral aneurysms. Neurosurgery 2008;62:396.

111. Nornes H. The role of intracranial pressure in the arrest of hemorrhage in patients with ruptured intracranial aneurysm. J Neurosurg 1973;39:226.

112. van Gijn J, Hijdra A, Wijdicks EF, et al. Acute hydrocephalus after aneurysmal subarachnoid hemorrhage. J Neurosurg 1985;63:355.

113. Pare L, Delfino R, Leblanc R. The relationship of ventricular drainage to aneurysmal rebleeding. J Neurosurg 1992;76:422.

114. Kawai K, Nagashima H, Narita K, et al. Efficacy and risk of ventricular drainage in cases of grade V subarachnoid hemorrhage. Neurol Res 1997;19:649.

115. Ochiai H, Yamakawa Y. Continuous lumbar drainage for the preoperative management of patients with aneurysmal subarachnoid hemorrhage. Neurol Med Chir (Tokyo) 2001;41:576.

116. McIver JI, Friedman JA, Wijdicks EF, et al. Preoperative ventriculostomy and rebleeding after aneurysmal subarachnoid hemorrhage. J Neurosurg 2002;97:1042.

117. Gurian JH, Martin NA, King WA, et al. Neurosurgical management of cerebral aneurysms following unsuccessful or incomplete endovascular embolization. J Neurosurg 1995;83:843.

118. Donaghy R, Yasargil MG. Microvascular surgery. St. Louis (MO): CV Mosby; 1967.

119. Mehdorn HM. Cerebral revascularization by EC-IC bypass—present status. Acta Neurochir Suppl 2008;103:73.

120. Peerless SJ, Hampf CR. Extracranial to intracranial bypass in the treatment of aneurysms. Clin Neurosurg 1985;32:114.

121. Sundt TM Jr, Piepgras DG, Marsh WR, et al. Saphenous vein bypass grafts for giant aneurysms and intracranial occlusive disease. J Neurosurg 1986;65:439.

122. Ausman JI, Diaz FG, Sadasivan B, et al. Giant intracranial aneurysm surgery: the role of microvascular reconstruction. Surg Neurol 1990;34:8.

123. Lawton MT, Hamilton MG, Morcos JJ, et al. Revascularization and aneurysm surgery: current techniques, indications, and outcome. Neurosurgery 1996;38:83.

124. Martin NA. Arterial bypass for the treatment of giant and fusiform intracranial aneurysms. Tech Neurosurg 1998;4:153.

125. Tanaka Y, Kobayashi S, Kyoshima K, et al. Multiple clipping technique for large and giant internal carotid artery aneurysms and complications: angiographic analysis. J Neurosurg 1994;80:635.

126. Clatterbuck RE, Galler RM, Tamargo RJ, et al. Orthogonal interlocking tandem clipping technique for the reconstruction of complex middle cerebral artery aneurysms. Neurosurgery 2006;59:ONS347.

127. Lanzino G, Spetzler RF. Clip wrapping for partial avulsion of the aneurysm neck. Technical note. J Neurosurg 2003;99:931.

Hydrocephalus After Aneurysmal Subarachnoid Hemorrhage

Anand V. Germanwala, MD[a],*, Judy Huang, MD[b],
Rafael J. Tamargo, MD[b]

KEYWORDS

- Hydrocephalus • Fenestration
- Subarachnoid hemorrhage • Aneurysm

Hydrocephalus often complicates the initial injurious effects of subarachnoid hemorrhage (SAH) (**Fig. 1**). In 1928, Bagley[1] was the first to suggest that ventricular dilatation could be a consequence of SAH. Most studies report an overall 20% to 30% incidence of hydrocephalus after SAH.[2–4] Although debate still exists over its pathophysiology, this condition typically presents acutely but can also occur in a delayed fashion, rarely even months after the initial hemorrhage. Its clinical sequelae can be devastating and lead to further neurologic deterioration and longer hospital stays. Early recognition and treatment, however, can lead to improved patient outcomes. Several strategies have been developed to minimize the need for placement of either temporary intraventricular catheters (IVCs) or permanent shunts. Intraoperative techniques used to reestablish normal cerebrospinal fluid (CSF) flow and resorption include fenestration of the lamina terminalis and thorough irrigation of blood out of the arachnoid cisterns. Postoperative techniques used to encourage CSF reabsorption in patients with IVCs or lumbar drains involve a steady, daily increase in the pop-off pressures, which is guided by recorded intracranial or thecal pressures, CSF output volume, and the patient's neurologic status. In patients without IVCs or lumbar drains but with persistent symptoms, serial lumbar punctures are necessary. Endovascular treatment of aneurysms may be associated with a higher rate of shunt-dependent hydrocephalus. In some institutions permanent shunting rates have been reduced to approximately 7%.

ETIOLOGY

The exact mechanism by which hydrocephalus develops after SAH remains poorly understood, although altered CSF dynamics in the acute and chronic states have been extensively studied. Although it is generally accepted that hydrocephalus after SAH is of the "communicating" type,[5] it is likely that this condition has communicating and noncommunicating components. Decreased absorption of CSF at the arachnoid granulations is defined as communicating hydrocephalus and an anatomic obstruction, as noncommunicating. Traditionally, if all 4 ventricles are equally dilated on CT scan, then hydrocephalus is presumed to be of the communicating type. This interpretation does not take into account that if the obstruction occurs at the foramina of Luschka and Magendie (ie, the outflow of the fourth ventricle), a noncommunicating or obstructive type of hydrocephalus may be misinterpreted radiologically as being communicating, given that all the ventricles are dilated. It is generally assumed that fibrosis of

[a] Division of Neurosurgery, University of North Carolina School of Medicine, 170 Manning Drive, Campus Box #7060, Chapel Hill, NC 27599-7060, USA
[b] Department of Neurosurgery, Johns Hopkins University School of Medicine, 600 North Wolfe Street, Meyer 8-181, Baltimore, MD 21287, USA
* Corresponding author.
E-mail address: anand_germanwala@med.unc.edu

Neurosurg Clin N Am 21 (2010) 263–270
doi:10.1016/j.nec.2009.10.013

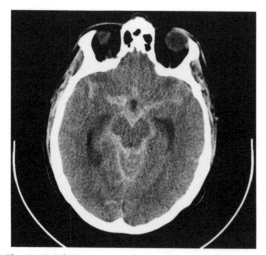

Fig. 1. Axial CT scan demonstrating acute SAH and enlarged third ventricle and temporal horns.

the leptomeninges and arachnoid granulations from blood product deposition causes impaired CSF flow and decreased absorption.[6,7]

There is increasing evidence, however, that hydrocephalus after SAH may be caused primarily by fibrosis and partial obstruction of the fourth ventricular outflow and secondarily by impaired CSF absorption. Based on this understanding, creation of an anterior third ventriculostomy has been proposed to facilitate CSF fluid dynamics with increased blood clearance, decreased leptomeningeal fibrosis, and better balance between CSF production and resorption.[5] In the authors' experience, the overall shunt rate in patients undergoing fenestration of the lamina terminalis can be reduced to 2.3%, whenever possible. The efficacy of lamina terminalis fenestration, however, has yielded conflicting results in other series, and a multi-center, randomized, controlled trial will most likely be necessary to determine the overall effectiveness of this technique.[8,9]

The type of hydrocephalus may be a function of the site of hemorrhage and not of the temporal breakdown of blood in the subarachnoid space.[10,11] This hypothesis may explain why ruptured posterior circulation aneurysms are associated with higher rates of hydrocephalus as compared with ruptured anterior circulation aneurysms.[12] Posterior circulation aneurysmal rupture may be more likely to cause impaired CSF egress from the fourth ventricle and an obstructive pattern of hydrocephalus. Alternatively, anterior circulation aneurysmal rupture may cause hydrocephalus primarily by fibrosis of the leptomeninges and arachnoid granulations and result in a communicating pattern in the acute and delayed states. It is evident that the pathophysiology of chronic

hydrocephalus remains poorly understood and that several hypotheses exist regarding its cause.[11]

DIAGNOSIS

Acute hydrocephalus, which develops 48 to 72 hours after SAH, occurs in approximately 20% of patients.[13] Most patients with aneurysmal SAH present with headache, nausea, and vomiting, which are symptoms attributable to the presence of acute blood in the subarachnoid space but are also compounded by hydrocephalus. Subacute hydrocephalus, which develops 3 to 7 days after the hemorrhage, is rare and has a frequency of 2% to 3%.[3] Because the clinical diagnosis of hydrocephalus after SAH is difficult, its recognition is based primarily on radiographic findings, specifically CT scans.

Although several ventricular measurements based on CT studies have been used to establish the diagnosis of hydrocephalus, currently, the preferred marker for this condition is the bicaudate index. Historically, there has been an evolution of radiological markers for hydrocephalus. In 1979, Vassilouthis and Richardson[14] measured the ratio between the width of the lateral ventricles at the foramen of Monro and the inner diameter of the skull at the same level. A ratio less than 1:6.4 was considered normal and a ratio more than 1:4 represented marked ventricular dilatation, suggestive of hydrocephalus. In 1970, Galera and Greitz[15] compared the maximum width of the frontal horns to that of the skull at the same axial level. Other studies have focused on volumetric measurements, suggesting that linear measurements are less accurate.[16] Zatz and colleagues[17] reported that the best correlation between ventricular volume and linear measurements existed with the width of the third ventricle. However, they concluded that the empiric radiographic evaluation by a radiologist is more accurate than any linear ratio in diagnosing hydrocephalus. Currently, the preferred system for the objective diagnosis of hydrocephalus is based on the bicaudate index (**Fig. 2**).

Using data from 2 separate control groups showing the distribution of bicaudate values in patients without neurologic disease,[18,19] Gijn and colleagues[20] proposed that hydrocephalus should be diagnosed when the bicaudate index was more than the age-corrected 95th percentile (**Table 1**).

In this manner, atrophic changes that result in ventriculomegaly and are not the result of increased ventricular CSF pressures are taken into account. They then prospectively studied 174 consecutive patients with SAH and found

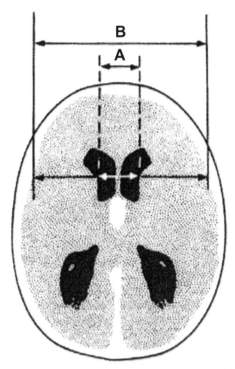

Fig. 2. Axial CT scan demonstrating method for determining bicaudate index (A, B). (A) is the width of the frontal horns at the level of the caudate nuclei; (B) is the diameter of the brain at the same level. (*Reproduced from* Van Gijn J, Hijdra A, Wijdicks EF et al. Acute hydrocephalus after aneurysmal subarachnoid hemorrhage. J Neurosurg 1985;63(3):355–62; with permission.)

that 20% (34 of 174) had bicaudate indices greater than the 95th percentile for their age. Using similar criteria, Hasan and colleagues[3] reported a consecutive series of 473 patients with SAH and found an incidence of acute hydrocephalus in 19% of patients (91 of 473). Several large retrospective series have confirmed these findings.

Chronic hydrocephalus (presenting later than one week after SAH) develops in an additional 10% to 20% of patients.[21] Although the cause may be different, this diagnosis must be entertained in the setting of progressive neurologic decline. As a general rule, SAH patients who regress clinically weeks to months after discharge should have a follow-up CT scan and clinical evaluation to rule out delayed hydrocephalus.

PREDICTIVE FACTORS

Experimental studies have shown that the injection of blood into the subarachnoid space results in intracranial pressure (ICP) elevation higher than that caused by infusion of an equivalent volume of saline. This effect is generally attributed to increased CSF outflow resistance at the level of the subarachnoid space or the arachnoid granulations caused by blood components, such as erythrocytes and proteins.[2] The infusion of heparinized blood causes only a transient rise in ICP, implying that fibrin formation and deposition in the subarachnoid space and arachnoid granulations play an important role in this process.[2,22] Such studies have partially elucidated the complex changes resulting from the presence of blood in the subarachnoid space, and have supported clinical and radiographic variables associated with hydrocephalus.

Clinically, the most important prognostic feature associated with the development of hydrocephalus is the neurologic condition of the patient at the time of presentation. Data from 3521 aneurysmal SAH cases in the Cooperative Aneurysm Study show that several factors were related to symptomatic hydrocephalus, which are listed in **Table 2**.[12] Among these, a poor level of

---

Table 1
Upper 95% confidence value for ventriculocranial ratio stratified by age, as proposed by Gijn and colleagues

Age (Years)	Upper 95% Confidence Value
<30	0.16
<50	0.18
<60	0.19
<80	0.21
<100	0.25

Van Gijn J, Hijdra A, Wijdicks EF, et al. Acute hydrocephalus after aneurysmal subarachnoid hemorrhage. J Neurosurg 1985;63(3):355–62.

Table 2
Admission variables predicting clinical hydrocephalus

Variable	P Value
CT Hydrocephalus	<.001
CT intraventricular hemorrhage	<.001
Consciousness level	<.001
Pre-SAH hypertension	<.001
Age	<.001
CT SAH	=.005
Posterior circulation aneurysm	=.012
Postoperative hypertension	=.024

Reproduced from Graff-Radford NR, Torner J, Adams Jr HP, et al. Factors associated with hydrocephalus after subarachnoid hemorrhage. A report of the Cooperative Aneurysm Study. Arch Neurol 1989;46(7):744–52; with permission.

consciousness and the presence of an intraventricular hemorrhage had a high statistical correlation. In a separate cohort study of 3120 patients, radiographic ventriculomegaly, ventilation on admission, aneurysms in the posterior circulation, and giant aneurysms were all predictors of shunt-dependent hydrocephalus.[23] Higher Fisher grades, and angiographic vasospasm on SAH day 7 have also been associated with hydrocephalus after SAH.[24]

TREATMENT

Reports of the proportion of patients with aneurysmal SAH who require permanent shunting are highly variable. In part, this variability is probably a result of treating neurosurgeons basing their decision to pursue permanent shunting on the presence of radiographic hydrocephalus alone or pursuing shunting only when symptomatic hydrocephalus is evident. Another important determining feature is when this decision is made during the course after the initial hemorrhage. For instance, according to the report of 473 patients with aneurysmal SAH by Hasan and colleagues,[3] 19% of their patients had radiographic hydrocephalus, but only two-thirds approximately were symptomatic, resulting in a rate of symptomatic hydrocephalus of only 13%. Furthermore, nearly half of their patients with symptomatic hydrocephalus improved spontaneously in the early stages, resulting in a final rate of persistent, symptomatic hydrocephalus of approximately 7%. Such findings are similar to those reported 10 years earlier by Vassilouthis and Richardson.[14] Hasan and colleagues noted a similar incidence of radiographic hydrocephalus in a group of 46 patients with SAH and negative arteriograms, but only one of these 46 patients (2%) developed symptomatic hydrocephalus.

Nevertheless, there is a minority of aneurysmal SAH patients in whom either temporary or permanent CSF diversion is of benefit. Hasan and colleagues noted improvement in 78% of the 32 patients treated with external ventricular drainage or a shunt. Raimondi and colleagues[25] saw improvement in 86% of 21 patients. Although initial studies noted high rates of infection with external ventricular drainage (50% in the Hasan series), precautions such as subcutaneous tunneling of the catheter, administering prophylactic antibiotics at the time of IVC placement, minimizing the duration of drainage to 5 days or less, and maintaining a closed drainage system have reduced infection rates to well below 10%. In a large study focusing on drainage days (DD) with external ventricular or lumbar drains, an overall infection rate was 6.3 per 1000 DD for ventricular drains and 19.9 per 1000 DD for lumbar drains, with an overall device-associated meningitis rate of 8.6 infections per 1000 DD.[26] Patients with poor grades (Hunt and Hess IV or V) typically require temporary CSF diversion.

Repeat rupture of an unsecured aneurysm is a major concern associated with placement of an IVC and continuous external ventricular drainage. Early studies reported a 43% incidence of rebleeding associated with CSF diversion in patients with unsecured aneurysms.[3] In another series in which ventricular drainage was pursued only when ICP was greater than 25 mmHg, a 17% rate of rebleeding was noted.[27] Patients with poor grades (III-V) have a higher incidence of rebleeding (25% vs 9.2% in patients with good grades).[28,29] Recent studies, however, have questioned whether CSF diversion via ventriculostomy or lumbar drainage increases the risk of rebleeding.[30] Perhaps this corresponds to improved control of ICP after ventriculostomy and lumbar drain placement and the natural history of unsecured ruptured aneurysms.

Temporary CSF diversion can be accomplished by insertion of an IVC (ventriculostomy), insertion of a lumbar drain, or with serial lumbar punctures. The need for permanent shunting can be reduced using several intraoperative maneuvers, such as fenestration of the lamina terminalis, opening the arachnoid cisterns, and thorough removal of subarachnoid clots. There is controversy over prolonged temporary CSF diversion increasing the incidence of shunt dependency.[31,32] Permanent CSF diversion procedures include ventriculoperitoneal shunting (VPS) (and its ventriculopleural and ventriculoatrial variants) and lumboperitoneal shunting (LPS). Currently the criteria for permanent CSF diversion are as varied as the ways of achieving it. Although the decision for permanent shunt placement is highly physician-dependent, a prolonged course of CSF diversion, persistent elevated ICPs, high drainage volumes, and persistent poor neurologic condition are criteria that justify permanent CSF diversion (**Fig. 3**).

Endovascular embolization for the treatment of intracranial aneurysms has become increasingly common, and it may be associated with a higher rate of shunt-dependent hydrocephalus. A large single-institutional review and meta-analysis comparing the risk of shunt dependence in patients with ruptured intracranial aneurysms treated by surgical clipping or endovascular coiling concluded that clipping of ruptured aneurysms may be associated with a lower incidence of shunt dependency.[24] In 385 patients treated at a single institution, those undergoing endovascular coiling had a higher shunting rate of 19.6% versus that of

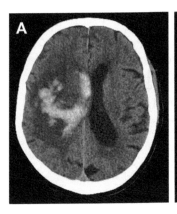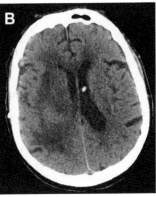

Fig. 3. (*A*) and (*B*) Initial CT scan revealing acute intraparenchymal and intraventricular hemorrhage (*left*). The patient was found to have a ruptured right internal carotid artery terminus aneurysm and underwent endovascular embolization. Follow-up CT scans showed persistent ventricular dilatation. A follow-up CT scan reveals the ventriculostomy catheter tip, decreased ventriculomegaly, and blood resolution (*right*). The patient required permanent CSF diversion with a ventriculoperitoneal shunt.

the surgical group, which was 17.4%. The overall shunt-dependent rate in this study was 18.4%. Although this difference was not statistically significant, combining this data with that of 4 other large series, for a total of 1718 patients, revealed a statistically significant higher rate of shunt dependence of 20.9% in endovascular patients, as opposed to 17.4% in surgical patients. Perhaps, clearing the subarachnoid clot and opening of the cisterns may lead to better CSF circulation and a reduced incidence of shunt dependence. A summary of the characteristics of the studies included in the meta-analysis is listed in **Table 3**.

MANAGEMENT STRATEGIES

The authors have summarized their strategy for the management of hydrocephalus after aneurysmal SAH (**Fig. 4**). At the authors' institutions, the rate of VPS placement after aneurysmal SAH has decreased to about 7%. They attribute this low rate to intraoperative fenestration of the lamina terminalis and a strict postoperative protocol in which postoperative external CSF drainage is minimized and CSF absorption is encouraged. Patients taken

to the operating room with a preoperatively placed IVC typically do not leave the operating room with the IVC. During surgery, the authors create an anterior third ventriculostomy by fenestration of the lamina terminalis whenever this structure is accessible, open the arachnoid cisterns, and irrigate out the subarachnoid clot. Fenestration of the lamina terminalis is always accomplished during frontosphenotemporal (pterional) approaches, but is obviously not possible during suboccipital, interhemispheric, or subtemporal approaches. Although, on occasion, an intraoperative IVC is placed for additional brain relaxation, this is removed after intraoperative fenestration of the lamina terminalis.

In the intensive care unit, patients are observed for evidence of symptomatic hydrocephalus. The intraoperative creation of a third ventriculostomy transforms any postoperative hydrocephalus into the communicating type. If progressive hydrocephalus is observed clinically or radiographically, serial lumbar punctures or placement of a lumbar drain catheter is performed. In rare instances, an IVC is placed in the unit postoperatively. In such cases, the pop-off is raised by 5mmHg every

Table 3
Summary characteristics of studies included in the meta-analysis, as described by de Oliveira and colleagues

Series	Number of Patients	Treatment Ratio Number of Clip/Coil	Total Shunt Rate (%)	Shunt Rate (%) Clip/Coil (*P* Value)
Gruber and colleagues[33]	187	125/62	21.4	23/18 (0.45)
Dorai and colleagues[34]	718	684/34	21.0	20/47 (0.001)
Dehdashti and colleagues[35]	245	180/65	15.5	14/19 (0.53)
Varelas and colleagues[36]	183	135/48	6.6	4.4/12.5 (0.16)
De Oliveira and colleagues[24]	385	212/173	18.4	17.4/19.6 (0.59)

Data from de Oliveira JG, Beck J, Setzer M, et al. Risk of shunt-dependent hydrocephalus after occlusion of ruptured intracranial aneurysms by surgical clipping or endovascular coiling: a single-institution series and meta-analysis. Neurosurgery 2007;61(5):924–33 [discussion: 33–4].

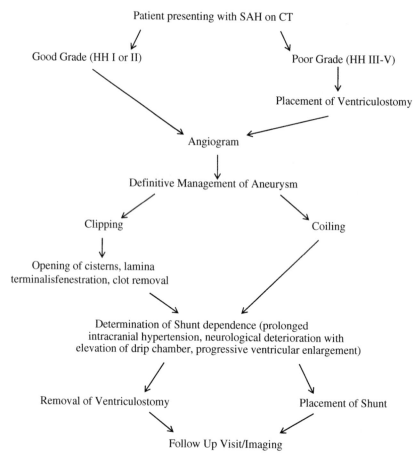

Patient presenting with SAH on CT

Good Grade (HH I or II)

Poor Grade (HH III-V)

Placement of Ventriculostomy

Angiogram

Definitive Management of Aneurysm

Clipping

Coiling

Opening of cisterns, lamina terminalisfenestration, clot removal

Determination of Shunt dependence (prolonged intracranial hypertension, neurological deterioration with elevation of drip chamber, progressive ventricular enlargement)

Removal of Ventriculostomy

Placement of Shunt

Follow Up Visit/Imaging

Fig. 4. Management strategies for patients with aneurysmal SAH.

24 hours, with close monitoring of ICP measurements, total CSF output, and the patient's neurologic condition. Once a pop-off of 20mmHg is reached and seems to be tolerated for 24 to 48 hours, the IVC is clamped. Provided that patients tolerate clamping for an additional 24 to 48 hours, a CT scan is obtained as a baseline and the IVC (or lumbar drain catheter) is removed. Further symptomatic hydrocephalus is managed with subsequent lumbar punctures. Either prolonged IVC dependence or the extended need for lumbar punctures then leads to insertion of a VPS or LPS.

A review of the literature reveals a broad range of shunting rates for aneurysmal SAH. Placement of a shunt depends on the biologic manifestations of hydrocephalus and the neurosurgeon's approach to this problem. The authors' inclination to minimize the rate of shunt placement may require patients to spend a few more days in the intensive care unit or undergo serial lumbar punctures. Although temporarily inconvenient, such steps may help avoid lifelong shunt dependency, a state that most patients and neurosurgeons prefer to avoid.

SUMMARY

Hydrocephalus after SAH has been recognized for over 80 years. Although the cause of this problem is not fully understood, more is known about this alteration of CSF dynamics from acute subarachnoid blood since Bagley's initial description. Although further clinical and experimental work is necessary to grasp the complex pathophysiology of hydrocephalus after SAH, ongoing awareness of this delayed complication and rapid intervention in the form of either temporary or permanent CSF diversion are required to minimize the devastating effects that can result from this condition.

REFERENCES

1. Bagley C Jr. Blood in the cerebrospinal fluid. Resultant functional and organic alterations in the central nervous system. A. Experimental data. Arch Surg 1928;17:18–38.
2. Brinker T, Seifert V, Stolke D. Acute changes in the dynamics of the cerbrospinal fluid system during

experimental subarachnoid hemorrhage. Neurosurgery 1990;27:369–72.

3. Hasan D, Vermeulen M, Wijdicks EF, et al. Management problems in acute hydrocephalus after subarachnoid hemorrhage. Stroke 1989;20(6):747–53.

4. Heros RC. Acute hydrocephalus after subarachnoid hemorrhage. Stroke 1989;20(6):715–7.

5. Komotar RJ, Olivi A, Rigamonti D, et al. Microsurgical fenestration of the lamina terminalis reduces the incidence of shunt-dependent hydrocephalus after aneurysmal subarachnoid hemorrhage. Neurosurgery 2002;51(6):1403–12 [discussion: 1412–3].

6. Kosteljanetz M. CSF dynamics in patients with subarachnoid and/or intraventricular hemorrhage. J Neurosurg 1984;60(5):940–6.

7. Torvik A, Bhatia R, Murthy VS. Transitory block of the arachnoid granulations following subarachnoid hemorrhage. A postmortem study. Acta Neurochir (Wien) 1978;41(1–3):137–46.

8. Komotar RJ, Hahn DK, Kim GH, et al. The impact of microsurgical fenestration of the lamina terminalis on shunt-dependent hydrocephalus and vasospasm after aneurysmal subarachnoid hemorrhage. Neurosurgery 2008;62(1):123–32 [discussion: 132–4].

9. Komotar RJ, Hahn DK, Kim GH, et al. Efficacy of lamina terminalis fenestration in reducing shunt-dependent hydrocephalus following aneurysmal subarachnoid hemorrhage: a systematic review. J Neurosurg 2009;111(1):147–54.

10. Greenberg M. Handbook of neurosurgery. 5th edition. New York (NY): Thieme Medical Publishers; 2001. p. 759.

11. McCormick P. Elevated intracranial pressure, ventricular drainage, and hydrocephalus after subarachnoid hemorrhage. Subarachnoid hemorrhage: pathophysiology and management. In: Neurosurgical Topics. Park Ridge (IL): AANS; 1997. p. 82.

12. Graff-Radford NR, Torner J, Adams HP Jr, et al. Factors associated with hydrocephalus after subarachnoid hemorrhage. A report of the Cooperative Aneurysm Study. Arch Neurol 1989;46(7):744–52.

13. MacDonald RL, Weir B. Perioperative management of subarachnoid hemorrhage. In: Youmans Neurological Surgery, vol. 2. 5th edition, 2004. p. 1823.

14. Vassilouthis J, Richardson AE. Ventricular dilatation and communicating hydrocephalus following spontaneous subarachnoid hemorrhage. J Neurosurg 1979;51(3):341–51.

15. Galera R, Greitz T. Hydrocephalus in the adult secondary to the rupture of intracranial arterial aneurysms. J Neurosurg 1970;32(6):634–41.

16. Penn RD, Belanger MG, Yasnoff WA. Ventricular volume in man computed from CAT scans. Ann Neurol 1978;3:216–23.

17. Zatz LM, Jernigan TL, Ahumada AJ. Changes on computed cranial tomography with aging: intracranial fluid volume. Am J Neuroradiol 1982;3:1–11.

18. Earnest MP, Heaton RK, Wilkinson WE, et al. Cortical atrophy, ventricular enlargement and intellectual impairment in the aged. Neurology 1979;29(8):1138–43.

19. Meese W, Kluge W, Grumme T, et al. CT evaluation of the CSF spaces of healthy persons. Neuroradiology 1980;19(3):131–6.

20. Van Gijn J, Hijdra A, Wijdicks EF, et al. Acute hydrocephalus after aneurysmal subarachnoid hemorrhage. J Neurosurg 1985;63(3):355–62.

21. Vale FL, Bradley EL, Fisher WS. The relationship of subarachnoid hemorrhage and the need for postoperative shunting. J Neurosurg 1997;86:462–6.

22. Blasberg R, Johnson D, Fenstermacher J. Absorption resistance of cerebrospinal fluid after subarachnoid hemorrhage in the monkey; effects of heparin. Neurosurgery 1981;9:686–91.

23. O'Kelly CJ, Kulkarni AV, Austin PC, et al. Shunt-dependent hydrocephalus after aneurysmal subarachnoid hemorrhage: incidence, predictors, and revision rates. J Neurosurg 2009;111(5):1029–35.

24. de Oliveira JG, Beck J, Setzer M, et al. Risk of shunt-dependent hydrocephalus after occlusion of ruptured intracranial aneurysms by surgical clipping or endovascular coiling: a single-institution series and meta-analysis. Neurosurgery 2007;61(5):924–33 [discussion: 933–4].

25. Raimondi AJ, Torres H. Acute hydrocephalus as a complication of subarachnoid hemorrhage. Surg Neurol 1973;1:23–6.

26. Scheithauer S, Bürgel U, Ryang YM, et al. Prospective surveillance of drain-associated meningitis/ventriculitis in a neurosurgery and a neurologic intensive care unit. J Neurol Neurosurg Psychiatr 2009;80(12):1381–5.

27. Voldby B, Enevoldsen EM. Intracranial pressure changes following aneurysmal rupture. J Neurosurg 1982;56:784–9.

28. Richardson AE, Jane JA, Payne PM. Assessment of the natural history of anterior communicating aneurysms. J Neurosurg 1964;21:266–74.

29. Adams HP Jr, Kassell NF, Torner JC. Early management of aneurysmal subarachnoid hemorrhage. A report of the Cooperative Aneurysm Study. J Neurosurg 1981;54:141–5.

30. Hellingman CA, van den Bergh WM, Beijer IS, et al. Risk of rebleeding after treatment of acute hydrocephalus in patients with aneurysmal subarachnoid hemorrhage. Stroke 2007;38(1):96–9.

31. Connolly ES Jr, Kader AA, Frazzini VI, et al. The safety of intraoperative lumbar subarachnoid drainage for acutely ruptured intracranial aneurysm: technical note. Surg Neurol 1997;48(4):338–42.

32. Auer LM, Mokry M. Disturbed cerebrospinal fluid circulation after subarachnoid hemorrhage and acute aneurysm surgery. Neurosurgery 1990;26(5):804–8.

33. Gruber A, Reinprecht A, Bavinzski G, et al. Chronic shunt-dependent hydrocephalus after early surgical and early endovascular treatment of ruptured intracranial aneurysms. Neurosurgery 1999;44(3):503–9.

34. Dorai Z, Hynan LS, Kopitnik TA, et al. Factors related to hydrocephalus after aneurysmal subarachnoid hemorrhage. Neurosurgery 2003; 52(4):763–9.

35. Dehdashti AR, Rilliet B, Rufenacht DA, et al. Shunt-dependent hydrocephalus after rupture of intracranial aneurysms: a prospective study of the influence of treatment modality. J Neurosurg 2004;101(3): 402–7.

36. Varelas P, Helms A, Sinson G, et al. Clipping or coiling of ruptured cerebral aneurysms and shunt-dependent hydrocephalus. Neurocrit Care 2006;4(3):223–8.

Endovascular Treatment of Aneurysmal Subarachnoid Hemorrhage

Monica Pearl, MD, Lydia Gregg, MA, CMI,
Philippe Gailloud, MD*

KEYWORDS

- Aneurysm • Intracranial • Subarachnoid hemorrhage
- Endovascular treatment

Intracranial aneurysms are common entities whose natural history and definitive management remain controversial. Their prevalence varies according to study design but is estimated at approximately 2.3% in the general population.[1,2] The most dreaded complication related to intracranial aneurysms is rupture leading to subarachnoid hemorrhage (SAH), a devastating condition still associated with a 30-day mortality rate of 30% to 40%,[3–5] despite a consistent decline over the past 3 decades.[6,7] The annual risk of rupture is 1.3%.[8] Only one-third of patients surviving an aneurysmal SAH remain functionally independent.[7,9] The primary goal in managing patients presenting with aneurysmal SAH is to prevent a new rupture of the aneurysm, which is associated with an even higher mortality rate. Surgical and endovascular methods are available to achieve this goal. This article reviews endovascular management of ruptured intracranial aneurysms.

Surgical clipping has been the gold standard of treatment for more than 70 years, since Walter Dandy first applied a silver clip to the neck of an unruptured internal carotid artery aneurysm at the The Johns Hopkins Hospital in 1937.[10] The surgical approach to intracranial aneurysms was then refined by the adaptation of microsurgical techniques to the neurosurgical field by Yasargil.

The concept of endovascular treatment of intracranial aneurysms, drawing on work performed by Serbinenko[11] in the 1970s, was initially based on the use of balloons inflated within the aneurysmal cavity. In 1991, Guglielmi and coworkers published the first description of the endovascular application of detachable platinum coils (the Guglielmi Detachable Coil) to induce thrombosis and obliteration of intracranial aneurysms in humans. After Food and Drug Administration approval was granted in 1995,[12] the use of endovascular coiling has steadily increased and has been adopted as an alternative technique for the treatment of ruptured and unruptured intracranial aneurysms. Only two randomized, prospective studies comparing endovascular coiling and surgical clipping have been reported. The first one is a single-center study published in 1999, which found no significant difference in the obliteration rates at 12 months in 109 patients with SAH randomly assigned to surgical clipping or endovascular coiling.[13] The second, the International Subarachnoid Aneurysm Trial (ISAT), compared clipping versus coiling in 2143 patients with ruptured intracranial aneurysms. Patients treated endovascularly were at a lower risk of death or dependence at 1 year compared with the surgical group, with an absolute risk reduction of 7.4%, which was maintained for up to 7 years.[14] The

Division of Interventional Neuroradiology, The Johns Hopkins School of Medicine, 600 North Wolfe Street, Nelson Building, B-100, Baltimore, MD 21287, USA
* Corresponding author.
E-mail address: pgaillo1@jhmi.edu

Neurosurg Clin N Am 21 (2010) 271–280
doi:10.1016/j.nec.2009.10.004
1042-3680/10/$ – see front matter © 2010 Published by Elsevier Inc.

neurosurgery.theclinics.com

risk of rehemorrhage was low but more common after coiling than clipping. The neurosurgical community found these results controversial, pointing to possible selection biases detrimental to the surgical group and to the level of expertise of the neurosurgeons performing the surgical treatments (general vs vascular neurosurgeons). Questions concerning the durability and long-term efficacy of coil embolization and protection against rerupture were also raised. Despite these drawbacks, the ISAT did support the notion that endovascular therapy is a valid alternative to surgical clipping.

ENDOVASCULAR TECHNIQUES

Endovascular techniques for the treatment of intracranial aneurysms with conservation of the parent artery, also known as constructive therapies, include standard coil embolization, coil embolization with balloon remodeling or stent assistance, and balloon-assisted liquid polymer embolization (**Fig. 1**A, B, and C). The use of covered stents (or stent grafts) has been proposed as an option for large, fusiform, or wide-necked aneurysms, primarily located in the carotid and vertebral arteries, where the risk of occluding functionally important side branches is relatively low (see **Fig. 1**D). The long-term patency of stent grafts placed in relatively small vessels, such as the internal carotid artery, is another potential drawback of this approach and remains currently unknown.[15] Stents with a tight mesh or stents covered with semipermeable membranes (collectively known as flow diverters) may represent an improvement over conventional stent grafts in terms of parent artery and side branches patency. These stents may expand the indications of stent grafting to intracranial lesions, although their use in ruptured aneurysms needs to be carefully evaluated. Parent artery occlusion, also referred to as deconstructive therapy, remains a valid alternative option for nonsurgical candidates whose aneurysms are not amenable to constructive treatment methods.

The clinical condition of patients, the aneurysm location and morphology (in particular the diameter of the neck and its relation to the parent artery), and the presence of branches arising from the sac or the neck are important considerations when choosing the most appropriate treatment plan. The aneurysm neck, in particular its size and relation to the parent artery and potential side branches, is the key feature in determining if coil embolization is an appropriate treatment option. Standard coil embolization is considered feasible for aneurysms with a small neck (<4 mm), a dome-to-neck ratio equal or greater than two, and in the absence of important branches arising from the sac or the neck.[16] Coil embolization is achieved primarily with platinum coils. Although a careful analysis of the aneurysm morphology is essential to planning efficient therapy, aneurysms with a seemingly unfavorable configuration can occasionally respond well to simple coiling (**Fig. 2**). Advances made in platinum coil technology have tried to address incomplete aneurysm occlusion, which increases the risk of coil compaction and aneurysm recanalization. Reported rates of recanalization are approximately 21% to 28.6% but can be as high as 60% for giant aneurysms.[17–19] Recently developed hybrid, or biologically active, coils are chemically pretreated to enhance their thrombogenicity[20] in an effort to try decreasing the recanalization rate.[21] Currently available modified coils include polyglycolic acid/lactide copolymer–coated coils (Matrix, Boston Scientific, Natick, MA, USA; Cerecyte, Micrus, Sunnyvale, CA, USA; and Nexus, Micro Therapeutics, Irvine, CA, USA) and hydrogel-coated coils (HydroCoil, MicroVention, Aliso Viejo, CA, USA).[22] Other types of coated or active devices, such as coils with radioactive components or coils coated with biologic material, such as collagen or cells, are in experimental phases. Matrix coils comprise an inner core of platinum covered with a biodegradable polymer (polyglycolide/polylactide) designed to accelerate aneurysm fibrosis, neointima formation, and inflammation.[21] The safety of these coils for aneurysm treatment is similar to that of bare platinum coils.[23,24] Higher rates of recanalization (32%, from 26.1% for small aneurysms with small necks to 75% for large aneurysms)[21,25] and thromboembolic events (up to 20% vs 2.5%–11%),[26,27] however, are reported with Matrix coils versus bare platinum coils. Progressive resorption of the polymer coat leading to loss of volume and instability is a possible explanation for the high recurrence rates associated with these coils.[28] A recently published study of 152 patients with ruptured and unruptured aneurysms treated exclusively with Matrix coils showed similar results with no better recanalization rates than those previously reported for bare platinum coils (recanalization rates: 31.1% for aneurysms <10 mm and 56% for aneurysms >10 mm, with more frequent recanalization in ruptured aneurysms).[29] HydroCoils are standard platinum coils coated with an expandable hydrogel material that results in delayed progressive coil expansion on contact with blood.[30] These coils are supposed to provide superior aneurysm volume filling to bare platinum coils[31] and to promote healing and endothelialization at the aneurysm neck.[31,32] Despite these features,

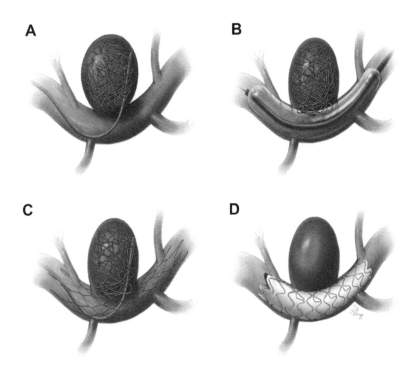

Fig. 1. Endovascular treatment of intracranial aneurysms: constructive techniques. (*A*) Coil embolization: the microcatheter was placed within the aneurysmal cavity, which was progressively filled (packed) with detachable microcoils of various diameters, length, and geometric configurations (helical, 2-D, 3-D, etc). Dense packing resulting in exclusion of the aneurysm from the circulation was obtained with a volume of coil material not exceeding 40% of the total aneurysm volume, the residual space being filled with thrombus. Standard coil embolization requires a favorable aneurysm geometry, particularly in regard to the sac-to-neck ratio. A low ratio (ie, a wide neck aneurysm) does not hold the coils within the aneurysmal cavity, jeopardizing the patency of the parent artery. (*B*) Balloon remodeling: inflation of a compliant microballoon across the aneurysm neck concomitantly to coil deployment allows treating lesions with unfavorable sac-to-neck ratio. The balloon was sequentially inflated and deflated in order to assist the placement of each coil. (*C*) Stent-assisted coiling: the deployment of a stent prior to aneurysm catheterization and coiling offers assistance for wide neck aneurysms without the need for iterative parent artery obliteration but leaves a permanent intravascular device that requires antiplatelet therapy and carries a still uncharacterized risk of delayed flow impairment (acute or subacute in-stent thrombosis, chronic in-stent stenosis from endothelial hyperplasia). Stent and balloon remodeling assistance can be combined for the treatment of dysplatic or fusiform aneurysms. (*D*) Stent graft/flow diverters: stent grafts can potentially interrupt the flow within the aneurysmal cavity without placement of intra-aneurysmal material. Such an approach is rapid (low radiation exposure) and solves the mass effect issues sometimes associated with dense packing of aneurysms located in the immediate vicinity of fragile structures, such as the optic nerve. Drawbacks of currently available stent grafts include poor trackability, unknown long-term patency of the parent artery, and, more importantly for neurovascular applications, the risk of side branches occlusion. Some of these issues may be addressed by the new generations of devices (flow diverters) with a semi-permeable architecture currently under development or in early clinical evaluation. (**Fig. 1**A *data from* Piotin M, Mandai S, Murphy KJ, et al. Dense packing of cerebral aneurysms: an in vitro study with detachable platinum coils. AJNR Am J Neuroradiol 2000;21(4):757–60.)

recanalization rates remain high, up to 27% for large aneurysms.[33] More concerning, however, are reported cases of aseptic meningitis and delayed hydrocephalus,[22,33,34] which seem specific to the HydroCoil as no cases have so far been described with polyglycolic acid/lactide copolymer–coated coils alone,[23] although some have occurred when Matrix coils were used in combination with HydroCoils.[35] Delayed perianeurysmal inflammation with dramatic neurologic dysfunction (bilateral visual loss) has been reported after embolization with HydroCoils.[36] Perianeurysmal inflammation leading to visual loss has also been described in cases of paraclinoid aneurysms treated with standard platinum or coated coils.[37] The factors leading to these various coil-related

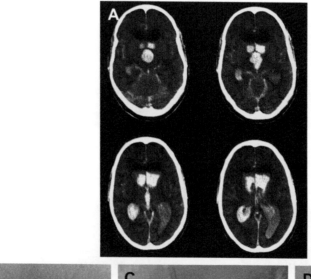

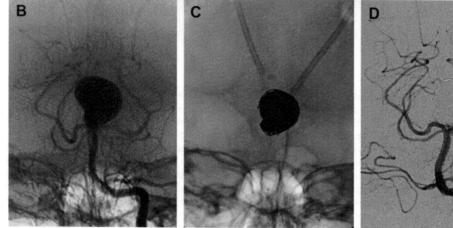

Fig. 2. A 45-year-old comatose patient with SAH and IVH. (*A*) Head CT documenting diffuse SAH and IVH. The patient was transferred to the authors' institution for further management. (*B*) DSA, transfacial view, showing a large basilar tip aneurysm. (*C*) Nonsubtracted image of the pack of microcoils (bare platinum coils). (*D*) DSA, transfacial view after treatment. Mild irregularity is observed at the neck, but there is no residual opacification of the aneurysmal cavity. At the 2-year follow-up visit, her neurologic examination was notable only for memory and cognitive changes.

events have not yet been elucidated, and more information is needed regarding the role of coils, clot burden, aneurysm size, and inflammatory mediators in the development of these complications.

Recent advances in stent technology have led to the development of flexible self-expanding nitinol stents (or reconstruction devices) (Neuroform, Boston Scientific Neurovascular, Natick, MA, USA; Enterprise, Cordis Neurovascular, Miami Lakes, FL, USA; and LEO, Balt, Montmorency, France) dedicated to intracranial aneurysm therapy, specifically for the treatment of complex and wide-necked aneurysms. Advantages of these self-expanding intracranial stents over the balloon expandable stents previously used for

assisted coiling include improved trackability, which helps navigate tortuous intracranial vasculature (although this is true only for the latest generation of self-expanding stents); improved deliverability; and decreased vessel injury during deployment.[38] Variations in stent design include open-cell (Neuroform)[39] versus closed-cell design (Enterprise and LEO),[40,41] low radial force (Neuroform)[39] versus high radial force (LEO)[40] versus low radial force/high compression resistance (Enterprise), and stent recoverability after partial deployment (a characteristic inherent to the closed-cell design, with up to 70% of stent length for the Enterprise[38] and up to 90% of the stent length for the LEO).[40] Despite several technical differences in stent design, these devices have been safe and effective in assisting the treatment of cerebral aneurysms.[40–42] The major argument against the use of these devices for the management of patients with aneurysmal SAH is linked to the need for concurrent antiplatelet therapy. A recent series of patients treated with stent-assisted coiling had a higher rate of hemorrhagic complications in the group presenting with SAH: two patients had a fatal outcome believed related to antiplatelet therapy, one from a massive intraventricular hemorrhage (IVH) secondary to an external ventricular drain change, the other from a parenchymal hemorrhage of unknown origin. The risk of parenchymal hemorrhage in patients taking antiplatelet therapy, however, may be independent of their having suffered a SAH. In the authors' experience, one patient with a nonruptured clinoid segment aneurysm was successfully treated with stent-assisted coiling, having suffered a nonfatal contralateral occipital lobe hemorrhage 2 days after the procedure. The goal of antiplatelet therapy is to reduce the risk of thromboembolic complications related to the stent placement itself and to the subsequent presence of an intraluminal foreign body, at least until the stent structure is covered by a layer of endothelial cells. Although protocols may slightly vary according to institutional and operator preferences, patients scheduled for elective therapy are typically placed under a combination of oral antiplatelet agents

several days prior to the procedure. In the authors' practice, patients are asked to take clopidogrel (75 mg) and aspirin (325 mg) daily starting 5 days before stent placement. Patients already taking these medications for other purposes are given an additional loading dose of clopidogrel (300 mg) the day preceding treatment. Such a drug regimen is not possible in patients presenting with aneurysmal SAH. There is no clear consensus about antiplatelet therapy in patients with SAH. As an example, the approach adopted at the authors' institution for ruptured wide-necked aneurysms that benefit from stent-assisted coiling is described. These aneurysms are divided into lesions that likely can be secured initially with partial coiling only but require a follow-up procedure for complete treatment and lesions unlikely to be secured with coiling only. This evaluation is based on the morphology of the aneurysm as depicted with 3-D digital subtraction angiography (DSA). In aneurysms that can be secured initially with partial coiling, the immediate goal is to ensure that the risk of re-rupture is eliminated (ie, that no residual flow is left within the aneurysmal cavity, in particular at its dome). This initial treatment may be helped by the use of the balloon remodeling technique and may even achieve definitive therapy (**Fig. 3**). The residual component, if any, is then addressed at a later date with the assistance of a stent, using

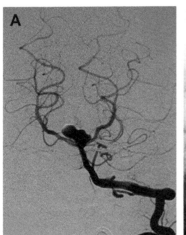 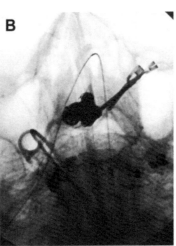 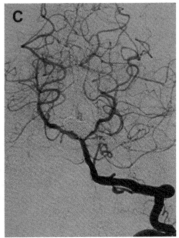

Fig. 3. A 49-year-old woman with a history of ruptured, surgically treated posterior communicating aneurysm, presenting with a new aneurysmal SAH. (*A*) DSA, left vertebral injection, anteroposterior view, showing an irregular, wide-necked aneurysm of the basilar tip. Coiling alone was attempted first. After successful deployment of several coils, coils loops starts protruding into the basilar artery and right P12 segment. A microballoon (Hyper-Form [4 mm × 7 mm], ev3 [ev3 Neurovascular, Irvine, CA, USA]) was advanced into the distal basilar artery, and the coiling was completed (using a remodeling technique described by Moret and colleagues[43]). (*B*) Nonsubtracted image of the pack of microcoils (bare platinum coils). (*C*) DSA, left vertebral injection, anteroposterior view, confirming the absence of residual flow within the aneurysm. Follow-up angiography at 8 months was unchanged, and the patient was neurologically intact.

standard antiplatelet preparation. Even when this first approach has been elected, a stent may be deployed if it becomes obvious that adequate treatment will not be achieved with coiling alone (**Fig. 4**). In situations where it seems likely that adequate treatment will not be achieved by coiling alone, a stent may be used as first intention therapy. In such instances, a microcatheter is placed within the aneurysmal cavity first, in order to secure access for subsequent coiling (jailing technique). The use of the jailing technique in this instance principally prevents the unlikely but potentially catastrophic situation in which a stent is deployed but the aneurysm cannot be

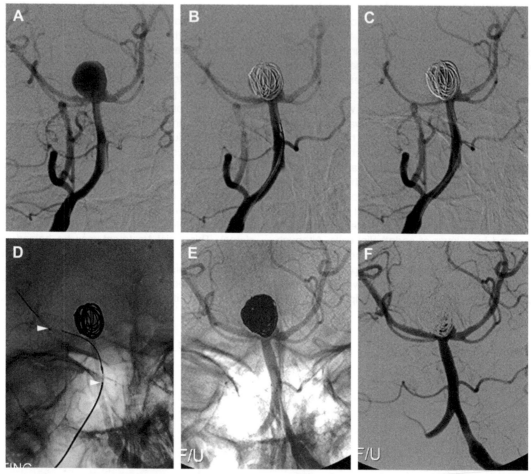

Fig. 4. A 54-year-old lethargic patient with diffuse SAH and IVH. After transfer to the authors' institution, a ventricular shunt was placed and angiography obtained. (*A*) DSA, right vertebral injection, transfacial view, documenting a basilar tip aneurysm. The angiographic projections and the 3-D reconstructions showed that the left posterior cerebral artery (PCA) was arising from the base of the aneurysm itself, with no detectable posterior communicating artery on that side. (*B*) DSA, right vertebral injection, transfacial view, after placement but before detachment of the first microcoil (Guglielmi Detachable Coil 18, Boston Scientific, Natick, Massachusetts). Both PCAs are patent. (*C*) DSA, right vertebral injection, transfacial view. After detachment of the first coil, the configuration of the coil pack was slightly different and the right PCA no longer patent. The decision was made to deploy a stent across the neck of the aneurysm into the right PCA. (*D*) DSA, left vertebral injection, transfacial view. A second microcatheter has been advanced into the right PCA. The proximal and distal markers of the stent (Enterprise, Cordis Neurovascular, Miami Lakes, FL, USA) are visible on this nonsubtracted image (*white arrowheads*). (*E*) DSA, left vertebral injection, nonsubtracted transfacial view, showing the pack of coils at the end of the procedure. The left aspect of the aneurysm base was not packed in order to preserve the patency of the left PCA. (*F*) DSA, left vertebral injection, transfacial view. This final angiographic control confirms the patency of both PCAs. It also shows residual aneurysmal neck, from which the left PCA takes origin. It was believed that the aneurysm was at this point secured and, further, would be performed at a later date, if needed, possibly with the assistance of a second stent. The patient was discharged home on day 16 neurologically intact.

subsequently catheterized. The stent is then advanced and deployed using a standard technique (**Fig. 5**). In the authors' practice, antiplatelet therapy is administered only when the stent has been successfully deployed. In the absence of injectable aspirin (eg, as in the United States), the authors' regimen consists aspirin (600 mg) administered rectally and clopidogrel (450 mg) delivered via a nasogastric tube. Intravenous heparin (initial dose 5000 IU intravenous bolus, monitored and adjusted using activated clotting time) is added after detachment of the first microcoil within the aneurysmal cavity. A concern with this approach lies in the potential need for subsequent placement of a ventricular shunt under antiplatelet therapy. In order to avoid, as much as

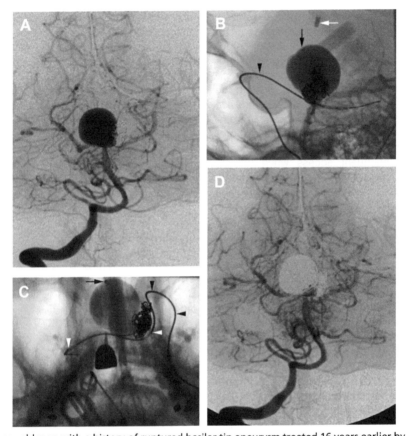

Fig. 5. A 58-year-old man with a history of ruptured basilar tip aneurysm treated 16 years earlier by endovascular coiling. The patient was transferred to the authors' institution for management of a new SAH. At admission, he was in acute respiratory failure and cardiac distress (ejection fraction of 15%). He underwent angiography once his vital functions were believed stable enough for transport. (A) DSA, right vertebral injection, transfacial view, documenting a basilar tip aneurysm. The 3-D reconstructions showed that both PCAs were originating from the base of the aneurysm. The compacted coil pack from the initial treatment can be seen along the left lateral aspect of the aneurysmal sac. The decision was made to proceed with stent-assisted coiling as first intention therapy. (B) DSA, right vertebral injection, lateral view. A microcatheter has first been placed within the aneurysmal cavity (*black arrow*). A second microcatheter has then been advanced across the neck of the aneurysm into the right PCA via the left internal carotid and posterior communicating arteries (*black arrowhead*). Note presence of a ventricular shunt (*white arrow*). (C) DSA, right vertebral injection, transfacial view, showing the microcatheter within the aneurysm cavity (*black arrow*), the second microcatheter through the left posterior communicating artery (*black arrowheads*), passing across the neck of the aneurysm. The proximal and distal markers of the stent (Enterprise, Cordis Neurovascular, Miami Lakes, FL, USA) are visible on this nonsubtracted view. Note also the compacted coil pack from the initial treatment performed 14 years before. (D) DSA, right vertebral injection, transfacial view, final angiographic control showing some residual neck at the base of the aneurysm, from which the left PCA takes origin. Both PCAs are patent. It was believed that the aneurysm was secured at this point and that the residual base could be addressed, if needed, at a later date. Unfortunately, the patient subsequently developed severe hemodynamic instability and metabolic imbalance with diffuse bilateral cerebral edema resistant to medical management, including barbiturate coma. He died 3 days after treatment from a cardiac arrest.

possible, such a situation, a CT scan is obtained immediately prior to the procedure and a shunt placed if ventricular enlargement is observed.

Several flow-diverting devices are in development or in early clinical evaluation phases. These new devices clearly carry promises for the endovascular management of intracranial aneurysms. It is, however, too early to define with certainty their exact role, in particular in regard to the treatment of aneurysmal SAH. As discussed previously, the use of antiplatelet therapy in the setting of SAH remains controversial, an issue possibly more significant for flow diverters, which might carry higher thromboembolic risks due to their intrinsic physical characteristics. Among the potential drawbacks or still unresolved features of these new devices in the setting of SAH are the delay between device deployment and aneurysm obliteration/thrombosis, the absence of structural elements reinforcing the aneurysm wall (no coils), the potential difficulty of subsequent access when primary occlusion fails, the preserved patency of important surrounding small arteries, and the durability of the achieved therapy. These points are illustrated in two recent publications concerning one of these emerging flow-diverting devices (Pipeline, Chestnut Medical Technologies, Menlo Park, CA, USA), a device made of a braided mesh cylinder composed of platinum and cobalt chromium microfilaments offering, after deployment, an approximately 30% to 35% surface coverage. This coverage is supposed to create significant flow disruption while remaining porous enough to maintain patency of the parent artery and adjacent branch vessels covered by the stent. One of these publications describes passage of contrast into the cavity of a midbasilar artery aneurysm that can still be observed by angiography 48 hours after a the placement of seven more partially overlapping devices.[44] In the other publication, two patients with fusiform aneurysms were each treated with three devices, resulting in aneurysm obliteration in one case and in flow reduction in the other, for which treatment was completed by adjunct coiling.[45] Although encouraging, these results raise questions about the preserved patency of perforating branches when several devices have to be used in a concentric manner and the risk of rebleeding during the latency period between deployment and actual aneurysm thrombosis, if the devices were used for the treatment of aneurysmal SAH.

SUMMARY

Endovascular therapy is now a well-accepted alternative to surgical clipping for ruptured and nonruptured intracranial aneurysms. The current state-of-the-art endovascular techniques for the treatment of aneurysmal SAH include coiling alone and coiling assisted by the balloon remodeling technique. The use of newly developed self-expandable stents seems tempting, as their safety and efficacy have been demonstrated for the treatment of nonruptured aneurysms. The important role played by antiplatelet therapy, prior and after stent deployment, however, renders their use for the treatment of ruptured aneurysms controversial. Although a recent publication warns about this specific application as carrying a higher risk of hemorrhagic complication, the size of the reported series does not allow drawing significant conclusions at this time.

New flow-diverting devices currently in development or early clinical evaluation carry great promise for the treatment of nonruptured aneurysms. As is the case with stent-assisted coiling, the role that these new devices will play in the management of aneurysmal SAH remains unclear at this time.

REFERENCES

1. Rinkel GJ, Djibuti M, Algra A, et al. Prevalence and risk of rupture of intracranial aneurysms: a systematic review. Stroke 1998;29(1):251–6.
2. Rinkel GJ. Natural history, epidemiology and screening of unruptured intracranial aneurysms. J Neuroradiol 2008;35(2):99–103.
3. Lavados PM, Sacks C, Prina L, et al. Incidence, 30-day case-fatality rate, and prognosis of stroke in Iquique, Chile: a 2-year community-based prospective study (PISCIS project). Lancet 2005; 365(9478):2206–15.
4. Pajunen P, Paakkonen R, Hamalainen H, et al. Trends in fatal and nonfatal strokes among persons aged 35 to > or = 85 years during 1991-2002 in Finland. Stroke 2005;36(2):244–8.
5. Kleindorfer D, Broderick J, Khoury J, et al. The unchanging incidence and case-fatality of stroke in the 1990s: a population-based study. Stroke 2006; 37(10):2473–8.
6. Ingall TJ, Whisnant JP, Wiebers DO, et al. Has there been a decline in subarachnoid hemorrhage mortality? Stroke 1989;20(6):718–24.
7. Hop JW, Rinkel GJ, Algra A, et al. Case-fatality rates and functional outcome after subarachnoid hemorrhage: a systematic review. Stroke 1997;28(3): 660–4.
8. Juvela S, Porras M, Poussa K. Natural history of unruptured intracranial aneurysms: probability of and risk factors for aneurysm rupture. J Neurosurg 2008;108(5):1052–60.

9. van Gijn J, Rinkel GJ. Subarachnoid haemorrhage: diagnosis, causes and management. Brain 2001; 124(Pt 2):249–78.

10. Dandy WE. Intracranial aneurysm of the internal carotid artery: cured by operation. Ann Surg 1938; 107(5):654–9.

11. Serbinenko FA. [Balloon occlusion of saccular aneurysms of the cerebral arteries]. Vopr Neirokhir 1974;Jul-Aug(4):8–15 [in Russian].

12. Guglielmi G, Vinuela F, Dion J, et al. Electrothrombosis of saccular aneurysms via endovascular approach. Part 2: preliminary clinical experience. J Neurosurg 1991;75(1):8–14.

13. Vanninen R, Koivisto T, Saari T, et al. Ruptured intracranial aneurysms: acute endovascular treatment with electrolytically detachable coils—a prospective randomized study. Radiology 1999;211(2):325–36.

14. Molyneux AJ, Kerr RS, Yu LM, et al. International subarachnoid aneurysm trial (ISAT) of neurosurgical clipping versus endovascular coiling in 2143 patients with ruptured intracranial aneurysms: a randomised comparison of effects on survival, dependency, seizures, rebleeding, subgroups, and aneurysm occlusion. Lancet 2005;366(9488): 809–17.

15. Saatci I, Cekirge HS, Ozturk MH, et al. Treatment of internal carotid artery aneurysms with a covered stent: experience in 24 patients with mid-term follow-up results. AJNR Am J Neuroradiol 2004; 25(10):1742–9.

16. Alexander MJ. Endovascular treatment of cerebral aneurysms in children. In: Alexander MJ, Spetzler RF, editors. Pediatric neurovascular disease: surgical, endovascular, and medical management. New York: Thieme; 2006. p. 145–51.

17. Murayama Y, Nien YL, Duckwiler G, et al. Guglielmi detachable coil embolization of cerebral aneurysms: 11 years' experience. J Neurosurg 2003;98(5):959–66.

18. Sanai N, Quinones-Hinojosa A, Gupta NM, et al. Pediatric intracranial aneurysms: durability of treatment following microsurgical and endovascular management. J Neurosurg 2006;104(Suppl 2):82–9.

19. Piotin M, Spelle L, Mounayer C, et al. Intracranial aneurysms: treatment with bare platinum coils–aneurysm packing, complex coils, and angiographic recurrence. Radiology 2007;243(2):500–8.

20. Eddleman C, Nikas D, Shaibani A, et al. HydroCoil embolization of a ruptured infectious aneurysm in a pediatric patient: case report and review of the literature. Childs Nerv Syst 2007;23(6):707–12.

21. Kimchi TJ, Willinsky RA, Spears J, et al. Endovascular treatment of intracranial aneurysms with matrix coils: immediate posttreatment results, clinical outcome and follow-up. Neuroradiology 2007; 49(3):223–9.

22. Kang HS, Han MH, Lee TH, et al. Embolization of intracranial aneurysms with hydrogel-coated coils: result of a Korean multicenter trial. Neurosurgery 2007;61(1):51–8 [discussion: 58–9].

23. Kang HS, Han MH, Kwon BJ, et al. Short-term outcome of intracranial aneurysms treated with polyglycolic acid/lactide copolymer-coated coils compared to historical controls treated with bare platinum coils: a single-center experience. AJNR Am J Neuroradiol 2005;26(8):1921–8.

24. Lubicz B, Leclerc X, Gauvrit JY, et al. Endovascular treatment of intracranial aneurysms with matrix coils: a preliminary study of immediate post-treatment results. AJNR Am J Neuroradiol 2005;26(2):373–5.

25. Fiorella D, Albuquerque FC, McDougall CG. Durability of aneurysm embolization with matrix detachable coils. Neurosurgery 2006;58(1):51–9 [discussion: 51–9].

26. Taschner CA, Leclerc X, Rachdi H, et al. Matrix detachable coils for the endovascular treatment of intracranial aneurysms: analysis of early angiographic and clinical outcomes. Stroke 2005;36(10):2176–80.

27. Workman MJ, Cloft HJ, Tong FC, et al. Thrombus formation at the neck of cerebral aneurysms during treatment with Guglielmi detachable coils. AJNR Am J Neuroradiol 2002;23(9):1568–76.

28. Murayama Y, Tateshima S, Gonzalez NR, et al. Matrix and bioabsorbable polymeric coils accelerate healing of intracranial aneurysms: long-term experimental study. Stroke 2003;34(8):2031–7.

29. Piotin M, Spelle L, Mounayer C, et al. Intracranial aneurysms coiling with matrix: immediate results in 152 patients and midterm anatomic follow-up from 115 patients. Stroke 2009;40(1):321–3.

30. Cloft HJ. HydroCoil for Endovascular Aneurysm Occlusion (HEAL) study: periprocedural results. AJNR Am J Neuroradiol 2006;27(2):289–92.

31. Gaba RC, Ansari SA, Roy SS, et al. Embolization of intracranial aneurysms with hydrogel-coated coils versus inert platinum coils: effects on packing density, coil length and quantity, procedure performance, cost, length of hospital stay, and durability of therapy. Stroke 2006;37(6):1443–50.

32. Ding YH, Dai D, Lewis DA, et al. Angiographic and histologic analysis of experimental aneurysms embolized with platinum coils, Matrix, and HydroCoil. AJNR Am J Neuroradiol 2005;26(7):1757–63.

33. Berenstein A, Song JK, Niimi Y, et al. Treatment of cerebral aneurysms with hydrogel-coated platinum coils (HydroCoil): early single-center experience. AJNR Am J Neuroradiol 2006;27(9):1834–40.

34. Im SH, Han MH, Kwon BJ, et al. Aseptic meningitis after embolization of cerebral aneurysms using hydrogel-coated coils: report of three cases. AJNR Am J Neuroradiol 2007;28(3):511–2.

35. Meyers PM, Lavine SD, Fitzsimmons BF, et al. Chemical meningitis after cerebral aneurysm treatment using two second-generation aneurysm coils: report of two cases. Neurosurgery 2004;55(5):1222.

36. Pickett GE, Laitt RD, Herwadkar A, et al. Visual pathway compromise after hydrocoil treatment of large ophthalmic aneurysms. Neurosurgery 2007; 61(4):E873–4 [discussion: E874].

37. Schmidt GW, Oster SF, Golnik KC, et al. Isolated progressive visual loss after coiling of paraclinoid aneurysms. AJNR Am J Neuroradiol 2007;28(10):1882–9.

38. Higashida RT, Halbach VV, Dowd CF, et al. Initial clinical experience with a new self-expanding nitinol stent for the treatment of intracranial cerebral aneurysms: the Cordis Enterprise stent. AJNR Am J Neuroradiol 2005;26(7):1751–6.

39. Howington JU, Hanel RA, Harrigan MR, et al. The Neuroform stent, the first microcatheter-delivered stent for use in the intracranial circulation. Neurosurgery 2004;54(1):2–5.

40. Lubicz B, Leclerc X, Levivier M, et al. Retractable self-expandable stent for endovascular treatment of wide-necked intracranial aneurysms: preliminary experience. Neurosurgery 2006;58(3):451–7 [discussion: 451–7].

41. Weber W, Bendszus M, Kis B, et al. A new self-expanding nitinol stent (Enterprise) for the treatment of wide-necked intracranial aneurysms: initial clinical and angiographic results in 31 aneurysms. Neuroradiology 2007;49(7):555–61.

42. Biondi A, Janardhan V, Katz JM, et al. Neuroform stent-assisted coil embolization of wide-neck intracranial aneurysms: strategies in stent deployment and midterm follow-up. Neurosurgery 2007;61(3): 460–8 [discussion: 468–9].

43. Moret J, Cognard C, Weill A, et al. [Reconstruction technic in the treatment of wide-neck intracranial aneurysms. Long-term angiographic and clinical results. Apropos of 56 cases]. J Neuroradiol 1997; 24:30–44 [in French].

44. Fiorella D, Kelly ME, Albuquerque FC, et al. Curative reconstruction of a giant midbasilar trunk aneurysm with the pipeline embolization device. Neurosurgery 2009;64(2):212–7 [discussion: 217].

45. Fiorella D, Woo HH, Albuquerque FC, et al. Definitive reconstruction of circumferential, fusiform intracranial aneurysms with the pipeline embolization device. Neurosurgery 2008;62(5):1115–20 [discussion: 1120–1].

Endovascular Management of Cerebral Vasospasm

Ben McGuinness, MBChB, FRANZCR[a],
Dheeraj Gandhi, MBBS, MD[a,b],*

KEYWORDS

- Vasospasm • Endovascular • Angioplasty
- Interventional • Subarachnoid hemorrhage
- Angiography

Cerebral vasospasm causes significant morbidity and mortality in patients with subarachnoid hemorrhage (SAH). The management of these patients is challenging and requires the multidisciplinary input of intensive care, neurosurgical, and endovascular specialists. Angiographic vasospasm occurs in approximately 70% of all aneurysmal SAH, but clinical neurological manifestations occur in only one third of these cases.[1] Up to 15% of patients surviving the initial subarachnoid hemorrhage will suffer stroke or death as a result of vasospasm.[2,3] Vasospasm rarely occurs before day 4; it tends to peak at day 7, and it may last up to 2 weeks after the initial hemorrhage.

Most cases of vasospasm can be managed medically. Medical strategies for treating vasospasm include hemodynamic augmentation to improve cerebral perfusion pressure and medical therapy to prevent or reduce cerebral vasospasm. A combination of volume expansion, hemodilution, and induced hypertension (Triple H therapy) has been used extensively, but its value has not been tested rigorously.[4] Currently, oral nimodipine is recommended for patients with aneurysmal SAH. Other, newer agents being evaluated include albumin, statins, magnesium sulphate infusion, and clazosentan (endothelin-1 antagonist).[4] Detailed discussion of medical therapy is beyond the scope of this article. Instead, it will focus on the endovascular therapy of vasospasm and the role of radiological imaging in the appropriate selection of patients who are likely to benefit from this form of treatment.

The clinical diagnosis of vasospasm often is based on detailed neurologic examination. The monitoring of patients at risk for clinical vasospasm requires constant neurological examination by intensive care specialists and the decision making of an experienced, multidisciplinary physician team. The diagnosis of symptomatic vasospasm requires identification of new focal motor deficits or sudden changes in mental status in at-risk patients. These new deficits should not be easily attributed to other causes such as development of hydrocephalus, systemic infection, seizures, or ongoing delirium. Although clinical examination is very useful, it is not always reliable. A significant proportion of patients with SAH may be neurologically impaired or comatose at baseline. In such patients, a meaningful neurological examination may not be obtainable.

IMAGING ASSESSMENT

Diagnostic imaging assessment of a patient with SAH in the vasospasm window serves many functions. These include ruling out other

[a] Division of Interventional Neuroradiology, Department of Radiology, Johns Hopkins Hospital, 600 North Wolfe Street, Nelson B-100, Baltimore, MD 21287, USA
[b] Division of Interventional Neuroradiology, Department of Neurology and Neurosurgery, Johns Hopkins Hospital, 600 North Wolfe Street, B100, Baltimore, MD 21287, USA
* Corresponding author. Division of Interventional Neuroradiology, Department of Neurology and Neurosurgery, Johns Hopkins Hospital, 600 North Wolfe Street, B100, Baltimore, MD 21287.
E-mail address: dgandhi2@jhmi.edu

Neurosurg Clin N Am 21 (2010) 281–290
doi:10.1016/j.nec.2009.10.007

pathologies, detecting the presence of vasospasm, and assessing its severity. In a patient with acute neurological deterioration, imaging assessment is essential to triage those patients appropriate for aggressive medical or endovascular therapy. Many different imaging modalities have been used, including transcranial Doppler (TCD) ultrasound, single photon emission computed tomography (SPECT) cerebral blood flow studies, positron emission tomography (PET), magnetic resonance angiography (MRA), magnetic resonance perfusion, stable xenon-enhanced computed tomography (CT), CT angiography, and CT perfusion. In a patient with suspected symptomatic vasospasm, noncontrast CT is a first-line study at most institutions. It can easily rule out other causes for deterioration such as hydrocephalus and rehemorrhage. In addition, a developing hypodensity in the vascular territory of clinical concern could indicate an established infarction. In such patients, aggressive endovascular therapy would be unlikely to be effective, and, in fact, it can be potentially harmful, as it can cause further morbidity or mortality from reperfusion hemorrhage.[5,6] Clearly, the relative size of this infarct needs to be weighed against the benefit of intervening to prevent infarction in a larger area of at-risk parenchyma (the so-called penumbra).[7]

TCD is used in many institutions and has the advantage of being a portable noninvasive study that can be performed at the bedside in the intensive care unit (ICU) setting. The TCD results correlate well with angiographic findings if the vessel under investigation is insonated adequately (**Fig. 1**). Its value, however, is rather limited in patients with poor acoustic windows. The sensitivity of TCD varies depending on the vessel affected by vasospasm, with relatively low sensitivity for supraclinoid internal carotid and anterior cerebral arteries (ACA).[4] TCD has been shown to be specific but not sensitive for vasospasm of the middle cerebral artery (MCA) when compared with angiography, and it is poorly predictive of developing secondary cerebral infarction.[8,9] In addition to limitations imposed by poor acoustic window, the utility of TCD is hampered further by operator dependence and inability to study the distal vessels.

Use of imaging modalities such as magnetic resonance imaging (MRI)/MRA/magnetic resonance perfusion, PET, SPECT, and xenon CT that assess cerebral vasculature or brain perfusion often require the patient to remain still for prolonged periods. These techniques are not universally available and are often not practical for routine clinical use in these very sick patients. In recent years, a combination of CT angiography (CTA) and CT perfusion (CTP) has emerged as an important tool. It is very helpful in triaging patients with suspicion of vasospasm into those who should have aggressive medical management and others who should undergo early endovascular therapy. It is an attractive technique as it is a fast, readily available, relatively inexpensive, and practical imaging modality well suited to ICU patients. This can be combined easily with noncontrast head CT and performed on most commercially available scanners. Modern multidetector scanners are capable of rapidly assessing the caliber of the intracranial arteries using CTA and the brain parenchymal perfusion (CTP) with the use of 50 to 100 cc bolus of iodinated contrast (**Figs. 2** and **3**). Multidetector CTA has a very high accuracy of 98% to 100% for detecting severe vasospasm when compared with digital subtraction angiography.[10–12] Lower degrees of accuracy for mild–moderate vasospasm (57% to 85%) have been reported. Supraclinoid internal carotid artery (ICA) and very distal intracranial arteries are slightly difficult areas to assess on the CTA studies.[10,12] The addition of CTP, however, however improves the accuracy of diagnosis of distal vasospasm by demonstrating tissue-level perfusional abnormalities despite the absence of proximal vasospasm on CTA.

CTP provides several quantitative parameters of cerebrovascular hemodynamics. These include MTT, CBV and CBF.[13] MTT is defined as the average transit time of blood through a given brain region, measured in seconds. CBV is defined as the total volume of blood in a given volume of brain, usually measured in milliliters per 100 grams of brain tissue. CBF is the volume of blood moving through a given volume of brain per unit time, measured in milliliters per 100 grams of brain tissue per minute.

MTT or time to peak (TTP) maps have been shown to be the most sensitive in detecting early auto-regulation changes in cerebral ischemia, and these maps should be interrogated first when reading a CTP study.[10,14] In the authors' experience, if these maps are normal and symmetrical, then clinically significant vasospasm is highly unlikely. Abnormality on these maps, however, mandates close and careful inspection of the CBV and CBF maps to further characterize the severity of the perfusional defect. Three patterns of CT perfusional abnormality can be identified with progressive severity.[10,15,16]

1. Elevated MTT/TTP with normal CBF and normal-to-increased CBV: indicates perfusional abnormality that is adequately compensated for by auto-regulation

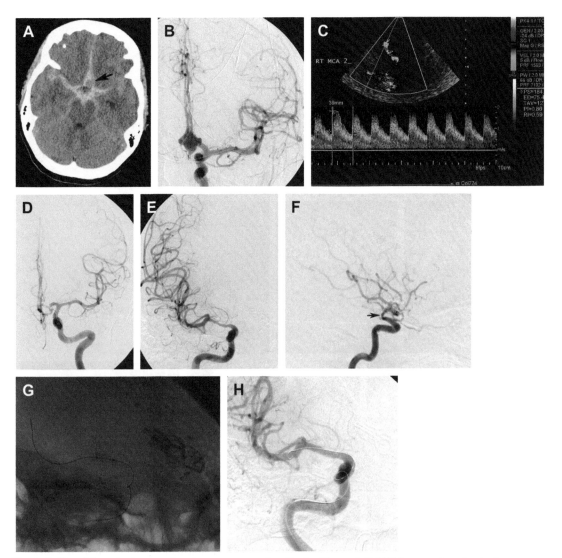

Fig. 1. Utility of Doppler in assessing the vasospasm. A patient with grade 3 SAH from ruptured anterior communicating artery. This aneurysm was clipped. (*A*) Initial CT scan demonstrates a diffuse subarachnoid blood. A small filling defect in the anterior interhemispheric fissure is suggestive of an aneurysm (*arrow*). (*B*) A digital subtraction angiography (DSA) study confirms the presence of a complex anterior communicating artery predominantly opacified from the left internal carotid artery (ICA) injection. Bilateral A2 segments fill from the left ICA injection, and the right A1 segment was hypoplastic or atretic. (*C*) The patient had a waxing and waning course in the ICU. A Doppler study on the sixth day demonstrated findings suggestive of severe vasospasm. This image shows the right middle cerebral artery (MCA) and the peak velocities in this vessel are markedly elevated. (*D*) The left ICA angiogram demonstrates occlusion of the aneurysm and some narrowing of the distal left A1 segment. There is, however, no flow limitation; therefore this vessel was not treated. (*E*) Anteroposterior (AP) and lateral (*F*) angiograms of the right ICA demonstrating severe spasm in the left supraclinoid carotid (*arrow*) and the proximal right MCA. (*G*) Inflation of a hyperform balloon in the right MCA M1 segment during the angioplasty. The patient also underwent ICA angioplasty. (*H*) After angioplasty, the caliber of the ICA and MCA has improved significantly, and there is good augmentation of flow. The patient made a complete recovery.

2. Elevated MTT/TTP with reduced CBF and normal-to-increased CBV: indicates perfusional abnormality with reversible cerebral ischemia (penumbra) (see **Figs. 2** and **3**)

3. Elevated MTT/TTP with reduced CBF and matched reduced CBV: indicates perfusional abnormality with irreversible cerebral ischemia.

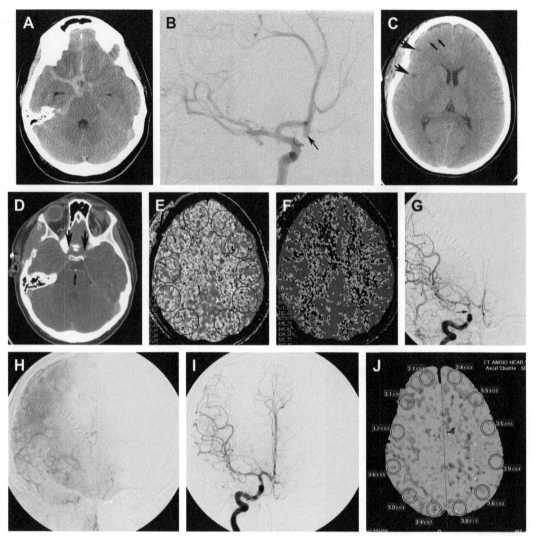

Fig. 2. This middle-aged female patient presented with a diffuse subarachnoid hemorrhage from a ruptured anterior communicating artery aneurysm. (*A*) Initial head CT shows diffuse subarachnoid blood in the basal cisterns. (*B*) An oblique angiogram of the right ICA demonstrates a small, inferiorly pointing anterior communicating artery aneurysm at the junction of the right A1 and A2 segments (*arrow*). This was treated with surgical clipping. (*C*) The patient developed new-onset weakness of left upper and lower extremities on day 8 from the initial SAH. A noncontrast CT demonstrates tiny new hypodensities in the right MCA distribution (*large arrows*) and questionable blurring of gray–white junction in the right frontal region (*small arrows*). (*D*) A CTA study (axial multiplanar reformat) demonstrates severe narrowing of bilateral supraclinoid ICAs (*large arrows*), as well as moderate narrowing of the basilar artery (*small arrow*). (*E*) A CTP study was obtained simultaneously. A mean transit time demonstrates asymmetry between the right and the left hemispheres with prolongation of mean transit times in the anterior cerebral artery (ACA) and MCA distributions (right hemisphere > left hemisphere). (*F*) Corresponding cerebral blood flow maps demonstrate decreased cerebral blood flow, again more severe on the right side. (*G*) A DSA image of the right ICA confirms very severe abnormalities in the caliber of the proximal vessels with profound reduction in caliber of the ICA (*arrow*) and severe narrowing of the MCA and ACA. Similar but slightly less severe abnormalities were present contralaterally (not shown). (*H*) A parenchymal phase of the right ICA angiogram shows heterogenous appearance with paucity of contrast staining, especially in the ACA distribution. The findings of DSA correlate very well with CTP findings. (*I*) After angioplasty, the vessel caliber of the ICA, MCA, and ACA is markedly improved with prompt opacification of the distal branches of ACA and MCA. Similar findings were seen on the left side (not shown). (*J*) A CTP scan the following day (mean transit time [MTT] map shown here) shows reversal of prior abnormalities and symmetrical, normal mean transit times in bilateral hemispheres.

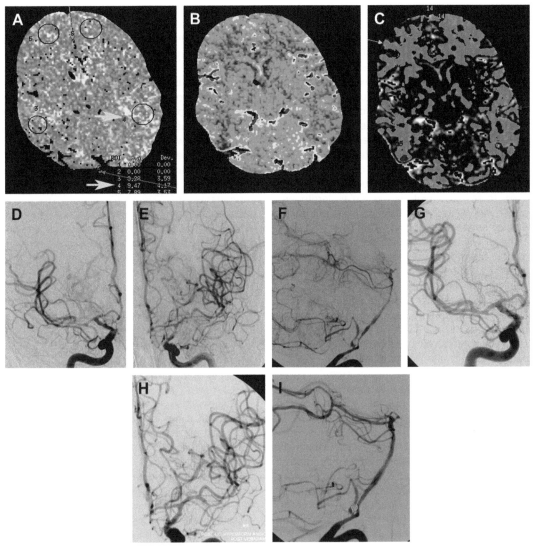

Fig. 3. A patient with diffuse SAH from right posterior inferior cerebellar artery (PICA) aneurysm that was treated with coil embolization. She subsequently developed increased somnolence and right-sided weakness. (*A*) MTT maps reveal bilateral and global prolongation of MTTs for example region of interest 4 (*large arrows*) and show MTT of 9.47 seconds. (*B*) cerebral blood flow (CBF) maps show similar global reduction in CBF. (*C*) Tissue classification map shows areas of reduced CBF but preserved cerebral blood volume (CBV) in yellow (representing ischemic penumbra) and areas of reduced CBF with significantly reduced CBV in purple (indicating likely irreversible ischemia). This map therefore shows that most of the brain is potentially salvageable ischemic penumbra, and aggressive intervention is indicated. Right internal carotid (*D*), left internal carotid (*E*), and vertebral angiograms (*F*), respectively show severe proximal vasospasm involving supraclinoid ICA bilaterally, M1 segments bilaterally, left A1 segment, V4 segment vertebral artery, basilar artery, and proximal posterior cerebral arteries bilaterally. (*G, H, I*) Corresponding angiograms following angioplasty of all involved segments shows marked improvement in caliber. Apart from some small cerebellar infarcts, the patient made an excellent recovery.

This constitutes a relative contraindication to aggressive therapy. Endovascular treatment targeted to this area is not advisable, as this region likely will progress to established cerebral infarction and will be at risk for reperfusion hemorrhage.

MTT and TTP have been shown to be sensitive and early predictors of secondary cerebral infarction in patients with vasospasm.[9,11,17] These CT perfusion changes occur a median of 3 days prior to the development of established infarct on noncontrast CT.[9] Wintermark and colleagues found MTT to have a negative predictive value for cerebral vasospasm of 99% and that the combination of CTA with an MTT threshold of greater than 6.4 seconds was the most accurate in the diagnosis of cerebral vasospasm.[11] In addition, a cortical regional CBF value of less than 39.3 mL/100 g/min was the most accurate (95%) indicator for the need for endovascular therapy.

Although CTA and CTP are excellent imaging tools, they also have a few limitations. Current limitations include metallic artifact from coils or clips preventing evaluation, problems with contrast bolus timing, and restricted range of parenchymal coverage on perfusion maps. Although the posterior fossa is usually not included on CTP, a range usually can be selected that includes a large part of all three supratentorial vascular territories. Further widespread availability of the latest multidetector scanner technology (256 and 320 slice scanners) will allow complete brain coverage. In addition, the problem of metallic artifacts is being addressed with new, dual-source CT technology.

Patients that are triaged as candidates for endovascular therapy will undergo initial emergent catheter angiography. Vasospasm found on angiography typically is divided into proximal and distal. Most literature divides severity of vasospasm arbitrarily into mild, moderate, and severe based on varying degrees of stenosis.[10,12,18] A useful example is that described by Kassell and colleagues,[18] with four grades: no stenosis or mild (<50%), moderate (50%), and severe (>50%) stenosis. The location of vasospasm determines the method of endovascular treatment employed. Proximal vasospasm should be treated with balloon angioplasty whenever possible. Intra-arterial (IA) vasodilators are used for distal spasm that is not amenable to balloon angioplasty or for vessels considered not safe for angioplasty, for example vasospasm in a vessel segment recently treated with surgical clipping of an aneurysm. The authors also use IA vasodilators as a complement to angioplasty.

INTRA-ARTERIAL INFUSION OF VASODILATORS

Papaverine and calcium channel blockers have been used extensively for IA infusion for pharmacological treatment of cerebral vasospasm. In general, the efficacy of these agents is modest at best and usually of limited duration. For these reasons, their use generally is limited to predominantly distal vasospasm that cannot be treated with angioplasty, mild proximal spasm where angioplasty is not indicated, and other instances where angioplasty is not possible because of anatomical or technical factors. In addition, vasodilators may be used prior to angioplasty to reduce vasomotor tone of the vessel. In the authors' experience (Gandhi D,

unpublished data, 2004–2009), the use of calcium channel blockers prior to angioplasty decreases the risk of acute vessel rupture. IA calcium channel blockers are probably the most widely used agents currently in the United States.

Papaverine is an alkaloid of the opium group, and it has been used for a long time as a nonspecific vasodilator in vasospasm via a direct action on smooth muscle. Its use now is largely of historical interest, with most operators preferring the more favorable safety profile of calcium channel blockers. Papaverine had a reported angiographic improvement of around 75% with a modest clinical improvement of 25% to 52%.[6,18,19] The use of papaverine largely has been abandoned because of the common recurrence of vasospasm requiring repeated treatment and complications reported with its use including

> Raised intracranial pressure (ICP)
> Seizures
> Hypotension
> Transient brainstem depression
> Worsening of vasospasm
> Monocular blindness if infused proximal
> to ophthalmic artery origin.[6,19,20]

IA nimodipine is not available in the United States, but it has been used throughout Europe and Australasia. In a study by Biondi and colleagues[21] of 25 patients with symptomatic vasospasm, there was clinical improvement in 19 (76%) with IA nimodipine. After follow-up of 3 to 6 months, 18 patients (72%) had a favorable clinical outcome. Successful dilatation of infused vessels, however, occurred in only 13 out of 30 (43%) procedures, raising some question as to the cause and effect. The dose used is up to 3 mg per vascular territory at a rate of 1 mg over 10 to 15 minutes to minimize hypotension. Verapamil is another agent used in some centers, although it has been less effective than nicardipine in reversing angiographic vasospasm in the authors' experience (Gandhi D, unpublished data, 2004–2006). Feng and colleagues[22] reported neurological improvement in 29% of 17 patients with vasospasm treated with an average dose of 3 mg. The safety profile was excellent, with just minimal reduction in mean arterial pressure (average of 5 mm Hg) and no evidence of raised intracranial pressure. There is some experimental evidence that demonstrates that nicardipine has greater efficacy than verapamil for endothelin-induced vasospasm.[23]

Nicardipine is a dihydropyridine calcium channel blocker that has more selective effects on vascular smooth muscle than cardiac muscle. Badjatia and colleagues[24] reported on use of IA nicardipine in 18 patients with vasospasm. There was angiographic and TCD improvement in all patients. Clinical improvement occurred in 42% of patients, and clinically significant improvement in TCD parameters was sustained for 4 days. There was one adverse event where there was an increase in ICP leading to termination of the nicardipine infusion. A series of 20 treatments in 11 patients by Tejada and colleagues[25] showed effective angiographic response in all patients (defined as 60% increase in arterial diameter of the most severely decreased in caliber vessel compared with the very first angiographic run). There was clinical improvement in GCS or resolution of focal symptoms in 10 of 11 (91%) patients. Linfante and colleagues[26] reported on the use of IA nicardipine for 22 patients with symptomatic vasospasm refractory to medical management. They found a 95% significant angiographic improvement rate in these patients. A recent study has confirmed significant improvement in CT perfusion parameters of CBF and MTT following IA treatment with nicardipine.[27] Some previous literature showed discordance between clinical and angiographic outcome following endovascular treatment. The use of CT perfusion for assessing treatment effect may be helpful in these situations, as it is able to show perfusional changes at the microvascular and parenchymal level. These changes may not be evident on inspection of the larger, more proximal arteries using conventional angiography.[21,27,28]

IA nicardipine is currently the drug of choice at the authors' institution. The authors closely monitor the arterial pressures, heart rate, electrocardiogram, and oxygen saturation during the nicardipine infusion. The cerebrospinal fluid (CSF) waveform and CSF pressures also are recorded for the patients who have a ventriculostomy catheter in place. The authors administer the drug very slowly (0.5 to 1 mg/min) and titrate the dose carefully with the arterial pressures during its infusion. If a drop of mean arterial pressure greater than 15 mm Hg or systolic pressure drop of greater than 25 mm Hg is identified, the infusion is halted temporarily. Temporary cessation of infusion often results in gradual return of the arterial pressures to the baseline values, when the infusion can be resumed. A control angiogram is obtained after 3 to 5 mg of the agent has been infused in the affected territory. Modest reduction in blood pressure has been reported with the use of IA nicardipine, and vasopressor support occasionally is needed. Reported systolic blood pressure reductions have been between 10% and 35% or mean systolic reductions of 17 to 23mmHg.[25,26,29]

Duration of effect seems favorable when compared with other IA agents, although retreatment is required in some patients.[25]

TRANSLUMINAL BALLOON ANGIOPLASTY

Zubkov and colleagues[30] first described the use of angioplasty in cerebral vasospasm in 1984. The use of this technique has increased steadily over the last two decades with introduction of dedicated neurovascular balloon technology. These balloons can be navigated distally because of their improved trackability and improved safety profiles. Angioplasty is the only method of endovascular treatment that has been shown by numerous subsequent retrospective case series to produce durable clinical improvement. This, however, comes at the cost of needing a specialist with neuroendovascular skills and the small risk of additional serious complications.

> Vessels amenable to angioplasty are the proximal intradural arteries, including
> Supraclinoid ICA
> MCA (M1 and M2 segments)
> ACA (A1 and less commonly A2 segments)
> Intracranial segment of vertebral arteries (VA)
> Basilar and posterior cerebral artery (P1 and P2 segments) (see **Fig. 3**).

It is essential to review the prior (baseline) angiograms in detail before considering an angioplasty for intracranial vasospasm. On the prior studies, careful assessment of vessel morphology and diameter should have been performed. Special note should be made of segments that are congenitally hypoplastic (most commonly A1 segments and intradural vertebral arteries) lest they are confused with arteries affected with vasospasm. Inflating a balloon in congenitally hypoplastic vessels can result in acute vessel rupture. This catastrophic complication can be prevented by review of the prior studies.

As far as possible, softer, dedicated intracranial balloons should be used for intracranial angioplasty to minimize the possibility of vessel rupture. The authors' preference is to use a conformable balloon like Hyperglide (ev3 Endovascular Incorporated, Plymouth, MN, USA) or Hyperform (ev3 Neurovascular, Irvine, CA, USA). These balloons are extremely trackable and can be navigated over a very atraumatic, 0.010 in X-pedion microwire (ev3 Neurovascular). A slight disadvantage of this balloon system is the lack of a continuous flush through the balloon and occasionally problems with steerability in tortuous arteries that form acute angles with more proximal vessels (eg, into the A1 segment). In difficult cases, a microcatheter can be placed first in the vessel to be angioplastied. This microcatheter is then exchanged for the balloon over a 0.010 in exchange length X-Celerator microwire (ev3 Neurovascular). Occasionally, the authors have used the small-diameter Gateway balloon system (Boston Scientific, Natick, MA, USA) for patients with difficult anatomy. New angioplasty armamentarium is likely to be available in the near future with an increasing range of available sizes of balloons, as well as introduction of newer, over-the-wire balloons. One always should keep in mind that the goal of angioplasty is to improve vessel caliber to augment flow rather than to achieve a picture-perfect result. The authors tend to slightly underinflate the balloon compared with projected normal diameter of the vessel. This gives an additional safety mechanism and decreases the possibility of acute rupture of a vessel. As a rule, the authors do not inflate a balloon at the site of recent surgical clipping of an aneurysm. Fatal rupture of a vessel has been reported by others during angioplasty close to a clipped aneurysm.[31]

A recent review of the literature found reports in the English language on 530 patients undergoing angioplasty for SAH-related vasospasm. Of these 530 patients, 62% improved clinically, with a range of 11% to 93%.[32] The largest series is by Eskridge and colleagues,[33] who reported on retrospective series of 50 consecutive cases (170 vessel segments) using a silicone microballoon (Target Therapeutics, Incorporated, Fremont, CA/Boston Scientific, USA). A significant proportion of patients (61%) showed sustained early neurological improvement within 72 hours, while 6% deteriorated. Two patients (4%) died immediately from vessel rupture. Other larger series have been by Bejjani and colleagues (31 patients with 72% neurological improvement), Higashida and colleagues[5,7,34] (28 patients with 61% neurological improvement), and Fuji and colleagues (19 patients with 63% neurological improvement). Firlik and colleagues[28] showed a 92% clinical improvement rate in 13 patients and also demonstrated quantitative improvement in CBF following angioplasty on Xenon-CT. Other studies have reported lower rates of clinical improvement, but some of these are confounded by the combined use of papaverine and angioplasty.[35,36] A more recent retrospective series of 38 patients by Jestaedt and colleagues[37] showed a clear benefit of angioplasty for reduction in CT evidence of infarct; however, clinical outcome was not assessed. They angioplastied the terminal ICA or MCA in 57 vessels but used 61 untreated anterior cerebral arterial segments with severe spasm as the control. Infarction by CT occurred in 7% of MCA territories compared with 38% of ACA territories.

Similar to acute stroke treatment, endovascular management of vasospasm is time-critical. Prompt referral, assessment, and intervention are essential if angioplasty is to achieve maximum clinical benefit. In one series, 71% of patients angioplastied within a 2-hour window showed sustained clinical improvement compared with 40% in the group treated beyond the 2-hour window, despite both showing good initial angiographic improvement.[38] In addition, Bejjani and colleagues[7] found a higher chance of dramatic clinical improvement in their series if angioplasty was performed within 24 hours of neurological deterioration. Prophylactic balloon angioplasty has been proposed, but it has failed to show a statistically significant improvement in clinical outcome at 3 months in Fisher grade 3 SAH.[39]

Complications of balloon angioplasty include catastrophic vessel rupture, thromboembolism, and reperfusion hemorrhage into an infarct.[5,28,30,31,33] The vessel rupture rate varies from 0 to 7.7%, with an average of 1.1% and major complications overall in up to 5%.[32] The improvements in compliant balloon technology likely mean that the risk of vessel rupture today is in the lower end of this reported range. The decision to angioplasty for vasospasm in the setting of an untreated ruptured aneurysm requires careful consideration of the small risk of rehemorrhage against severity of the vasospasm and the possibility of performing coiling of the aneurysm at the same time as angioplasty.[7,33]

SUMMARY AND RECOMMENDATIONS

Cerebral vasospasm causes significant morbidity in patients with SAH who survive the initial ictus. Prompt imaging evaluation and institution of therapy can be highly effective in improving outcomes in these sick patients. Endovascular therapy should be used early and emergently in those shown on imaging triage to have findings suggestive of severe vasospasm or perfusion impairment despite medical management. Perfusion scans, if available, should be assessed carefully for evidence of significant established irreversible ischemia. For proximal vasospasm, wherever technically possible, balloon angioplasty should be used, as this is the only method that shows durable clinical improvement. IA vasodilators are used for distal vasospasm and as an adjunct to angioplasty. The sustained efficacy of IA vasodilators, however, is less well established, and repeated treatments may be necessary.

REFERENCES

1. Kassell NF, Sasaki T, Colohan AR, et al. Cerebral vasospasm following aneurysmal subarachnoid hemorrhage. Stroke 1985;16(4):562–72.

2. Kassell NF, Torner JC, Haley EC Jr, et al. The International Cooperative Study on the timing of aneurysm surgery. Part 1: overall management results. J Neurosurg 1990;73(1):18–36.

3. Mayberg MR. Cerebral vasospasm. Neurosurg Clin N Am 1998;9(3):615–27.

4. Zubkov AY, Rabinstein AA. Medical management of cerebral vasospasm: present and future. Neurol Res 2009;31(6):626–31.

5. Higashida RT, Halbach VV, Dowd CF, et al. Intravascular balloon dilatation therapy for intracranial arterial vasospasm: patient selection, technique, and clinical results. Neurosurg Rev 1992;15(2):89–95.

6. Firlik KS, Kaufmann AM, Firlik AD, et al. Intra-arterial papaverine for the treatment of cerebral vasospasm following aneurysmal subarachnoid hemorrhage. Surg Neurol 1999;51(1):66–74.

7. Bejjani GK, Bank WO, Olan WJ, et al. The efficacy and safety of angioplasty for cerebral vasospasm after subarachnoid hemorrhage. Neurosurgery 1998;42(5):979–86 [discussion: 986–7].

8. Lysakowski C, Walder B, Costanza MC, et al. Transcranial Doppler versus angiography in patients with vasospasm due to a ruptured cerebral aneurysm: a systematic review. Stroke 2001;32(10):2292–8.

9. Pham M, Johnson A, Bartsch AJ, et al. CT perfusion predicts secondary cerebral infarction after aneurysmal subarachnoid hemorrhage. Neurology 2007;69(8):762–5.

10. Binaghi S, Colleoni ML, Maeder P, et al. CT angiography and perfusion CT in cerebral vasospasm after subarachnoid hemorrhage. AJNR Am J Neuroradiol 2007;28(4):750–8.

11. Wintermark M, Ko NU, Smith WS, et al. Vasospasm after subarachnoid hemorrhage: utility of perfusion CT and CT angiography on diagnosis and management. AJNR Am J Neuroradiol 2006;27(1):26–34.

12. Anderson GB, Ashforth R, Steinke DE, et al. CT angiography for the detection of cerebral vasospasm in patients with acute subarachnoid hemorrhage. AJNR Am J Neuroradiol 2000;21(6):1011–5.

13. Konstas AA, Goldmakher GV, Lee TY, et al. Theoretic basis and technical implementations of CT perfusion in acute ischemic stroke, part 1: theoretic basis. AJNR Am J Neuroradiol 2009;30(4):662–8.

14. Wintermark M, Fischbein NJ, Smith WS, et al. Accuracy of dynamic perfusion CT with deconvolution in detecting acute hemispheric stroke. AJNR Am J Neuroradiol 2005;26(1):104–12.

15. Wintermark M, Reichhart M, Cuisenaire O, et al. Comparison of admission perfusion computed tomography and qualitative diffusion- and perfusion-weighted magnetic resonance imaging in acute stroke patients. Stroke 2002;33(8):2025–31.

16. Wintermark M, Reichhart M, Thiran JP, et al. Prognostic accuracy of cerebral blood flow measurement by perfusion computed tomography, at the time of emergency room admission, in acute stroke patients. Ann Neurol 2002;51(4):417–32.

17. Kanazawa R, Kato M, Ishikawa K, et al. Convenience of the computed tomography perfusion method for cerebral vasospasm detection after subarachnoid hemorrhage. Surg Neurol 2007; 67(6):604–11.

18. Kassell NF, Helm G, Simmons N, et al. Treatment of cerebral vasospasm with intra-arterial papaverine. J Neurosurg 1992;77(6):848–52.

19. McAuliffe W, Townsend M, Eskridge JM, et al. Intracranial pressure changes induced during papaverine infusion for treatment of vasospasm. J Neurosurg 1995;83(3):430–4.

20. Clouston JE, Numaguchi Y, Zoarski GH, et al. Intra-arterial papaverine infusion for cerebral vasospasm after subarachnoid hemorrhage. AJNR Am J Neuroradiol 1995;16(1):27–38.

21. Biondi A, Ricciardi GK, Puybasset L, et al. Intra-arterial nimodipine for the treatment of symptomatic cerebral vasospasm after aneurysmal subarachnoid hemorrhage: preliminary results. AJNR Am J Neuroradiol 2004;25(6):1067–76.

22. Feng L, Fitzsimmons BF, Young WL, et al. Intra-arterially administered verapamil as adjunct therapy for cerebral vasospasm: safety and 2-year experience. AJNR Am J Neuroradiol 2002;23(8):1284–90.

23. Lavine SD, Wang M, Etu JJ, et al. Augmentation of cerebral blood flow and reversal of endothelin-1-induced vasospasm: a comparison of intracarotid nicardipine and verapamil. Neurosurgery 2007; 60(4):742–8 [discussion: 748–9].

24. Badjatia N, Topcuoglu MA, Pryor JC, et al. Preliminary experience with intra-arterial nicardipine as a treatment for cerebral vasospasm. AJNR Am J Neuroradiol 2004;25(5):819–26.

25. Tejada JG, Taylor RA, Ugurel MS, et al. Safety and feasibility of intra-arterial nicardipine for the treatment of subarachnoid hemorrhage-associated vasospasm: initial clinical experience with high-dose infusions. AJNR Am J Neuroradiol 2007; 28(5):844–8.

26. Linfante I, Delgado-Mederos R, Andreone V, et al. Angiographic and hemodynamic effect of high concentration of intra-arterial nicardipine in cerebral vasospasm. Neurosurgery 2008;63(6):1080–6 [discussion: 1086–7].

27. Nogueira RG, Lev MH, Roccatagliata L, et al. Intra-arterial nicardipine infusion improves CT perfusion-measured cerebral blood flow in patients with subarachnoid hemorrhage-induced vasospasm. AJNR Am J Neuroradiol 2009;30(1):160–4.

28. Firlik AD, Kaufmann AM, Jungreis CA, et al. Effect of transluminal angioplasty on cerebral blood flow in the management of symptomatic vasospasm following aneurysmal subarachnoid hemorrhage. J Neurosurg 1997;86(5):830–9.

29. Avitsian R, Fiorella D, Soliman MM, et al. Anesthetic considerations of selective intra-arterial nicardipine injection for intracranial vasospasm: a case series. J Neurosurg Anesthesiol 2007;19(2):125–9.

30. Zubkov YN, Nikiforov BM, Shustin VA. Balloon catheter technique for dilatation of constricted cerebral arteries after aneurysmal SAH. Acta Neurochir (Wien) 1984;70:65–79.

31. Linskey ME, Horton JA, Rao GR, et al. Fatal rupture of the intracranial carotid artery during transluminal angioplasty for vasospasm induced by subarachnoid hemorrhage. Case report. J Neurosurg 1991;74(6):985–90.

32. Hoh BL, Ogilvy CS. Endovascular treatment of cerebral vasospasm: transluminal balloon angioplasty, intra-arterial papaverine, and intra-arterial nicardipine. Neurosurg Clin N Am 2005;16(3):501–16, vi.

33. Eskridge JM, McAuliffe W, Song JK, et al. Balloon angioplasty for the treatment of vasospasm: results of first 50 cases. Neurosurgery 1998;42(3):510–6 [discussion: 516–7].

34. Fujii Y, Takahashi A, Yoshimoto T. Effect of balloon angioplasty on high-grade symptomatic vasospasm after subarachnoid hemorrhage. Neurosurg Rev 1995;18(1):7–13.

35. Coyne TJ, Montanera WJ, Macdonald RL, et al. Percutaneous transluminal angioplasty for cerebral vasospasm after subarachnoid hemorrhage. Can J Surg 1994;37(5):391–6.

36. Polin RS, Hansen CA, German P, et al. Intra-arterially administered papaverine for the treatment of symptomatic cerebral vasospasm. Neurosurgery 1998; 42(6):1256–64 [discussion: 1264–7].

37. Jestaedt L, Pham M, Bartsch AJ, et al. The impact of balloon angioplasty on the evolution of vasospasm-related infarction after aneurysmal subarachnoid hemorrhage. Neurosurgery 2008;62(3):610–7 [discussion: 610–7].

38. Rosenwasser RH, Armonda RA, Thomas JE, et al. Therapeutic modalities for the management of cerebral vasospasm: timing of endovascular options. Neurosurgery 1999;44(5):975–9 [discussion: 979–80].

39. Zwienenberg-Lee M, Hartman J, Rudisill N, et al. Effect of prophylactic transluminal balloon angioplasty on cerebral vasospasm and outcome in patients with Fisher grade III subarachnoid hemorrhage: results of a phase II multicenter, randomized, clinical trial. Stroke 2008;39(6): 1759–65.

The Role of Transcranial Doppler Ultrasonography in the Diagnosis and Management of Vasospasm After Aneurysmal Subarachnoid Hemorrhage

Scott A. Marshall, MD[a,b,*], Paul Nyquist, MD, MPH[a,c], Wendy C. Ziai, MD, MPH[a,c]

KEYWORDS

- Transcranial Doppler • Vasospasm
- Subarachnoid hemorrhage • Lindegaard Index

Aneurysmal subarachnoid hemorrhage and its accompanying sequelae are management challenges for the neurosurgeon and neurointensivist. Transcranial Doppler ultrasonography (TCD) has emerged as a tool used extensively by many centers for the surveillance and monitoring of vasospasm after aneurysmal subarachnoid hemorrhage (SAH).[1] The overall management of the primary and secondary complications of SAH is complex, and the use of appropriate tools and diagnostic strategies is helpful. TCD has emerged as an inexpensive, noninvasive tool used not only for bedside monitoring of intracerebral hemodynamic changes seen with SAH. TCD can also be used to evaluate other neurologic conditions in the Neurosciences Critical Care Unit such as

The views and opinions herein belong solely to the authors. They do not nor should they be construed as belonging to, representative of, or being endorsed by the Uniformed Services University of the Health Sciences, the US Army, The Department of Defense, or any other branch of the federal government of the United States.

[a] Division of Neurosciences Critical Care, Departments of Anesthesiology Critical Care Medicine, Johns Hopkins University School of Medicine, Meyer 8-140, 600 North Wolfe Street, Baltimore, MD 21287, USA
[b] Department of Neurology, Uniformed Services University of the Health Sciences, 4301 Jones Bridge Road, Bethesda, MD 20814, USA
[c] Departments of Neurosurgery and Neurology, Johns Hopkins University School of Medicine, Meyer 8-140, 600 North Wolfe Street, Baltimore, MD 21287, USA
* Corresponding author. Department of Neurology, Uniformed Services University of the Health Sciences, 4301 Jones Bridge Road, Bethesda, MD 20814.
E-mail address: scott.marshall@amedd.army.mil

Neurosurg Clin N Am 21 (2010) 291–303
doi:10.1016/j.nec.2009.10.010
1042-3680/10/$ – see front matter © 2010 Published by Elsevier Inc.

intra- and extracranial vascular stenosis, arteriovenous malformations, intraoperative emboli, venous sinus thrombosis, ischemic stroke, sickle cell disease, and brain death.[2–4] This article provides a brief review of the pathophysiology of vasospasm, and other devices used to detect vasospasm. Also reviewed are the indices and technical aspects of TCD ultrasonography, the interpretation of data obtained from TCD studies, and TCD-based management algorithms for vasospasm.

VASOSPASM AFTER SUBARACHNOID HEMORRHAGE

The diminution of blood flow transiting through the cerebral vasculature seen after aneurysmal SAH due to vasoconstriction is referred to as vasospasm.[5,6] Arterial spasm after SAH was originally described by Ecker, and has since been the subject of decades of laboratory research and clinical investigation.[7] Various definitions of vasospasm are employed, including vasospasm seen on digital subtraction angiography or computed tomography angiography referred to as "angiographic vasospasm" and "clinical vasospasm," which includes "delayed ischemic neurologic deficit" (DIND) and "delayed cerebral ischemia." (DCI) DIND and DCI refer to clinical signs of transient or permanent neurologic deficits occurring remotely from the initial SAH or surgery, after other complications of SAH potentially causing neurologic deficits have been excluded.[5] The exact cause of vasospasm is not clearly understood, but it is thought that extra-arterial blood products surrounding the arterial wall trigger a cascade of events at the cellular level, that culminate in vasoconstriction.[1,4,5] Other factors involved include decreased vascular autoregulation, reversible vasculopathy, and relative hypovolemia.[8,9] A further review of the current pathophysiology of vasospasm is presented in this edition of *Neurosurgical Clinics*. Vasospasm occurs most intensely adjacent to the subarachnoid clot, but can occur distantly from the majority of the subarachnoid blood, and is predicted by clot volume, age, location, and density of the SAH seen on the initial computed tomography (CT) scan.[10,11] In the past, the most likely cause of mortality after SAH was from aneurysmal rerupture in the early period after SAH. Due to more aggressive early surgical and endovascular treatment of ruptured aneurysms, this has now been replaced by hydrocephalus and vasospasm.[12,13]

The incidence of angiographic vasospasm after aneurysmal subarachnoid hemorrhage has been estimated to occur in 50% to 70% of patients with aneurysmal SAH, with approximately 50% of those exhibiting symptoms of clinical vasospasm.[14] A review of angiography studies of more than 2700 cases of aneurysmal SAH found the average incidence to be approximately 67%, with the highest incidence occurring between days 10 and 17 after SAH.[15] Vasospasm classically is reported to occur from days 4 to 14 after aneurysmal SAH, but variations on this rule abound.[1,5,12–14,16,17] The incidence of *early* angiographic vasospasm, detected within 48 hours of aneurysm rupture, occurs in 10% to 13% of SAH patients and is associated with prior aneurysmal SAH, large aneurysms, intraventricular hemorrhage, and with reduced morbidity at 3 months.[18] The impact of clinical vasospasms on outcome has been established, with both morbidity and mortality estimates ranging from 10% to 20%.[15,19]

MODALITIES USED FOR MONITORING CEREBRAL VASOSPASM

It should be emphasized that vasospasm is a clinical diagnosis, and radiographic studies and other markers of brain perfusion support this diagnosis through evidence of diminished vessel caliber. Left unchecked, patients with vasospasm may progress from diffuse neurologic signs such as confusion, increasing somnolence, and combativeness to focal neurologic deficits suggestive of infarction. Radiographic findings often precede such clinical deficits, and thus offer the opportunity to intervene to prevent neurologic injury. To this effect, in 1982 Aaslid and colleagues[20,21] provided the first descriptions of the use of TCD for such purposes, by monitoring flow in intracranial arteries and later used TCD in the assessment of arterial vasospasm. Much work has been done on the use of this technology in the evaluation of cerebral blood flow, due to its relative inexpensiveness, bedside availability, and noninvasive nature. The gold standard for the diagnosis of cerebral vasospasm has remained digital subtraction angiography. Because of its expense, potential for severe complications, and the need to move the patient to the angiography suite, this test is impractical for use as a frequent monitor of vasospasm.[22] The major advantage of angiography is the potential for both diagnosis and therapeutic intervention, discussed elsewhere in this issue. Computed tomography angiography (CTA) has emerged as a potentially helpful tool in the evaluation of vasospasm, with relatively good sensitivity and specificity for discovery of severe vasospasm in the proximal arteries of the circle of Willis, and with a high negative predictive value.[23] Some have raised concern that sending a patient who has severe vasospasm to undergo CTA may delay definitive treatment with angioplasty or intra-arterial injection of antispasmodic agents.[5] CTA is relatively insensitive for mild and moderate vasospasm, and ideally requires a baseline study early on in the course of SAH for purposes of comparison.[24] Ionita and colleagues[22] reported that with strongly positive or strongly negative TCD findings and a correlative neurologic examination, obtaining a CTA was not of added value in the management of such patients. These investigators suggested that CTA's best role may be in a patient population with indeterminate TCD findings and an examination suggestive of vasospasm. Magnetic resonance angiography (MRA) has been used by some to assess for vasospasm after SAH, although it is a technology limited by logistics, acquisition time, motion, and hardware artifact.[25–27] Other emerging technologies employ an altogether different approach to the detection of vasospasm. Perfusion imaging such as MR perfusion, CT perfusion (CTP), single photon emission computed tomography (SPECT), positron emission tomography (PET), and diffusion-weighted MR imaging are being studied for use with this indication.[28–32] Of these technologies, a combination of CTA and CTP may be useful as a second-tier diagnostic study in cases where a high index of suspicion exists or TCDs are not reliable.[12] Continuous electroencephalography (EEG) is also under investigation as a means to detect subclinical cortical dysfunction related to inadequate cerebral perfusion from vasospasm. A recent study has shown this to be a beneficial mode of monitoring SAH patients, allowing for detection of subsequent vasospasm days before the detection of abnormalities by TCD.[33,34] Several logistical limitations to continuous EEG monitoring preclude widespread use of this technique currently, although further data correlating this technique to the development of vasospasm may make its use more widespread in the future.

TCD has become the most common screening tool for vasospasm monitoring due to its portability and noninvasive nature, and ease of repeat testing.[35] Many advocate frequent TCD monitoring with schedules ranging from every other day to twice daily, usually starting on the first day after SAH onset, ending with resolution of vasospasm.[1,5,16] TCD is also recommended for following the temporal course of angiographic vasospasm during its peak incidence.[36]

The efficacy of TCD as a monitor for vasospasm is controversial.[37] TCD is operator dependent, and limitations of insonation secondary to adequate acoustic windowing restrict its use in about 8% of patients.[12,38] Other limiting factors include the rate of false-negative studies and variability between technicians performing examinations.[39] These limitations may be overcome with new TCD techniques.[40]

Many studies have established TCD threshold velocities for vasospasm diagnosis. These studies usually incorporate TCD and angiographic comparisons. In such work, a relationship has been demonstrated between intracerebral vessel diameter on angiography and velocities measured with TCDs.[41,42] The underlying principle used for TCD estimations of cerebral blood velocity is based on variations of the Bernoulli equation. The velocity of blood flow in a conduit is inversely related to the diameter of that conduit. As the diameter of a blood vessel decreases, the blood velocity will increase. Although the vessel itself is not directly visualized with TCD ultrasonography, an indirect evaluation of the vessel diameter is achieved using the Doppler effect by calculating the Doppler shift, which is the difference between the frequencies of the transmitted and received ultrasound waves.[43,44] The following equation allows for the calculation of vessel flow velocities and gives an indirect indication of vessel diameter.[5]

$$f = 2 * f_0 * v/c$$

$$v = f * c/(2 * f_0)$$

where f_0 is transmitted ultrasound frequency (1.0–3.0 MHz in TCD)
    c is velocity of sound in blood (approximately 1540 m/s)
    v is velocity of blood flow.

INDICES AND TECHNICAL ASPECTS TCD ULTRASONOGRAPHY

TCD provides several indices that are useful when making clinical decisions regarding the management of vasospasm in SAH patients. The flow velocity (FV) is the most used metric and is further defined by the mean flow velocity (MFV), the peak systolic flow velocity (V_s), and the end-diastolic flow velocity (V_d). In clinical practice, the mean flow velocity (MFV = $\{V_s - V_d/3\} + V_d$) is typically reported, but additional information is used to calculate the resistance index (RI) and pulsatility index (PI). Both the RI and PI are presumptive measures of downstream vascular resistance, and serve as indicators of extravascular or intracranial pressure (equations 1, 2). Elevated RI and PI occur secondary to vascular stenosis, distal vasospasm, and elevated intracranial compliance.[45]

$$RI = (FVsystolic - FVdiastolic)/FVsystolic \quad (1)$$

$$\text{Gosling Pulsatility Index : } PI = (FVsystolic - FVdiastolic)/MFV \quad (2)$$

The Lindegaard index (LI) is an important method of correcting for increases in hyperdynamic systemic flow velocities, either physiologic or induced, in patients with SAH. To calculate the LI, the MFV of the middle cerebral artery (MCA) is compared with an ipsilateral extracranial vessel, namely the proximal internal carotid artery (ICA). This ratio (equation 3) helps to distinguish global hyperemia from vasospasm, especially in the setting of triple-H therapy.[41]

$$LI = MFV_{mca}/MFV_{ica} \quad (3)$$

An understanding of normal TCD velocities is vital to understanding TCD findings of vasospasm, and it is recognized that each major cerebral artery has its own range of normal values. Data from a large study with normal volunteers has proposed normal values for mean velocity and pulsatility index in the anterior and posterior circulation (**Tables 1–3**).[46] The velocities are reported for men and women separately, as many of these differences were found to be statistically significant. FV may vary between technicians acquiring TCD indices by as much as 7.5% on the same day and 13.5% on different days.[47] A combination of TCD velocities, Lindegaard ratios, clinical characteristics, and a spasm index (TCD velocities/hemispheric blood flow obtained from ^{133}Xe cerebral blood flow studies), called the Vasospasm probability index, has been proposed recently.[11]

The combination of Fisher grade, Hunt and Hess grade, and spasm index accurately detected clinical vasospasm in 92.9%. A model that included Fisher grade, Hunt and Hess grade, and Lindegaard ratio had an accuracy of 89.9% for detection of angiographic vasospasm. This study, along with others, suggests that the predictive value of TCD can be improved when used with other indicators. Another proposed "vasospasm risk index" found that a combination of high Fisher grade, early increase in the MCA MFV 110 cm/s or more recorded on or before post-SAH day 5, Glasgow Coma Scale score less than 14, and ruptured aneurysm of the anterior cerebral or internal carotid arteries translated into a high probability of identifying patients who would develop symptomatic vasospasm.[48,50]

An explanation of why TCD measurements alone may not correlate with angiographic or symptomatic vasospasm is likely based on the effect of decreased vessel lumen diameter on flow resistance in different hemodynamic situations. It has been postulated that with moderate vasospasm, cerebral autoregulation compensates for perfusion pressure reduction in the region of spasm (as long as arterial blood pressure [ABP] is above the lower limit of autoregulation), and flow velocity increases as lumen area falls, yielding good correlation between angiographic and TCD measured spasm.[51] This situation is depicted by region I on the Spencer curve (**Fig. 1**). In region II a plateau occurs whereby volume of flow is reduced and velocity remains high independent of diameter. Clinical vasospasm may occur because autoregulation is not effective. If ABP is increased (from A to B) with hypervolemic therapy,

Table 1
Normal reference TCD values for males

Insonated Vessel	MFV[a]		
	Age 20–39	Age 40–59	Age >60
ACA	54–62	51–61	45–55
MCA	66–74	62–69	55–62
PCA (P1)	48–53	41–48	40–45
PCA (P2)	43–49	40–45	39–45
Vertebral	37–43	29–36	30–35
Basilar	39–49	27–39	30–37

Abbreviations: ACA, anterior cerebral artery; MCA, middle cerebral artery; PCA, posterior cerebral artery; MFV, mean flow velocity.
[a] Range in cm/s.
Data from Martin PJ, Evans DH, Naylor AR. Transcranial color-coded sonography of the basal cerebral circulation. Reference data from 115 volunteers. Stroke 1994;25:390–6.

Table 2
Normal reference TCD values for females

Insonated Vessel	MFV[a]		
	Age 20–39	Age 40–59	Age >60
ACA	57–64	62–71	44–58
MCA	73–80	73–83	53–62
PCA (P1)	52–57	50–56	37–47
PCA (P2)	45–51	50–57	37–47
Vertebral	45–51	44–50	31–37
Basilar	51–58	47–56	29–47

Abbreviations: ACA, anterior cerebral artery; MCA, middle cerebral artery; PCA, posterior cerebral artery; MFV, mean flow velocity.
[a] Range in cm/s.
Data from Martin PJ, Evans DH, Naylor AR. Transcranial color-coded sonography of the basal cerebral circulation. Reference data from 115 volunteers. Stroke 1994;25:390–6.

volume flow increases and ischemic symptoms may improve, but the patient may paradoxically have much higher TCD velocities than in a normotensive setting. Here the correlation between TCD velocity and the degree of angiographic vasospasm is likely to be poor. Under conditions of critical stenosis (region III), additional reduction in lumen diameter results in lower TCD velocities, and reduction of flow to critical values with resultant neurologic deficits. Here TCD is unable to provide sufficient information to assess the hemodynamic state of the cerebral circulation.[51]

New imaging technology available for clinical use may make TCD more accurate and less subject to operator error. Power M-mode (PMD)/TCD facilitates the location of the acoustic temporal windows and allows viewing blood flow from multiple vessels at the same time.[1] The display that is used in PMD/TCD allows for color-coded information regarding the directionality of blood flow, and this has allowed for

PMD/TCD to be the most commonly used form of TCD performed currently at the bedside.[5] Transcranial color-coded duplex sonography (TCCS) allows 2-dimensional representation of the large cerebral arteries in color with outlining of parenchymal structures, in addition to color-coded flow directionality information.[5] In a prospective comparison of the accuracies of TCCS and TCD in the diagnosis of MCA vasospasm using same-day digital subtraction angiography as the reference standard, the accuracy of TCCS and TCD was similar, although improvements in sensitivity of TCCS in detecting MCA vasospasm was noted.[40] TCCS allowed for the detection of vasospasm at an earlier stage and at lower velocities (using a threshold of 120 cm/s), which may allow for more timely interventions to arrest the complications of vasospasm when it occurs. At higher velocities (threshold of 200 cm/s), conventional TCD and TCCS exhibited similar accuracy in the detection of vasospasm. However,

Table 3
Pulsatility index normal values

Insonated Vessel	Pulsatility Index		
	Age 20–39	Age 40–59	Age >60
ACA	0.78–0.85	0.73–0.79	0.87–0.97
MCA	0.82–0.87	0.79–0.83	0.93–1.02
PCA (P1)	0.8–0.88	0.75–0.82	0.91–1.02
PCA (P2)	0.79–0.86	0.75–0.8	0.91–1.03
Vertebral	0.79–0.85	0.74–0.82	0.89–0.99
Basilar	0.76–0.86	0.73–0.83	0.86–1.03

Abbreviations: ACA, anterior cerebral artery; MCA, middle cerebral artery; PCA, posterior cerebral artery.
Data from Martin PJ, Evans DH, Naylor AR. Transcranial color-coded sonography of the basal cerebral circulation. Reference data from 115 volunteers. Stroke 1994;25:390–6.

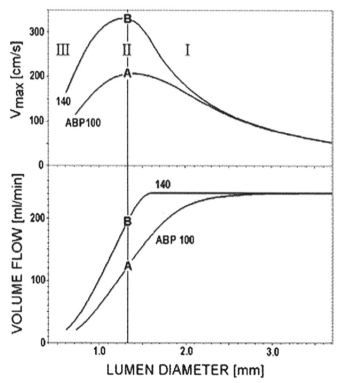

Fig. 1. "Spencer" curves (*above*) and volume flow as a function of lumen diameter (*below*) for 2 levels of arterial blood pressure (ABP). (*From* Aaslid R. Transcranial Doppler assessment of cerebral vasospasm. Eur J Ultrasound 2002;16(1–2):3–10; with permission.)

the investigators were unable to recommend universal additional capital investment of this technology by intensive care units (ICU) to routinely perform TCCS over traditional TCD. This question is currently being investigated.

INTERPRETATION OF DATA FROM TCD ULTRASONOGRAPHY

TCD studies generate a great deal of information, as they are performed daily to every other day in the Neurosciences ICU for patients with SAH.[1,5,16] These data can be interpreted based on absolute criteria for vasospasm, or used to see trends in the tempo of vasospasm over the course of several days.[37] Studies establishing the correlation between TCD mean flow velocities with decreases in vessel diameter on angiography have been most convincing for examinations of the MCA, but it is not acceptable to interpret flow velocity as cerebral blood flow or use TCD indices to estimate cerebral perfusion pressure.[1] Studies attempting to correlate these 2 parameters of perfusion have not been supportive.[52–54] Data comparing results of TCD and vasospasm seen on digital subtraction angiography give estimates for potential cutoff values for considering

vasospasm in different cerebral arteries (**Table 4**). One of the most important questions regarding the use of TCD is the proper placement of the reference standard. In the case of TCD, this concerns mostly the MFV.

Vasospasm in the anterior cerebral artery (ACA) may be difficult to detect with TCD, in part due to anatomic factors.[41] In a study by Suarez and colleagues[55] of 199 SAH patients, the correlation between elevated TCD flow velocities and symptomatic vasospasm was better in either the ICA (sensitivity: 80%; specificity: 77%) or MCA (64% and 78%) distributions compared with the ACA (45% and 84%).[56]

To improve the sensitivity of TCD of the ACA, Lindegaard and colleagues[41] had suggested that clinicians use both ACAs to access vasospasm on either side, because the collateralization of the ACAs by the anterior communicating artery (ACom) is so prominent. In any case, sensitivity has been a challenge in TCD studies of this vessel to detect vasospasm, and some investigators have suggested using not absolute velocity values but rather a relative increase in MFVs of greater than 50% change over subsequent examinations or a change of 50 cm/s in MFV over a 24-hour period.[57,58] The issue with accuracy of TCD for

Table 4
A composite of practical MFV and other parameters from TCD ultrasound indicating vasospasm after aneurysmal SAH

Insonated Vessel	Mild Vasospasm MFV, cm/s	Moderate Vasospasm MFV, cm/s	Severe Vasospasm MFV, cm/s	Intracranial MFV/ Extracranial MFV
ACA	φ	MFV >50% increase from baseline in 24 h	MFV >50% increase from baseline in 24 h	φ
ICA (terminal)	>120	>130	φ	φ
MCA	>120	>130	>200	>3 mild[a] >6 severe
PCA	φ	>110	>110	φ
Basilar	>60	>80	>115	>3 severe[b]
Vertebral	>60	>80	>80	φ

Abbreviations: ACA, anterior cerebral artery; MCA, middle cerebral artery; MFV, mean flow velocities; PCA, posterior cerebral artery; φ, limited data to guide recommendations.
[a] Middle cerebral artery/extracranial internal carotid artery.
[b] Basilar artery/extracranial vertebral artery.
Data from Refs.[22,49,51,57,62–65,71–73]

the ACA may be mostly technical and anatomic, as increasing the FV cutoff from 120 to 140 cm/s failed to increase sensitivity for detecting vasospasm in one study.[59] In that article, where TCD ultrasound was performed for 75 ACAs in 41 patients, TCD did have a specificity of nearly 100%, although in patients with postcommunicating ACA (A2 segment) vasospasm on angiography, no abnormal findings were evident on TCD. In this study, TCD insensitivity to angiographic vasospasm was explained by aneurysm location, with all false negatives occurring in patients with ACom aneurysms. This finding has been demonstrated in other studies, and is problematic given the frequency of aneurysms in this region.[60,61] In addition, others have reported a higher rate of cerebral ischemia in the setting of negative TCDs in the ACA vascular territory, although intraoperative ischemia may be confounding.[62]

The best data for correlating increased MFV with angiographic vasospasm exist for the MCA. Lindegaard and colleagues[41] proposed a cutoff of MFVs of 140 cm/s for detecting vasospasm in the MCA, based on their work with 51 patients. Langlois and colleagues[63] showed that a cutoff of 130 cm/s for the MCA had a sensitivity of 73% and a specificity of 100% for detecting vasospasm. In another study of 49 patients using a cutoff of at least 130 cm/s, specificity reached 100% for finding vasospasm in the MCA.[64] In a larger study of more than 100 patients, an MFV of less than 120 cm/s was able to reliably predict absence of vasospasm (negative predictive value of 94%) and MFV of greater than 200 cm/s reliably predicted moderate

to severe angiographic vasospasm (87% positive predictive value).[65] This study group recommended caution when interpreting intermediate velocities (ie, 120–200 cm/s). Others have used the Lindegaard ratio (intracranial MCA MFV/extracranial ICA MFV) to overcome issues related to cerebral hyperemia.[41] Lindegaard's original ratios indicating vasospasm were values greater than 10 in severe cases, with normal ranges from 1.1 to 2.3 and a median of 1.7.[41] A recent article used an LI of greater than 6 to reliably predict vasospasm in patients with clinical findings possibly indicating ischemia.[22] The LI is subject to variability because a small decrease in the ICA velocity may greatly overestimate the degree of vasospasm. This variability can be minimized by insonating the distal portion of the extracranial ICA as close as possible to the base of the skull (depth 40–50 mm).[51]

Other helpful corrections may be to standardize MCA MFVs to a patient's age and sex, although this has only been reported to have aided in the identification of mild arterial vasospasm, and has not been largely accepted in clinical practice.[66] It is recognized that a small percentage of patients develop only distal vasospasm (7.5%), which may be outside the range of TCD insonation.[67,68] For this reason the M2 segments should be evaluated for elevated velocities and bruits that may indicate distal spasm.[69]

ICA vasospasm in the terminal aspect of the vessel has been studied by several investigators. In a retrospective study, Creissard and Proust[70] reported sensitivities of 95% for the detection of vasospasm with an ICA aneurysm, if the MCA (M1) and the ICA are successfully insonated. A prospective study by the same investigators reported lower sensitivities for detection of vasospasm in the ICA.[61] Older work with 49 patients and 90 intracranial ICAs reported a specificity and positive predictive value of 100% when MFV values exceeded 130 cm/s in the intracranial ICA.[64]

Detection of vertebral or basilar artery vasospasm with TCD has different criteria than for the anterior circulation. In an article addressing the question of posterior circulation specifically, a cutoff velocity of 85 cm/s in the basilar artery predicted more frequent progression to cerebral ischemia, indicating that if this degree of vasospasm was diagnosed with TCD, interventions to reduce neurologic injury should be introduced earlier.[62] In a study correlating the relationship between basilar artery (BA) vasospasm and regional cerebral blood flow, the risk for delayed brainstem ischemia increased significantly when TCD BA FVs were greater than 115 cm/s.[71] **Fig. 2** shows an example of BA vasospasm on TCD. As mentioned earlier, a modified version of the LI for the posterior circulation is available. This study calculated normative values for the intracranial/extracranial vertebral artery (VA) FV ratio (IVA/EVA) and BA/extracranial VA FV ratio (BA/EVA), and evaluated 34 SAH patients with TCD and CT angiography (CTA).[72] A BA/EVA ratio of more than 2 was 100% sensitive and 95% specific for detection of BA vasospasm. In addition, the BA/EVA ratio showed close correlation with BA diameter and was greater than 3 in all patients with severe vasospasm.

TCD detection of vasospasm in the posterior cerebral artery (PCA) was studied by Wozniak and colleagues.[73] The difficulty with use of TCD for insonating the ACA and PCA was specifically addressed in this article. In a study of 84 PCAs in 53 patients, they reported sensitivity of 48% and specificity of 69% in technically adequate TCDs with an MFV cutoff value of 90 cm/s. If this value was increased to 110 cm/s, the specificity increased to 93% with sensitivity remaining low. A false-positive rate of 37% was attributed to anatomic factors, including occlusion as well as operator inexperience.[73] The PCA, like the ACA, has proven to be a difficult vessel for which to reliably establish TCD criteria for vasospasm.

Although TCD monitoring of vasospasm is usually started after aneurysm repair has occurred, there may be a role for early monitoring to establish increased risk of DCI. In a study of 199 patients with TCD examinations within 48 hours of SAH onset, 38% of patients had MCA elevation greater than 90 cm/s, which was associated with younger age, angiographic vasospasm on admission, and elevated white blood cell count.[74] DCI occurred in 19% of these patients, which was independently predicted by elevated admission MCA MFV of more than 90cm/s and poor clinical grade. These data suggest that transient vasospasm during the early phase of SAH may predict delayed arterial spasm and DCI.

LIMITATIONS OF TCD

Several factors known to affect TCD velocity measurements that may impact assessment during SAH include hematocrit, arterial carbon dioxide tension, the patient's level of consciousness, and the observer's level of experience.[75] It has been suggested that because vasospasm may be episodic, intermittent measurements may miss episodes of vasospasm.[76] One study of continuous TCD measurement of cerebral blood flow velocities revealed a significant moment-to-moment variability of the MCA MFV in both patients and volunteers, ranging from −38% to 78%, suggesting that either false-negative or false-positive results may occur in the diagnosis of vasospasm.[76] In this study, continuous TCD

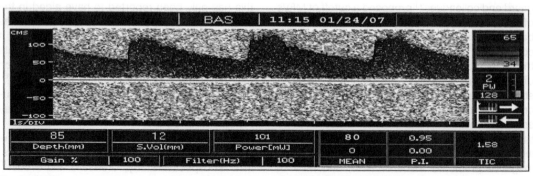

Fig. 2. Basilar artery vasospasm in a SAH patient with good correlation on cerebral angiography.

monitoring did not improve upon the sensitivity of intermittent TCD for detection of velocity evidence of vasospasm that was confirmed by angiography. At this time there seems to be no particular advantage of continuous TCD monitoring, although further study into how moment-to-moment variability affects detection of vasospasm has been suggested.[77]

MANAGEMENT ALGORITHMS

Our practice has evolved to use TCD ultrasonography in all patients with aneurysmal SAH by the performance of daily studies correlated with clinical examinations and physiologic data. Patients admitted with aneurysmal SAH are studied as soon as possible after digital subtraction angiography and securing of the aneurysm. In the setting of clinical stability, TCDs are continued daily while patients are maintained in a state of normovolemia and normonatremia. When a patient without new examination findings enters the window for increased risk of developing vasospasm, if TCD velocities increase to generally accepted levels for vasospasm for that vessel, fluid balance is shifted to maintaining a positive fluid state, and serum sodium is augmented with hypertonic saline if cerebral salt wasting develops. Patients are allowed to autoregulate blood pressure up to systolic pressures (SBP) of 200 mm Hg or mean arterial pressures (MAP) of 120 to 140 mm Hg, depending on the clinical status of the patient and other existing comorbidities. The placement of a pulmonary artery catheter or PiCCO-catheter may also be considered to optimize cardiopulmonary function and fluid management. If clinical suspicion for vasospasm increases with either increasing TCD values or clinical findings of potential ischemia, hypervolemic and hypertensive therapy is begun with either phenylephrine or norepinephrine and placement of a hemodynamic monitor. As an alternative, dobutamine or milrinone may be used in the setting of neurogenic stunned myocardium to augment cardiac output.

Depending on the clinical status of the patient and the reliability of the neurologic examination, other diagnostic imaging protocols may then be considered. The use of a perfusion study such as CT perfusion may be helpful in these cases, but if the suspicion is strong for clinical worsening then titration of MAP or SBP goals is warranted. Cerebral angiography, as both a diagnostic and therapeutic intervention, may be performed at this stage. TCD follow-up then may be vital in assessing the results of therapy and, along with the clinical examination, will aid in the timing of repeat angiography and will guide hemodynamic management.

OTHER USES OF TCD ULTRASONOGRAPHY

Several clinical applications of TCD exist currently in practice. TCD ultrasonography may be helpful in the setting of head trauma, as a marker of increased intracerebral pressure (ICP), assessment of cerebral autoregulation, brain death, ischemic stroke, intraoperative monitoring, and assessment of right to left shunt (ie, patent foramen ovale).[2–4,43,78] The utility of TCD in the Neurosciences ICU is primarily concerned with cerebral vasospasm and occlusive intracranial disease related to stroke, although new uses of TCD ultrasonography as a diagnostic, and even as a therapeutic tool, are increasing.

Evidence has emerged regarding the incidence of vasospasm after traumatic SAH or blast-related head injury.[6,62] This incidence has been reported to be higher in some populations with traumatic SAH than aneurysmal SAH, a concept that is not consistent with prior conventional teaching regarding vasospasm.[79] In a prospective cohort study of 299 patients with traumatic brain injury, hemodynamically significant vasospasm in the anterior circulation was found in 44.6% of the patients, whereas vasospasm in the BA (BA FV >90 cm/s) or hemodynamically significant vasospasm in the posterior circulation was found in 19% and 22.5% of patients, respectively.[80] The most common day of vasospasm onset was post injury day 2. Vasospasm resolved after 5 days in 50% of the patients with anterior circulation spasm and after 3.5 days in 50% of patients with posterior circulation spasm. It was recommended that TCD monitoring be used in the management of patients with traumatic brain injury. The use of TCD in sickle cell disease is widespread, and level IA evidence exists for use as a guide to help decide timing and frequency of transfusion therapy as a means to prevent stroke in this population.[81] Guidelines have been published as to insonation protocols and interpretation for performance of TCD in this setting in accordance with the STOP trial.[82]

The use of TCD in brain death may provide helpful additional information as confirmatory testing for this clinical diagnosis. Several centers use this as a standard practice, and recent work showed improved results with no false positives reported in a study of 184 patients with the inclusion of transcervical and transorbital carotid insonation in the brain death TCD protocol.[83] TCD has not to date been accepted as a formal ancillary test for diagnosis of brain death.

The correlation of TCD PI and intracranial pressure deserves discussion. ICP and PI have been shown in early work to share a direct correlation.[84]

The PI (equation 2) as a ratio is sensitive to changes in ICP, because downstream compression of arterioles due to high ICP will decrease the denominator of this equation (MFV), which is a surrogate measure of flow. This process is a result of the increased downstream vascular resistance created by compression of smaller arterioles, but not of the larger insonated arteries of the circle of Willis. Also, as increased ICP reduces compliance of the entire system, velocity variations due to the rigidity of arteries and reduced diastolic flow velocities will increase the numerator of this relationship. In turn, both of these factors will increase the index, and may indicate increasing ICP.[45] Follow-up prospective studies on this relationship have shown this correlation to be significant in a mixed population of neurosurgical patients who underwent TCD evaluation with an extraventricular drain in place.[45,85] This correlation has not gained acceptance as a surrogate for invasive ICP monitoring, although information provided by TCD ultrasonography may guide decisions to place invasive extraventricular drains, subdural monitors, or intraparenchymal monitors for suspicion of increased ICP in patients with severe neurologic illness or trauma.

The only current use of TCD as a therapeutic entity involves the management of ischemic stroke.[4] Patients enrolled in the Combined Lysis of Thrombus in Brain Ischemia Using Transcranial Ultrasound and Systemic rt-PA (CLOTBUST) trial had increased rates of recanalization when treated with recombinant tissue plasminogen activator (rt-PA) and TCD ultrasound monitoring, and showed a trend toward improved outcomes.[86,87] Complete recanalization within 2 h after rt-PA bolus occurred in 25% of patients treated with rtPA + TCD compared with 8% who received rt-PA alone. This result is thought to be due to better penetration of rt-PA into the blood clot due to concomitant ultrasound during clot lysis.[88,89] The administration of intra-arterial (IA) contrast microbubbles together with IA rt-PA and continuous TCD monitoring during bridging IA-rescue therapy for acute ischemic stroke has also shown enhanced thrombolytic effect and increased recanalization rates compared with rt-PA alone.[90] Intra-arterial rt-PA delivery may also be enhanced with delivery of low-intensity ultrasound at the site of the occlusion via the EKOS Micro-Infusion Catheter (1×7–2×1-MHz pulsed wave ultrasound) (EKOS catheter, IMS trial).[89] The EKOS catheter is also being tested as an intraventricular application for enhancement of thrombolytic treatment of intraventricular hemorrhage (SLEUTH trial).

SUMMARY

The utility of TCD in the Neurosciences ICU has grown substantially since its introduction in 1982. TCD currently maintains an important role in the day-to-day management and triage of more invasive and expensive diagnostic tests and subsequent intervention in the setting of vasospasm due to aneurysmal SAH. Limitations currently exist to the use of TCD as a lone marker of radiographic vasospasm but as the technology continues to advance, these shortcomings may be overcome. At this time issues remain particularly with regard to the diagnosis of vasospasm in ACA and PCA distribution in the presence of ACom aneurysms. Technical advances such as Power-M mode TCD and TCCS may help refine this test in the future. Complete TCD evaluations, including calculation of LI for the anterior circulation and a modified LI for the posterior circulation, may increase the specificity for vasospasm detected by TCD in the setting of cerebral hyperemia. Like many tools used in the ICU, TCD is best employed as part of the multimodality approach that incorporates radiographic, metabolic, and clinical findings to better manage patients with vasospasm from SAH.

REFERENCES

1. Saqqur M, Aygun D, Demchuck A. Role of transcranial Doppler in neurocritical care. Crit Care Med 2007;35(Suppl 5):s216–23.
2. Bassocchi M, Quaia E, Auiani C, et al. Transcranial Doppler: state of the art. Eur J Radiol 1998;27(Suppl 2):S141–8.
3. Lowe LH, Bulas DI. Transcranial Doppler monitoring and clinical decision making after subarachnoid hemorrhage. J Stroke Cerebrovasc Dis 2003;35:54–65.
4. Kincaid MS. Transcranial Doppler ultrasonography: a diagnostic tool of increasing utility. Curr Opin Anaesthesiol 2008;21:552–9.
5. Rigamonti A, Ackery A, Baker AJ. Transcranial Doppler monitoring in subarachnoid hemorrhage: a critical tool in critical care. Can J Anesth 2008; 55:112–23.
6. Armonda RA, Bell RS, Vo AH, et al. Wartime traumatic cerebral vasospasm: recent review of combat casualties. Neurosurgery 2006;59:1215–25.
7. Ecker A, Riewmanschneider PA. Arteriographic demonstration of spasm of the intracranial arteries. With special reference to saccular arterial aneurisms. J Neurosurg 1951;8:600–67.
8. Sarrafzadeh AS, Haux D, Ludemann L, et al. Cerebral ischemia in aneurysmal subarachnoid

hemorrhage: a correlative microdialysis-PET study. Stroke 2004;35:638–43.

9. Vajkoczy P, Horn P, Thome C, et al. Regional cerebral blood flow monitoring in the diagnosis of delayed ischemia following aneurysmal subarachnoid hemorrhage. J Neurosurg 2003;98:1227–34.

10. Reilly C, Amidei C, Tolentino J, et al. Clot volume and clearance rate as independent predictors of vasospasm after aneurysmal subarachnoid hemorrhage. J Neurosurg 2004;101(2):255–61.

11. Gonzalez NR, Boscardin WJ, Glenn T, et al. Vasospasm probability index: a combination of transcranial Doppler velocities, cerebral blood flow, and clinical risk factors to predict cerebral vasospasm after aneurysmal subarachnoid hemorrhage. J Neurosurg 2007;107:1101–12.

12. Zubkov AY, Rabinstien AA. Medical management of cerebral vasospasm: present and future. Neurol Res 2009;31(6):626–31.

13. Smith M. Intensive care management of patients with subarachnoid hemorrhage. Curr Opin Anaesthesiol 2007;20:400–7.

14. Keyrouz SG, Diringer MN. Prevention and therapy of vasospasm in subarachnoid hemorrhage. Crit Care 2007;11:220.

15. Dorsh NW, King MT. A review of cerebral vasospasm in aneurysmal subarachnoid hemorrhage. Part I: incidence and effects. J Clin Neurosci 1994;1:19–26.

16. Mascia L, Fedorko L, terBrugge K, et al. The accuracy of transcranial Doppler to detect vasospasm in patients with aneurysmal subarachnoid hemorrhage. Intensive Care Med 2003;29:1088–94.

17. Otten ML, Mocco J, Connolly ES, et al. A review of medical treatments of cerebral vasospasm. Neurol Res 2008;30:444–9.

18. Baldwin ME, Macdondald RL, Huo D, et al. Early vasospasm on admission angiography in patients with aneurysmal subarachnoid hemorrhage is a predictor for in hospital complications and poor outcome. Stroke 2004;35(11):2506–11.

19. Bleck TP. Rebleeding and vasospasm after SAH: new strategies for improving outcome. J Crit Illn 1997;12:572–82.

20. Aaslid R, Markwalder TM, Nornes H. Noninvasive transcranial Doppler ultrasound recording of flow velocity in basal cerebral arteries. J Neurosurg 1982;57:769–74.

21. Aaslid R, Huber R, Nornes H. Evaluation of cerebrovascular spasm with transcranial Doppler ultrasound. J Neurosurg 1984;60:37–41.

22. Ionita CC, Graffagnino C, Alexander MJ, et al. The value of CT angiography and transcranial Doppler sonography in triaging suspected cerebral vasospasm in SAH prior to endovascular therapy. Neurocrit Care 2008;9:8–12.

23. Anderson GB, Ashforth R, Steinke DE, et al. CT angiography for the detection of cerebral vasospasm in patients with acute subarachnoid hemorrhage. Am J Neuroradiol 2000;21(6):1011–5.

24. Sanelli PC, Ougorets I, Johnson CE, et al. Using CT in the diagnosis and management of patients with cerebral vasospasm. Semin Ultrasound CT MR 2006;27(3):194–206.

25. Heiserman JE. MR angiography for the diagnosis of vasospasm after subarachnoid hemorrhage. Is it accurate? Is it safe? Am J Neuroradiol 2000;21(9):1571–2.

26. Grandin CB, Cosnard G, Hammer F, et al. Vasospasm after subarachnoid hemorrhage: diagnosis with MR angiography. Am J Neuroradiol 2000;21(9):1611–7.

27. Gauvrit JY, Leclerc X, Ferre JC, et al. Imaging of subarachnoid hemorrhage. J Neuroradiol 2009;36(2):65–73.

28. Novak L, Emri M, Molnar P, et al. Regional cerebral (18)FDG uptake during subarachnoid hemorrhage induced vasospasm. Neurol Res 2006;28(8):864–70.

29. Sviri GE, Britz GW, Lewis DH, et al. Dynamic perfusion CT in the diagnosis of cerebral vasospasm. Neurosurgery 2006;59:319–25.

30. Yonas H. Cerebral blood measurements in vasospasm. Neurosurg Clin N Am 1990;1:307–18.

31. Condeltte-Auliac S, Bracard S, Anxionnat R, et al. Vasospasm after SAH: interest in diffusion weighted MR imaging. Stroke 2001;32:1818–24.

32. Jabre A, Babikian V, Powsner RA, et al. Role of single photon emission computed tomography and transcranial Doppler ultrasonography in clinical vasospasm. J Clionm Neurosci 2002;9:400–3.

33. Claassen J, Mayer SA. Continuous EEG monitoring in neurocritical care. Curr Neurol Neurosci Rep 2002;2:534–40.

34. Claassen J, Hirsch LJ, Dreiter KT, et al. Quantitative continuous EEG for detecting delayed cerebral ischemia in patients with poor grade subarachnoid hemorrhage. Clin Neurophysiol 2004;115:2699–710.

35. Daffertshofer M, Gass A, Ringleb P, et al. Transcranial low-frequency ultrasound-mediated thrombolysis in brain ischemia: increased risk of hemorrhage with combined ultrasound and tissue plasminogen activator: results of a phase II clinical trial. Stroke 2005;36(7):1441–6.

36. Sloan MA, Alexandrov AV, Tegeler CH, et al. Assessment: transcranial Doppler ultrasonography: report of the therapeutics and technology Assessment Subcommittee of the American Academy of Neurology. Neurology 2004;62(9):1469–81.

37. Bederson JB, Connolly ES, Batjer HH, et al. Guidelines for the management of aneurysmal subarachnoid hemorrhage: a statement for healthcare professionals from a special writing group of the stroke council, American Heart Association. Stroke 2009;40(3):994–1025.

38. Moppett IK, Majajan RP. Transcranial Doppler ultrasonography in anesthesia and intensive care. BJA 2004;93(5):710–24.

39. Lysakowski C, Walder B, Costanza MC, et al. Transcranial Doppler versus angiography in patients with vasospasm due to a ruptured cerebral aneurysm: a systematic review. Stroke 2001;32:2292–8.

40. Swiat M, Weigele J, Hurst RW, et al. Middle cerebral artery vasospasm: transcranial color-coded duplex sonography versus conventional nonimaging transcranial Doppler sonography. Crit Care Med 2009; 37(3):963–8.

41. Lindegaard KF, Nornes H, Bakke SJ, et al. Cerebral vasospasm after subarachnoid hemorrhage investigated by means of transcranial Doppler ultrasound. Acta Neurochir Suppl (Wien) 1988;42:81–4.

42. Sloan MA, Haley EC Jr, Kassell NF, et al. Sensitivity and specificity of transcranial Doppler ultrasonography in the diagnosis of vasospasm following subarachnoid hemorrhage. Neurology 1989;39: 1514–8.

43. Kassab MY, Majid A, Farooq MU, et al. Transcranial Doppler: an introduction for primary care physicians. J Am Board Fam Med 2007;20(1):65–71.

44. McGirt MJ, Blessing RP, Goldstein LB. Transcranial Doppler monitoring and clinical decision-making after subarachnoid hemorrhage. J Stroke Cerebrovasc Dis 2003;12(2):88–92.

45. Bellner J, Romner B, Reinstrup P, et al. Transcranial Doppler sonography pulsatility index (PI) reflects intracranial pressure (ICP). Surg Neurol 2004;62: 45–51.

46. Martin PJ, Evans DH, Naylor AR. Transcranial color-coded sonography of the basal cerebral circulation. Reference data from 115 volunteers. Stroke 1994; 25:390–6.

47. Maeda H, Etani H, Handa N, et al. A validation study on the reproducibility of transcranial Doppler velocimetry. Ultrasound Med Biol 1990;16:9–14.

48. Qureshi AI, Sung GY, Suri MAK, et al. Prognostic value and determinants of ultraearly angiographic vasospasm after aneurismal subarachnoid hemorrhage. Neurosurgery 1999;44:967–74.

49. Sloan MA, Burch CM, Wozniak MA, et al. Transcranial Doppler detection of vertebrobasilar vasospasm following subarachnoid hemorrhage. Stroke 1994; 25:2187–97.

50. Qureshi AI, Sung GI, Razumovsky AY, et al. Early identification of patients at risk for symptomatic vasospasm after aneurysmal subarachnoid hemorrhage. Crit Care Med 2000;28:984–90.

51. Aaslid R. Transcranial Doppler assessment of cerebral vasospasm. Eur J Ultrasound 2002;16(1–2):3–10.

52. Barwish RS, Ahn E, Amiridze NS. Role of transcranial Doppler in optimizing treatment of cerebral vasospasm in subarachnoid hemorrhage. J Intensive Care Med 2008;23(4):263–7.

53. Clyde BL, Resnick DK, Yonas H, et al. The relationship of blood velocity as measured by transcranial Doppler ultrasonography to cerebral blood flow as determined by stable xenon computed tomographic studies after aneurysmal subarachnoid hemorrhage. Neurosurgery 1996;38(5):896–904.

54. Romner B, Brandt L, Berntman L, et al. Simultaneous transcranial Doppler sonography and cerebral blood flow measurements of cerebrovascular CO_2-reactivity in patients with aneurysmal subarachnoid haemorrhage. Br J Neurosurg 1991;5(1):31–7.

55. Suarez JI, Qureshi AI, Yahia AB. Symptomatic vasospasm diagnosis after subarachnoid hemorrhage: evaluation of transcranial Doppler ultrasound and cerebral angiography as related to compromised vascular distribution. Crit Care Med 2002;30(6): 1348–55.

56. Barwish RS, Ahn E, Amiridze NS. Role of transcranial Doppler in optimizing treatment of cerebral vasospasm in subarachnoid hemorrhage. J Intensive Care Med 2008;23(4):263–7.

57. Grolimund P, Seiler RW, Aaslid R, et al. Evaluation of cerebrovascular disease by combined extracranial and transcranial Doppler sonography: experience in 1,039 patients. Stroke 1987;18:1018–24.

58. Grosset D, Straiton J, McDonald I, et al. Use of a transcranial Doppler to predict development of a delayed ischemic deficit after subarachnoid haemorrhage. J Neurosurg 1993;78:183–7.

59. Lennihan L, Petty GW, Fink ME, et al. Transcranial Doppler detection of anterior cerebral artery vasospasm. J Neurol Neurosurg Psychiatr 1993;56: 906–9.

60. International Subarachnoid Aneurysm Trial (ISAT) Collaborative Group. International Subarachnoid Aneurysm Trial (ISAT) of neurosurgical clipping versus endovascular coiling in 2143 patients with ruptured intracranial aneurysms: a randomised trial. Lancet 2002;360:1267–74.

61. Creissard P, Proust F, Langlois O. Vasospasm diagnosis: theoretical and real transcranial Doppler sensitivity. Acta Neurochir (Wien) 1995;136(3–4): 181–5.

62. Soustiel JF, Bruk B, Shik B, et al. Transcranial Doppler in vertebrobasilar vasospasm after subarachnoid hemorrhage. Neurosurgery 1998;43: 282–91.

63. Langlois O, Rabehaniona C, Proust F, et al. Diagnosis of vasospasm: comparison between arteriography and transcranial Doppler. A series of 112 comparative tests. Neurochirurgia 1992;38(3):138–40.

64. Burch CM, Wozniak MA, Sloan MA, et al. Detection of intracranial internal carotid artery and middle cerebral artery vasospasm following subarachnoid hemorrhage. J Neuroimaging 1996;6(1):8–15.

65. Vora YY, Suarez-Almazor M, Steinke DE, et al. Role of transcranial Doppler monitoring in the diagnosis

of cerebral vasospasm after subarachnoid hemorrhage. Neurosurgery 1999;44(6):1237–47.

66. Krejza J, Mariak Z, Lewko J. Standardization of flow velocities with respect to age and sex improves the accuracy of transcranial color Doppler sonography of middle cerebral artery spasm. Am J Roentgenol 2003;181(1):245–52.

67. Newell DW, Grady MS, Eskridge JM, et al. Distribution of angiographic vasospasm after subarachnoid hemorrhage: implications for diagnosis by transcranial Doppler ultrasonography. Neurosurgery 1990; 27:574–7.

68. Oertel M, Boscardin WJ, Obrist WD, et al. Posttraumatic vasospasm: the epidemiology, severity, and time course of an underestimated phenomenon: a prospective study performed in 299 patients. J Neurosurg 2005;103(5):812–24.

69. Mursch K, Bransi A, Vatter H, et al. Blood flow velocities in middle cerebral artery branches after subarachnoid hemorrhage. J Neuroimaging 2000;10:157–61.

70. Creissard P, Proust F. Vasospasm diagnosis: theoretical sensitivity of transcranial Doppler evaluated using 135 angiograms demonstrating vasospasm. Practical consequences. Acta Neurochir (Wien) 1994;131(1–2):12–8.

71. Sviri GE, Lewis DH, Correa R, et al. Basilar artery vasospasm and delayed posterior circulation ischemia after aneurysmal subarachnoid hemorrhage. Stroke 2004;35:1867–72.

72. Soustiel JF, Shik V, Shreiber R, et al. Basilar vasospasm diagnosis: Investigation of a modified "Lindegaard Index" based on imaging studies and blood velocity measurements of the basilar artery. Stroke 2002;33:72–7.

73. Wozniak MA, Sloan MA, Rothman MI, et al. Detection of vasospasm by transcranial Doppler sonography: the challenges of the anterior and posterior cerebral arteries. J Neuroimaging 1996;6:87–93.

74. Carrera E, Schmidt JM, Oddo M, et al. Transcranial Doppler ultrasound in the acute phase of aneurysmal subarachnoid hemorrhage. Cerebrovasc Dis 2009;27(6):579–84.

75. Manno EM. Transcranial Doppler ultrasonography in the neurocritical care unit. Crit Care Clin 1997;13: 79–104.

76. Venkatesh B, Shen Q, Lipman J. Continuous measurement of cerebral blood flow velocity using transcranial Doppler reveals significant moment-to-moment variability of data in healthy volunteers and in patients with subarachnoid hemorrhage. Crit Care Med 2002;30(3):563–9.

77. Bell RD, Benitez RP. Continuous measurement of cerebral blood flow velocity by using transcranial Doppler reveals significant moment-to-moment variability of data in healthy volunteers and in patients. Crit Care Med 2002;30(3):712–3.

78. White H, Venkatesh B. Applications of transcranial Doppler in the ICU: a review. Intensive Care Med 2006;32:981–94.

79. Soustiel JF, Shik V, Feinsod M. Basilar vasospasm following spontaneous and traumatic subarachnoid haemorrhage: clinical implications. Acta Neurochir (Wien) 2002;144:137–44.

80. Alexandrov AV. Ultrasound enhanced thrombolysis for stroke. Int J Stroke 2006;1(1):26–9.

81. Lee MT, Piomelli S, Granger S, et al. Stroke Prevention Trial in Sickle Cell Anemia (STOP): extended follow-up and final results. Blood 2006;108(3): 447–52.

82. Nichols FT, Jones AM, Adams RJ. Stroke prevention in sickle cell disease (STOP) study guidelines for transcranial Doppler testing. J Neuroimaging 2001; 11(4):354–62.

83. Conti A, Iacopino DG, Spada A, et al. Transcranial Doppler ultrasonography in the assessment of cerebral circulation arrest: improving sensitivity by transcervical and transorbital carotid insonation and serial examinations. Neurocrit Care 2009;10(3): 326–35.

84. Klingelhöfer J, Conrad B, Benecke R, et al. Evaluation of intracranial pressure from transcranial Doppler studies in cerebral disease. J Neurol 1988;235(3):159–62.

85. Voulgaris SG, Partheni M, Kaliora H, et al. Early cerebral monitoring using the transcranial Doppler pulsatility index in patients with severe brain trauma. Med Sci Monit 2005;11(2):CR49–52.

86. Alexandrov AV, Molina CA, Grotta JC, et al. CLOTBUST Investigators. Ultrasound-enhanced systemic thrombolysis for acute ischemic stroke. N Engl J Med 2004;351:2170–8.

87. Alexandrov VA, Babikian VL, Adams RJ, et al. The evolving role of transcranial Doppler in stroke prevention and treatment. J Stroke Cerebrovasc Dis 1998;7(2):101–4.

88. Francis CW, Blinc A, Lee S, et al. Ultrasound accelerates transport of recombinant tissue plasminogen activator into clots. Ultrasound Med Biol 1995;21: 419–24.

89. Tachibana K, Tachibana S. Albumin microbubble echo-contrast material as an enhancer for ultrasound accelerated thrombolysis. Circulation 1995; 92:1148–50.

90. Ribo M, Molina CA, Alvarez B, et al. Intra-arterial administration of microbubbles in continuous 2-MHz ultrasound insonation to enhance intra-arterial thrombolysis. J Neuroimaging 2009 [Epub ahead of print].

Noninvasive Imaging Techniques in the Diagnosis and Management of Aneurysmal Subarachnoid Hemorrhage

Scott A. Marshall, MD[a,b,c], Sudhir Kathuria, MBBS[d],
Paul Nyquist, MD, MPH[a,b], Dheeraj Gandhi, MBBS, MD[d,e,*]

KEYWORDS

- Subarachnoid hemorrhage • Vasospasm
- Aneurysmal subarachnoid hemorrhage
- Computed tomography angiography
- Transcranial Doppler • Magnetic resonance angiography
- Single photon emission computed tomography
- Positron emission tomography

Aneurysmal subarachnoid hemorrhage (aSAH), a devastating medical condition and its accompanying sequelae pose significant diagnostic and therapeutic challenges for the neurosurgeon, interventional neuroradiologist, and neurointensivist. The management of the primary and secondary complications of aSAH requires use of a multimodality approach in many cases, both for the diagnosis of aSAH as well as the radiographic diagnosis and management of vasospasm (VS). Currently, digital subtraction angiography (DSA) is the recognized gold standard for the diagnosis of both aSAH and VS, although it is not universally available. Moreover, it is resource intensive, costly, and has a small but not insignificant risk of neurologic complications, making the consideration of other modalities attractive.[1–5] We will present a review of the current literature

---

Disclaimer: The opinions and views expressed herein belong solely to those of the authors. They are not nor should they be implied as being endorsed by the Uniformed Services University of the Health Sciences, Department of the Army, Department of Defense, or any other branch of the federal government of the United States.

[a] Division of Neurosciences Critical Care, Department of Anesthesiology and Critical Care Medicine, Johns Hopkins University School of Medicine, 600 North Wolfe Street, Baltimore, MD 21287, USA
[b] Division of Neurosciences Critical Care, Department of Neurology and Neurosurgery, Johns Hopkins University School of Medicine, 600 North Wolfe Street, Baltimore, MD 21287, USA
[c] Department of Neurology, Uniformed Services University of the Health Sciences, Bethesda, MD, USA
[d] Division of Interventional Neuroradiology, Department of Radiology, Johns Hopkins Hospital, Johns Hopkins University School of Medicine, 600 North Wolfe Street, B100, Baltimore, MD 21287, USA
[e] Department of Neurology and Neurosurgery, Johns Hopkins Hospital, Johns Hopkins University School of Medicine, 600 North Wolfe Street, B100, Baltimore, MD 21287, USA
* Corresponding author. Department of Radiology, Johns Hopkins Hospital, Johns Hopkins University School of Medicine, 600 North Wolfe Street, B100, Baltimore, MD 21287.
E-mail address: dgandhi2@jhmi.edu

regarding the use of noninvasive imaging studies to aid in the diagnosis of ruptured intracerebral arterial aneurysms and VS, along with the current published data comparing the gold standard of DSA to these newer modalities.

IMAGING FOR THE DIAGNOSIS OF ANEURYSMAL SUBARACHNOID HEMORRHAGE

The initial diagnosis of aSAH is dependent on using a proper history, physical and neurologic examination, laboratory data, and radiographic studies. In the correct population, brain imaging with computed tomography (CT) and lumbar puncture (LP) are standard of care and commonly used when concern for aSAH exists.[6–8] Once the nontraumatic subarachnoid blood is found, then a combination of CT, magnetic resonance (MR) imaging, and/or conventional angiography are used to identify if it is secondary to a ruptured arterial aneurysm. If an aneurysm is confirmed, these modalities are further helpful in characterizing the nature of the aneurysm, identifying the ruptured aneurysm if multiple lesions are found, and to plan for operative or interventional techniques to secure the ruptured aneurysm.

Non–contrast-enhanced Computed Tomography

Noncontrast head CT plays an important role in the emergency evaluation of patients with acute headaches. Among the many causes of thunderclap headaches, a diagnosis of nontraumatic subarachnoid hemorrhage should be made emergently because of a possibility of an underlying ruptured aneurysm. The sensitivity of noncontrast CT to detect SAH in the acute period is greater than 90%; however, supplementary patient history and cerebrospinal fluid analysis maintains an important role in the diagnosis of SAH.[7–12] This may be especially important in subacute SAH presenting days after the initial symptomatic period, where conventional CT has decreased sensitivity for the detection of subarachnoid blood.[9]

Acute hemorrhage in the subarachnoid space appears as areas of hyperdensity in the basal cisterns, cerebral sulci, and/or the ventricles (**Fig. 1**). Despite its characteristic imaging appearance, a wide range of misdiagnosis rates have been reported in the literature. In a recent study, a misdiagnosis rate of 5% was reported for the CT diagnosis of SAH.[13] When clinical suspicion for aSAH exists, a detailed search pattern for blood should be adopted on CT. Careful attention should be paid to areas where a small amount of blood can be easily overlooked. These areas

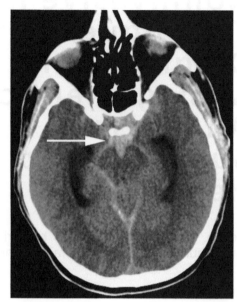

Fig. 1. Axial noncontrast CT image at the level of midbrain shows characteristic appearance of diffuse SAH with arrow pointing to blood collection in interpeduncular cistern suggestive of ruptured basilar tip aneurysm. Please note the early developing hydrocephalus with dilated bilateral temporal horns.

include posterior aspects of the sylvian fissures, interpeduncular cistern, deep cerebral sulci, occipital horns of the lateral ventricles, and the foramen magnum.

Occasionally, some entities can result in a false positive impression of SAH on CT scans. Crowding of structures at the basal aspect of the brain can create an appearance similar to SAH within the basal cisterns, a term called pseudo-subarachnoid hemorrhage. This finding is attributable to elevated intracranial pressure, apposition of pial surfaces, and resultant engorgement of pial veins.[14] Such an imaging appearance can be seen with conditions resulting in diffuse cerebral edema as well as intracranial mass lesions and severe obstructive hydrocephalus (**Fig. 2**). Awareness of this condition, the clinical context, and recognition of diffuse mass effect can help differentiate this entity from "true SAH." Layering of high-density exudates in the subarachnoid space in patients with meningitis as well as prior administration of intravenous contrast for unrelated radiographic examinations may also simulate the imaging features of SAH.[14]

Similar to clinical grading schemes for SAH, imaging-based grading systems have also been proposed. A popular imaging-based grading scheme was proposed by Fisher and colleagues.[15] It is based on the extent and appearance of SAH on CT, and is used to predict the

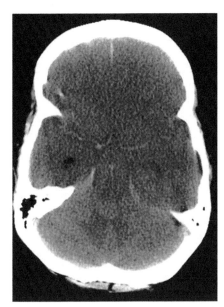

Fig. 2. Noncontrast CT with pseudo SAH due to diffuse severe hypoxia causing apparent hyperdensity in interpeduncular cistern and along the tentorium.

likelihood of developing VS (**Table 1**) and was later revised by Claassen and colleagues (**Table 2**).[16,17] Noncontrast CT can provide information to point toward the location of a ruptured aneurysm, especially important when multiple aneurysms are found to exist. Several studies have confirmed the ability in some cases of CT to predict the location of ruptured aneurysms found later on DSA.[18–22] There are several imaging findings that can help locate the site of ruptured aneurysm. The distribution of blood in the subarachnoid space and thickness of a localized clot can often help with such localization (**Fig. 3**).[14] For example, a large amount of blood along the interhemispheric fissure indicates anterior communicating artery aneurysms. Similarly, a large amount of blood in a sylvian fissure indicates middle cerebral artery aneurysm. Posterior fossa distribution of blood is

seen with basilar, superior cerebellar, and posterior inferior cerebellar artery (PICA) aneurysms. On occasion, one may be able to directly observe a ruptured aneurysm as a lucent area within the subarachnoid clot. However, even despite these helpful clues, correct determination of ruptured aneurysm may be difficult or impossible in many cases.

The ability of noncontrast CT to correctly identify the vascular location of aSAH was recently retrospectively studied by Karttunen and colleagues in 180 patients.[22] The entire cohort had a noncontrast CT done within 24 hours of SAH, and DSA was done within 48 hours of SAH. All patients studied had confirmed SAH, and were taken for surgical clipping. Initial noncontrast CT was able to correctly identify the site of aneurysmal rupture in general for middle cerebral artery (MCA) and anterior communicating artery (AcoA) aneurysms, but for aneurysms at other sites, accurate predictions were not possible in this study. The presence of a parenchymal hematoma, seen in 34% of the cohort, was a statistically significant predictor for evaluating the location of the ruptured aneurysm. The amount or distribution of the subarachnoid blood did not correlate well with the location of other aneurysms. A similar-sized retrospective study reported earlier that only anterior cerebral artery (ACA) or AcoA aneurysms were accurately predicted with noncontrast CT, and that MCA, internal carotid artery (ICA), and posterior circulation artery aneurysms were inconsistent or otherwise poorly predicted by noncontrast CT alone.[23] Classically, focal parenchymal hematomas of the skull base, medial temporal lobe, and intraventricular hemorrhage into the third ventricle have been associated with PICA aneurysms, posterior communicating (PCOM) aneurysms, and basilar artery aneurysms respectively.[24]

Perimesencephalic hemorrhage can have imaging appearance that can be confused with aSAH, although certain characteristics may help identify this benign condition. A location centered

Table 1		
Fisher grading system		
Grade	**CT Appearance of Subarachnoid Hemorrhage**	
1	None evident	
2	Less than 1 mm thick	
3	More than 1 mm thick	
4	Any thickness with associated parenchymal or intraventricular hematoma	

Data from Villablanca JP, Martin N, Jahan R, et al. Volume-rendered helical computerized tomography angiography in the detection and characterization of intracranial aneurysms. J Neurosurg 2000;93:254–64.

Table 2
Subarachnoid hemorrhage computed tomography rating scale[16]

Grade	CT Appearance of Subarachnoid Hemorrhage
0	No SAH or IVH
1	Minimal SAH, no IVH in both lateral ventricles
2	Minimal SAH with IVH in both lateral ventricles
3	Thick SAH, no IVH in both lateral ventricles
4	Thick SAH, with IVH in both lateral ventricles

around the anterior aspect of the midbrain, absence of large amounts of intraventricular blood, and potential extension to the posterior intrahemispheric or fissure or basal part of the sylvian fissure are characteristic imaging features of this condition. There is lack of parenchymal hematoma and a four-vessel angiogram is negative for aneurysm (**Fig. 4**)[25,26] (D. Gandhi, personal communication, 2009).

Computed Tomography Angiography

Much enthusiasm exists over the utility of CT angiography (CTA) as a less invasive diagnostic tool in the investigation of SAH found on noncontrast CT or LP. The advantages of CTA include its near uniform availability, safety profile, high spatial resolution, and limited time required to perform the test. Additionally, it can be obtained at the same sitting when the patient makes a trip to the CT scanner for the noncontrast CT. In recent years, multidetector CT (MDCT) technology is gaining popularity and has become widely available. MDCT scanners provide superior image resolution, extended z-axis coverage, and markedly reduced acquisition times. Additionally, with many centers increasingly using endovascular treatments over microsurgical clipping for treatment of aSAH, strain on limited angiographic resources for diagnostic purposes has increased.[1,27] It is hoped that diagnostic CTA may help offset some of the strain on this resource and increase use for therapeutic purposes.[28]

Several other advantages of the use of CTA in the setting of SAH that should be emphasized include its ability to demonstrate the precise relationship between bony structures of the skull and the aneurysm. Additionally, the relationship of the aneurysm to the brain structures and/or the hematoma can be studied, which is useful information for treatment planning, especially when craniotomy is being considered. The CTA may also help demonstrate other characteristics of the aneurysm that are less well studied on the DSA; for example, presence of endo-luminal thrombus

as well as calcification of the aneurysm wall. Preoperative knowledge of these aneurysm characteristics significantly aids in therapeutic decisions (**Figs. 5** and **6**).

Published reports of the sensitivity and specificity of CTA are encouraging its increasingly widespread use as a sole imaging modality for surgical or endovascular treatment planning of aSAH.[6,29–31] Wintermark and colleagues[31] published a report of the comparison of multislice CTA with DSA for 50 patients with aSAH. The sensitivity was 94.8% and the specificity was 95.2% for the detection on a per aneurysm basis and 99.0% and 95.2% on a per patient basis, respectively. In this study, a cut-off size of 2 mm was found as the inflection point in which multislice CTA became less able to detect intracerebral aneurysms, a finding that has since been replicated.[32,33] This is important, given that the slight majority of aneurysms implicated in SAH are 5 mm or smaller as reported in the International Subarachnoid Aneurysm Trial (ISAT) of more than 2000 patients.[34] Other studies have published sensitivities for the detection of aneurysms 5 to 12 mm in size of 90.6% and 100.0% for aneurysms larger than 12 mm.[35] This article showed a concerning low sensitivity at 83.3% for aneurysms smaller than 5 mm.[35] The overall sensitivity was reported at 89.5% compared with DSA. If the history and examination findings yield a high pretest probability of aSAH and the CTA fails to show an aneurysm, follow-up studies including DSA should be done.[1] Given this understanding, it may be reasonable to use CTA as the initial test for characterizing aSAH, with the understanding that a negative CTA in the setting of SAH is of very limited use.

The dose of intravenous contrast given during CTA is roughly 80 to 100 mL for many protocols[1] and compares very favorably when compared with a four-vessel DSA study. The radiation dose in CTA (100 mGy) has been estimated to be less than that of DSA.[1,36] The radiation from CT perfusion (CTP), if needed, adds in the range of 700 to 1400 mGy.[37] There have been reported cases of transient bandage-shaped hair loss after multiple

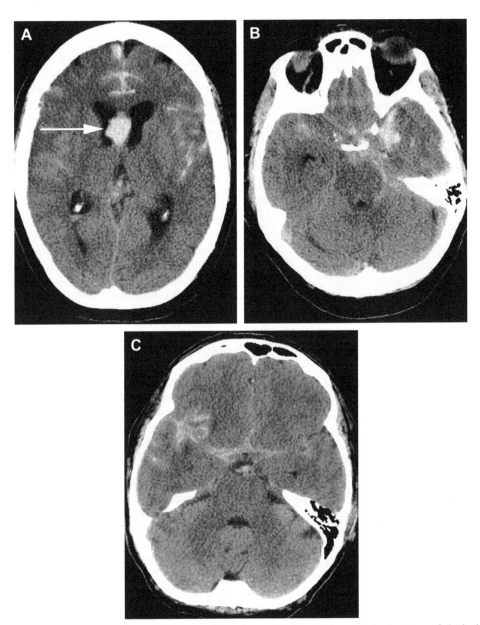

Fig. 3. Noncontrast CT images from different patients demonstrating that particular location of thick clot can often help in predicting the location of ruptured aneurysm: (*A*) Blood collection along interhemispheric fissure from ruptured ACOM aneurysm. (*B*) Focal collection along left side of suprasellar cistern from ruptured left PCOM aneurysm. (*C*) Blood pooling in right sylvian fissure from ruptured middle cerebral artery aneurysm. Please note the lucent center representing the actual aneurysm.

studies of perfusion CT combined with DSA or interventional procedures in a relatively short period of time. In these cases, the overall dose was estimated to be about 3 to 5 Gy to the skin.[38] The danger of excessive radiation exposure must be considered when patients are subjected to combination and repeated studies. There are many strategies available to reduce the radiation dose associated with CT and CTA protocols. Some of

these involve changes in the acquisition parameters such as kVp, gantry rotation time, milliampere, and pitch. These changes, however, are a compromise between image quality and radiation dose but can be optimized for desired information from the study and associated noise level that is acceptable for diagnostic purpose. More recent dose-reduction tools include dose modulation, in which the tube current is adjusted along

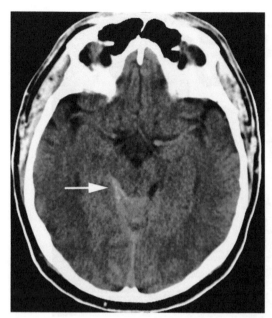

Fig. 4. Perimesencephalic SAH (*arrow*) along right side with no associated parenchymal hematoma. Subsequent DSA was negative for aneurysm.

with the image acquisition, according to patient's size and attenuation. This technique is capable of up to 60% dose reduction without significant image compromise.[36]

Despite the many advantages of CTA and rapid improvement in its quality, DSA is still considered the gold standard for evaluation of SAH. As discussed earlier, CTA has lower sensitivity for the detection of very small aneurysms. Additionally, normal variants like infundibular enlargements and tortuous vascular loops can be mistaken for intracranial aneurysm, resulting in a false positive CTA examination (**Fig. 7**). Therefore, if there is any doubt regarding the findings on CTA, one should have a low threshold for recommending further evaluation with a DSA. Several authors have identified clinical situations where CTA and DSA should be performed in concert, or perhaps DSA should be performed alone. This includes cases where bypass surgery may be required for large aneurysms, aneurysms with complex morphology, and cases where confirmation of the degree of development of the vein of Labbé is needed.[29,30,39–41] Additional concern exists over the concordance of arteriovenous malformation (AVM) and arterial aneurysms, owing to the failure of CTA to demonstrate an AVM in some series.[42] CTA used alone could potentially lead to an incomplete understanding of the vascular anatomy and poor surgical or endovascular planning in these cases.

Magnetic Resonance Imaging

The use of MRI to diagnose SAH and characterize aSAH has been partially limited to an ancillary use as a means to rule out other potential causes of SAH such as venous thrombosis or vasculitis.[43] The sensitivity of T2-weighted gradient echo (GRE) and fluid-attenuated inversion recovery (FLAIR) sequences is thought to increase over time, rather than decrease, as it does for CT.[44,45] In a study of MRI obtained in acute (<4 days from hemorrhage) versus subacute (4–14 days from hemorrhage) SAH, the sensitivity of T2-weighted GRE was 94% and 100%, respectively. FLAIR performed only slightly worse than GRE for the detection of acute or subacute SAH. More recently, available susceptibility weighted imaging (SWI) has the potential to further increase sensitivity for detecting hemorrhage over that of GRE. Nonetheless, MRI has a limited role in the initial or emergency department management of SAH because of logistics and time acquisition issues, although its sensitivity in the setting of acute evaluation of SAH has been further studied.[44–49] Fiebach and colleagues[44] published pilot data from a small series of patients who had a stroke protocol-based 8-minute MRI with 100% sensitivity of detecting SAH on proton density–weighted images. Diffusion-weighted imaging was also positive in 80% of the patients, and perfusion maps were normal in all patients.

Similarly, in a recent study by Yuan and colleagues,[9] similar MRI sequences were studied and compared with the sensitivity of CT and MR in acute (<5 days) and subacute (6–30 days) SAH. In the acute period, SAH was identified on FLAIR in 100% of cases, and on T2-weighted GRE sequences and noncontrast CT both in 90.9% of cases (**Fig. 8**). In the subacute period, FLAIR sensitivity was markedly reduced to 33%, whereas T2-weighted GRE was 100% sensitive and noncontrast CT found SAH in 45.5%. It appears that MRI may be of use in confirming suspected SAH, perhaps when other testing is unavailable or equivocal, or in the subacute phase as a supplement to CT when the sensitivity of CT is markedly reduced.

Magnetic Resonance Angiography

The use of 3D time-of-flight (TOF) magnetic resonance angiography (MRA) as a sole modality for diagnosis and characterization of cerebral aneurysms has been studied. In a large study of 205 consecutive patients with aSAH, a protocol using a 20-minute MRA during the acute period after SAH showed that the lesion could be identified and successful surgical planning undertaken

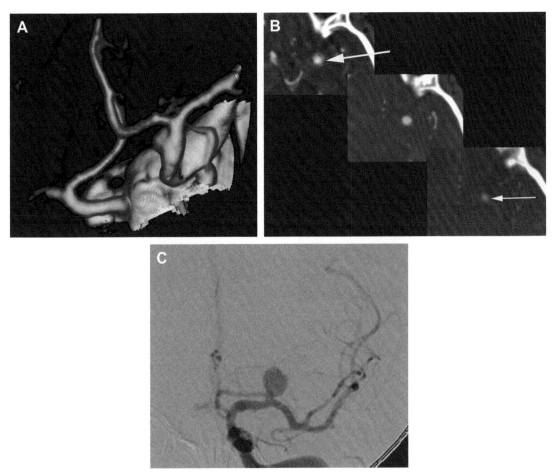

Fig. 5. (*A*) Reconstruction 3D CTA image showing precise location of aneurysm that is distal in relation to the anterior clinoid process, extremely useful information for surgical planning. (*B*) Axial source images from CTA showing thick rim of calcification around the base of contrast-filled aneurysm (*thick arrow*), which is not apparent and can be completely missed on subsequent DSA (*C*) of the same patient.

based on MRA, if the lesion was well characterized by this modality.[50] If an aneurysm was not identified, then DSA was done. One of the 205 patients studied had a false positive result, where a tortuous loop of the MCA was found at craniotomy. In a subset of approximately 16% of these patients, DSA was performed because of inconclusive findings on MRA. Seven asymptomatic aneurysms were found on MRA, all smaller than 5 mm in diameter. Importantly, the neuroradiologists interpreting the MRA data were not blinded to results of the initial noncontrast CT and thus were aided by noting a potential region of interest for the MR study. The authors concluded that DSA could be replaced by 3-dimensional (3D) TOF MRA as the initial diagnostic study in suspected aSAH.

Similar conclusions were made by Sato and colleagues[51] in a study of 108 patients with 3D TOF MRA. This article included both patients with ruptured aSAH and unruptured aneurysms. They concluded that MRA was accurate and useful as the primary imaging modality for the diagnosis of anterior circulation aneurysms of 5 mm diameter or larger. Interestingly, the authors also reported success with surgical planning and intervention without DSA.[51] In a systematic review, White and colleagues[52] reported a sensitivity of MRA in the detection of aneurysms 3 mm or larger of 90%, but this number fell precipitously for smaller aneurysms to a reported sensitivity of less than 40%. Logistics, image degradation as a result of patient movement, sedation issues inherent to MRI/A, and problems for use in high-grade patients make MRA impractical for many acutely neurologically ill patients with acute SAH. It remains unclear at this time whether further advances that may overcome these issues will

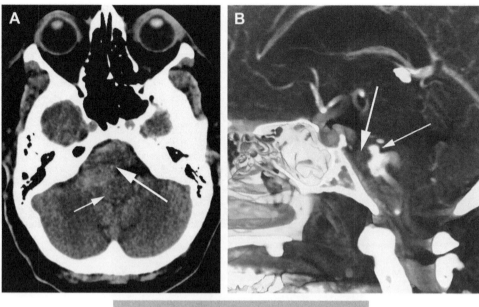

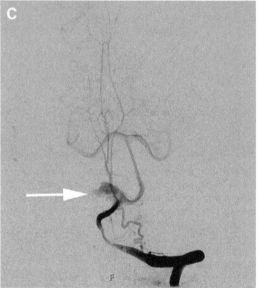

Fig. 6. (*A*) Large hyperdense mass (*large arrow*) located anterior to brainstem (*small arrow*) on this noncontrast CT is suggestive of thrombosed aneurysm. (*B*) Sagittal reformat image from CTA very nicely shows small patent portion of aneurysm filled with contrast (*small arrow*) and the larger thrombosed portion (*large arrow*) of aneurysm. (*C*) DSA also demonstrates the patent portion of the aneurysm (*arrow*) but completely fails to show the true configuration and size of the aneurysm. This important information is best provided by CTA and is critical for treatment planning.

make use of this helpful diagnostic tool more clinically relevant and widespread.[48,49]

IMAGING FOR DIAGNOSIS OF VASOSPASM AFTER ANEURYSMAL SUBARACHNOID HEMORRHAGE

Vasospasm refers to the diminution in cerebral blood flow seen after aneurysmal SAH owing to

the decreased caliber of intracranial arteries.[53,54] This was originally described by Ecker and Riewmanschneider,[55] and has since been the subject of much laboratory research and clinical investigation. Other terminology used includes VS seen only on DSA or CTA referred to as "angiographic vasospasm." Also used are the terms "delayed ischemic deficit" or "clinical vasospasm," and thus refer to VS that has become clinically

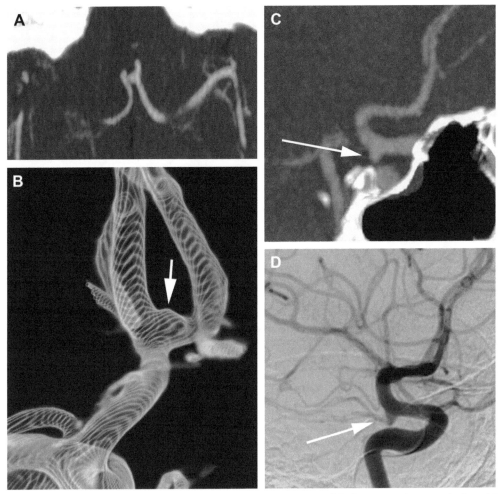

Fig. 7. False positive CTA as seen with this apparent ACOM aneurysm (*A*) that was subsequently found to be a dysplastic vessel segment on rotational DSA (*B*). In a separate patient, suspected PCOM aneurysm on CTA (*C*) was in fact an infundibulum (*D*) with clear visualization of its triangular shape and vessel continuation (*arrow*).

apparent resulting from decreased perfusion to a region of the brain with the development of a transient or permanent neurologic deficit.[53]

The exact cause of VS has not been clearly shown, but it is thought that extra-arterial blood products in contact with the arterial wall triggers a cascade of events at the cellular level that, in effect, culminates in vasoconstriction or overall reduced arterial vascular caliber.[53,56,57] Other factors involved include decreased vascular autoregulation, reversible vasculopathy, and relative hypovolemia.[58,59] A comprehensive review of the current imaging findings and endovascular management of VS is presented elsewhere in this edition of *Neurosurgical Clinics*. In the past, the most likely cause of mortality after SAH was from re-rupture of the aneurysm in the early period after SAH, although because of more aggressive early

surgical or endovascular treatment of ruptured aneurysms, this has now been replaced by complications of hydrocephalus and VS as the most common and serious causes of morbidity and mortality after SAH.[60,61]

The incidence of VS after aSAH is estimated at 50% to 70% of patients, with approximately 30% to 50% of those exhibiting symptoms of clinical VS.[62,63] A review of angiography studies of more than 2700 cases of aSAH found the average incidence to be approximately 67%, with the highest incidence occurring between day 10 and day 17 after SAH.[64] In our experience, the peak of VS occurs between day 7 and day 12 after the initial aSAH. The impact on outcome after the emergence of clinical VS (early or delayed) after SAH ranges from 10% to 20% mortality, along with similar increases in morbidity.[64,65] Clearly, VS is

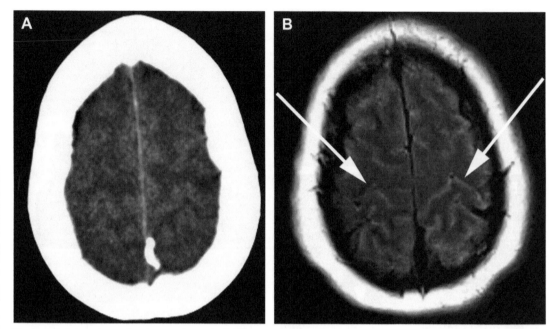

Fig. 8. (*A*) Subtle hyperdensity causing sulcal effacement suggestive of possible acute SAH. This is much better appreciated on FLAIR (*B*) as hyperintensity along the sulci. FLAIR is more sensitive than CT for diagnosing acute subarachnoid bleed.

of diagnostic importance in the management of aSAH, and the early radiographic recognition of VS may allow for institution of therapy and improved outcomes.

The gold standard for the diagnosis of cerebral VS is DSA, although its expense, small potential for neurologic complications, and the need to transfer the patient to the angiography suite make this impractical for use as a screening study for VS.[65] VS is a clinical diagnosis, and radiographic studies and other markers of brain perfusion establish anatomic evidence of diminished vessel caliber. Patients with VS may progress from nonfocal neurologic signs such as confusion, increasing somnolence, and combativeness to focal and localizable neurologic deficits. Radiographic findings often precede such clinical deficits, and thus offer the opportunity to potentially intervene to prevent neurologic injury.

Transcranial Doppler

The initial evidence was provided in 1982 for the use of transcranial Doppler (TCD) in monitoring flow in intracranial arteries and later for the use of this technology in the assessment of arterial VS.[66,67] Much work has been done on the use of TCD in the evaluation of cerebral blood flow, in part because of its relatively inexpensive cost, bedside availability, noninvasive nature, and lack of known adverse side effects from its use as

a diagnostic tool.[68,69] Currently, many advocate every other day to twice daily performance of TCD examinations of patients from the first day after presenting with SAH until no longer indicated.[54,70–74] It is also recommended for following the temporal course of angiographic VS during its peak incidence after SAH.[75] The validity of TCD as a monitor for VS has been, however, somewhat controversial.[76] It is an operator-dependent examination, and thin layers of skull that allow insonation by TCD to evaluate blood flow, known as acoustic windows, may be limited in about 8% of patients.[60,76] Limiting factors also include the high false negative rates of VS reported by some as well as the variability among technicians performing the examinations.[77] This may be overcome or lessened with new TCD techniques described in the followingparagraph.[77]

New such technology available for clinical use may make TCD more accurate, and less subject to operator error. This includes Power M-mode (PMD) TCD and transcranial color-coded duplex sonography (TCCS). PMD/TCD facilitates the location of the acoustic temporal window and allows viewing blood flow from multiple vessels at the same time.[56] The display that is used in PMD/TCD allows for color-coded information regarding the directionality of blood flow, and this has allowed for PMD/TCD to be the most commonly used form of TCD performed currently at the bedside.[53] TCCS has expounded on this improvement, with a 2D representation of the large arteries insonated in addition to color-coded flow directionality information.[53] A study using TCCS has been published recently, where the authors reported comparable accuracy of TCCS and TCD, although improvements in sensitivity of TCCS in detecting MCA VS were noted.[77] An interesting aspect of this study was that comparisons of conventional TCD and TCCS were done on the same patients on the day where DSA was performed. TCCS allowed for the detection of VS at an earlier stage and at lower velocities, which may allow for more timely interventions to potentially intervene and arrest the complications of clinical VS if it were to occur.

The sensitivity of TCD varies depending on the vessel affected by VS, with relatively low sensitivity for supra-clinoid internal carotid and anterior cerebral arteries.[9] In addition, VS of the second- and third-order arteries (small-vessel VS) cannot be studied with transcranial Doppler. TCD has been shown to be specific but not sensitive for VS of the middle cerebral artery when compared with angiography and it is poorly predictive of developing secondary cerebral infarction.[77–79]

Computed Tomography Angiography

CTA has emerged as a potential helpful tool in the evaluation of VS, with relatively good sensitivity and specificity in discovering severe VS of proximal arteries, and with a high negative predictive value in a normal study (**Fig. 9**).[80–82] Early work by Ochi and Takagi showed that CTA was potentially useful in the detection of VS.[82,83] One study interestingly performed CTA followed by DSA in both the patients with VS and without VS seen on CTA, and in this small series, the CTA results were confirmed.[79] Further studies showed that overall correlation between CTA and DSA for a diagnosis of VS was 0.757, but was improved in proximal artery locations and where there was either no spasm or severe spasm (>50% luminal reduction).[84,85] Where CTA performed well, correlation with DSA approached 1.0, and in proximal locations with mild (<30% luminal reduction) or moderate (30%–50% luminal reduction) VS, correlations with DSA were reported as 90% and 95%, respectively. More distal locations with mild or moderate VS were not as evident on CTA, and respective accuracies of 81% and 94% were reported. This has been replicated in other work by Chaudhary.[86]

In a recent article by Yoon and colleagues[84] a series of patients with clinical suspicion for VS underwent both postoperative multidetector-row CTA and DSA. Seventeen patients were studied and a total of 251 arterial segments analyzed. Of the 40 arterial segments with hemodynamically significant stenosis found on DSA, 39 of these lesions were identified with multidetector-row CTA yielding a sensitivity of 97.5%. Unlike prior reports, no difference was found in terms of diagnostic accuracy of distal compared with proximal

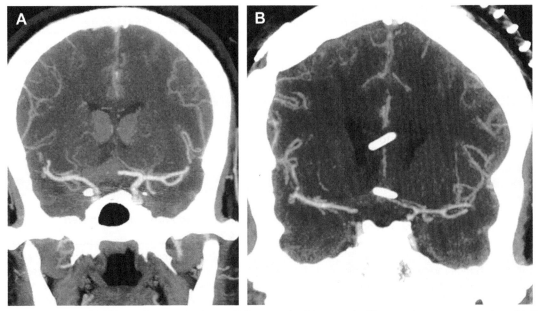

Fig. 9. CTA is good in diagnosing proximal vessel VS as seen in this example. Please note severe narrowing of left distal ICA, left proximal MCA, and left proximal ACA (*A*) compared with the normal caliber of these vessels in baseline CTA (*B*) obtained 4 days earlier.

arterial segments, and this has not been as clearly shown in other subsequent series.[86] There was a trend of overestimation of the degree of spasm by CTA noted; this mostly occurred in the anterior circulation and in the A1 and A2 segment of the ACA, specifically. The authors suggested that CTA would triage resources and allow planning for an interventional procedure such as angioplasty or intra-arterial infusions of vasodilators if findings suggested VS on CTA.[84]

It appears clear that CTA has a role in the diagnosis of VS after aSAH, likely in concert with DSA in select patients, and certainly in cases where CTA findings suggest VS and interventional techniques to arrest cerebral ischemia from VS are used. It seems reasonable, based on current data and with an understanding of the modalities limitations, to use CTA for this purpose as part of a multimodality approach to the diagnosis and treatment of VS after aSAH.

Computed Tomography Perfusion

Coupled with CTA, perfusion studies using CT have created much recent interest. Neither TCD nor DSA provide information about actual brain perfusion during the time period of VS, and this can be directly assessed with CT perfusion (CTP). CTP can provide several quantitative parameters of cerebrovascular hemodynamics. Several perfusion parameters can be obtained from this deconvolution-based technique, including mean transit time (MTT), cerebral blood volume (CBV), and cerebral blood flow (CBF).[87,88] MTT is defined as the average transit time of blood through a given brain region, measured in seconds. The total volume of blood in a given volume of brain, usually measured in milliliters per 100 g of brain tissue, is referred to as CBV. CBF is the volume of blood moving through a given volume of brain per unit time, measured in milliliters per 100 g of brain tissue per minute. MTT and time to peak (TTP) maps have been shown to be the most sensitive in detecting early autoregulation changes in VS and other causes of cerebral ischemia.[88,89] Experimental studies using preclinical models of SAH have shown CTP to reliably predict early mortality and the later development of moderate to severe VS.[90] In this study, MTT was the most reliable predictor of moderate to severe VS and early (within 48 hours) mortality in their model of SAH. Kanazawa and colleagues[91] studied 19 patients with aSAH in which CTP, CTA, and DSA were performed. The authors were able to suggest an MTT threshold that may serve as a criterion for cerebral ischemia and thus require mobilizing angiographic resources for intervention, but this threshold may be institution/equipment specific and requires more study. Binaghi and colleagues[88] published data that confirmed CTP's ability to identify severe VS, which warrants interventional angiographic procedures. All 27 patients in this study had clinical evidence of VS, such as new focal findings, mental status changes, or new aphasia. The DSA showed either mild or moderate VS in 48% and severe VS in 40% of the study subjects. The investigators used CTA as well as CTP, and DSA and CTA correlated with a reported sensitivity and specificity of CTA with DSA of 88% and 99%, respectively. CTP was reported to correctly diagnose the correct vascular territory supplied by the vessel exhibiting VS on DSA. Sensitivity of CTP was found to be 90% in severe VS, with successful detection of severe lesions in all but one patient. Sensitivities were lower for mild or moderate VS. In several of the patients, the decision to treat with interventional techniques was influenced by CTP (**Fig. 10**).

Of these technologies, a combination of CTA and CTP has been suggested as a useful paired diagnostic study.[60] Evidence exists that this combination approach is more effective than TCD in indicating which patients will require endovascular intervention.[92] Additionally, because any change in the examination of a patient with aSAH will prompt noncontrast CT imaging to assess for hydrocephalus, cerebral edema, or new SAH, a CT-based multimodality approach for imaging of VS seems quite practical.

Positron Emission Tomography

The use of positron emission tomography (PET) in the diagnosis of VS and subsequent cerebral ischemia has been investigated in aSAH induced VS.[93–96] PET may play a future role in the multimodal approach to this population and in a subset of these patients but its use is currently limited because of logistics and long acquisition times. Many in this patient population are worsening neurologically during their evaluation for radiographic or other evidence of VS, and are not able to tolerate prolonged diagnostic evaluation such as PET.[92]

Single-Photon Emission Computed Tomography

Single-photon emission computed tomography (SPECT) is able to demonstrate regional cerebral blood flow in patients with neurologic injury by evaluating uptake of radioactive tracer into the brain.[97] Changes in tissue perfusion reflecting functional VS have been seen with SPECT imaging.[98–99] Studies using this technology in the setting of aSAH and VS

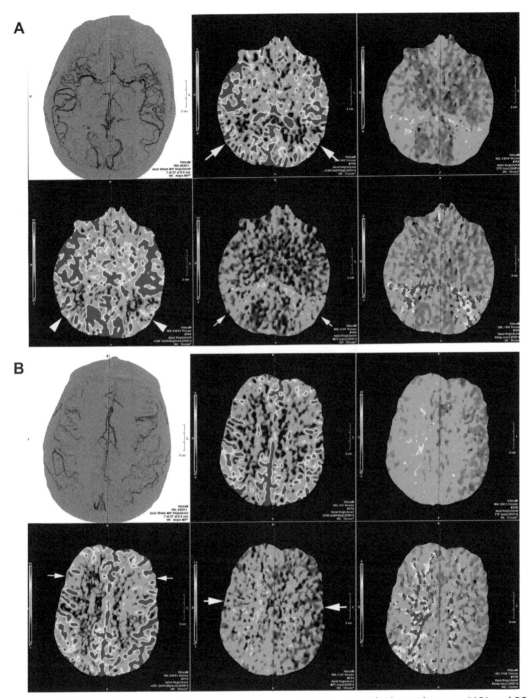

Fig. 10. (A) CTP images for suspected VS demonstrate increased MTT in watershed zone between MCA and PCA territory (*arrows* in middle lower image) with corresponding decreased rCBF (*arrowheads* in left lower image) and matched defect on rCBV (*arrows* in middle upper image). (B) CTP images from same study at slightly higher level shows increased MTT in large area of right MCA distribution compared with left (middle lower image) suggestive of VS and ischemia. rCBF shows lower values (*arrows* in left lower image) corresponding to already infracted watershed zone between anterior and middle cerebral artery. Subsequent DSA (C) demonstrates the expected significant spasm in right distal ICA and proximal MCA and ACA that was treated with intra-arterial nicardipine and balloon angioplasty. Posttreatment DSA (D) shows significant improvement in vessel caliber along with clinical improvement. Noncontrast CT image (E) obtained a few days later only showed watershed infarcts that were initially noticed during CTP images. Further infarcts were prevented using timely intervention.

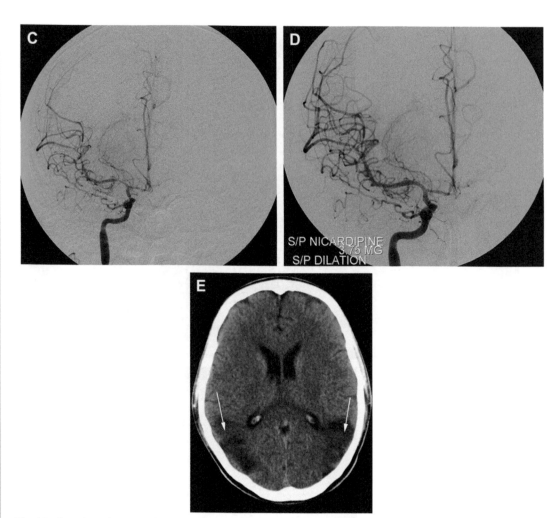

Fig. 10. (*continued*)

have been done, but SPECT has met with controversy over its relative clinical usefulness in this setting.[100–102] At this time, the clinical utility of SPECT in this setting remains unclear.

Magnetic Resonance Angiography

MRA has been used to assess for VS after aSAH, although its limitations include logistics, long time for acquisition, patient characteristics, motion and hardware artifact from surgical clips, or endovascular coils on TOF MRA.[48,49,90] Others have suggested that the most supported role of MRA in SAH is in the case where the SAH is unrelated to aneurysmal rupture, and MRI/MRA may aid in the exclusion of other etiologies.[43] MRA evaluation of cerebral vasoconstriction in other settings such as the reversible cerebral vasoconstriction syndrome unrelated to aSAH, migrainous infarctions, and acute mountain sickness, among others, has been helpful.[103–105] Longer than

a decade ago, Tamatani and colleagues[106] reported on the value of MRA to diagnose VS, and compared MRA findings with DSA in a population of 32 patients with aSAH. This study was complicated by poor image quality and inability to evaluate several segments owing to surgical aneurysmal clip or other artifact degrading the images and hampering interpretation. In a study addressing this issue of artifact and titanium-alloy aneurysm clips, data regarding safety and image quality data were provided, and the finding of VS was noted on MRA that was later confirmed on DSA.[107] This technology has not gained widespread acceptance for this purpose to date.

Perfusion-Weighted MRI

Perfusion-weighted MRI (MRP) has gained wide acceptance for use in the setting of stroke, and the use of MRP for detection of cerebral VS has been studied. Although MR technologies continued to be hampered by logistics, cost, and time constraints, protocols addressing specific issues with MR technology perhaps may lessen some of these issues in the future.[44,50,108,109] In a recent study using diffusion-weighted imaging (DWI), MRP, and DSA, infarct patterns associated with VS were identified. Interestingly, in the setting of moderate VS on DSA, perfusion and diffusion abnormalities were noted remote to areas of VS, implying again that the process of VS involves the cerebral circulation globally.[110] Ohtonari and colleagues[110] presented data recently where DWI, MRP, and SPECT were used to detect VS after aSAH. Seventeen patients were studied, and of the three patients with clinical findings of somnolence, focal neurologic signs, or aphasia, MRP revealed increased MTT with normal CBF and normal to elevated CBV. SPECT failed to show any abnormality during this same period. Medical therapy for VS was instituted, and none of the three patients had permanent infarcts in the area of MRP abnormality. Another paper used MRP and DSA to study 51 patients with aSAH both with and without angiographic evidence of VS. This study was not designed to show or predict ischemic injury as a result of VS, but it did reveal that MRP could clearly indicate impaired cerebral autoregulation via changes in CBV and CBF in the setting of aSAH with or without angiographic VS.[111]

In a recent retrospective review, Hertel and colleagues reported that of 20 patients studied with MRP, 19 showed evidence of perfusion abnormalities in the MTT or TTP maps, and 15 of these had clinical evidence of VS which localized to the region of hypoperfusion on MRP. DWI revealed abnormalities in areas smaller than the MRP abnormalities, indicating a diffusion/perfusion mismatch. The authors concluded that knowledge of this diffusion/perfusion mismatch would allow for interventions to prevent larger areas of ischemia developing in these patients.[109] In the case of this study, intra-arterial vasodilators were used to prevent perfusion abnormalities progressing to infarction in a subset of the population. No adverse events were reported resulting from the MR procedure. This data show promise for the use of MRP in this setting, although concern still exists for the potentially impractical nature of the use of MRP as a screening tool. Further prospective study may also help answer whether knowledge of a perfusion abnormality will result in better outcome by acute introduction of interventional techniques or medical management of VS.

SUMMARY

The management of aSAH and VS presents challenges to the neurosurgeon, neurointensivist, and interventional neuroradiologist. Newer and less invasive modalities for the diagnosis of aSAH and detection of VS are being increasingly used. The current data support use of several of these new techniques in a subset of this population of patients, although DSA still retains its place as the gold standard.

REFERENCES

1. Goddard AJP, Tan G, Becker J. Computed tomography angiography for the detection and characterization of intracranial aneurysms; current status. Clin Radiol 2005;60:1221–36.
2. Maurice-Williams RS. Subarachnoid haemorrhage: preoperative management. Subarachnoid haemorrhage. Bristol (England): Wright; 1987. p. 154–83.
3. Leffers AM, Wagner A. Neurologic complications of cerebral angiography. A retrospective study of complication rate and patient risk factors. Acta Radiol 2000;41:204–10.
4. Waugh JR, Sacharias N. Arteriographic complications in the DSA era. Radiology 1992;182:243–6.
5. Cloft HJ, Joseph GJ, Dion JE. Risk of cerebral angiography in patients with subarachnoid hemorrhage, cerebral aneurysm, and arteriovenous malformation. A meta-analysis. Stroke 1999;30:317–20.
6. Carstairs SD, Tanen DA, Duncan TD, et al. Computed tomographic angiography for the evaluation of aneurysmal subarachnoid hemorrhage. Acad Emerg Med 2006;13(5):486–92.
7. Cortelli P, Cevoli S, Nonino F, et al. Evidenced-based diagnosis of nontraumatic headache in the emergency department: a consensus statement of four clinical scenarios. Headache 2004;44(6):587–95.
8. American College of Emergency Physicians. Clinical policy: critical issues in the evaluation and management of patients presenting to the emergency department with acute headache. Ann Emerg Med 2002;39:108–22.
9. Yuan MK, Lai PH, Chen JY, et al. Detection of subarachnoid hemorrhage at acute and subacute/chronic stages: comparison of four magnetic resonance imaging pulse sequences and computed tomography. J Chin Med Assoc 2005;68(3):131–7.
10. Go S. Nontraumatic headaches in the emergency department: a systematic approach to diagnosis and controversies in two "big ticket" entities. Mo Med 2009;106(2):156–61.

11. Van Gijn J, Van Dongen KJ. The time course of hospitalis haemorrhage on computed tomograms. Neuroradiology 1982;23:153–6.

12. Adams HP, Kassel NF, Torner JC, et al. CT and clinical correlations in recent aneurismal subarachnoid hemorrhage: a preliminary report of the cooperative aneurysm study. Neurology 1983;33:981–8.

13. Ammerman JM. Pseudosubarachnoid hemorrhage: a zebra worth looking for. South Med J 2008;101:1200.

14. Provenzale JM, Hacein-Bey L. CT evaluation of subarachnoid hemorrhage: a practical review for the radiologist interpreting emergency room studies. Emerg Radiol 2009;16(6):441–51.

15. Fisher CM, Kistler JP, Davis JM. Relation of cerebral vasospasm to subarachnoid hemorrhage visualized by computerized tomographic scanning. Neurosurgery 1980;6:1–9.

16. Claassen J, Bernardini GL, Kreiter K, et al. Effect of cisternal and ventricular blood on risk of delayed cerebral ischemia after subarachnoid hemorrhage: the Fisher scale revisited. Stroke 2001;32:2012–20.

17. Pedersen HK, Bakke SJ, Hald JK, et al. CTA in patients with acute subarachnoid haemorrhage. A comparative study with selective, digital angiography and blinded, independent review. Acta Radiol 2001;42:43–9.

18. Villablanca JP, Martin N, Jahan R, et al. Volume-rendered helical computerized tomography angiography in the detection and characterization of intracranial aneurysms. J Neurosurg 2000;93:254–64.

19. Hino A, Fujimato M, Iwanoto Y, et al. False localization of rupture site in patients with multiple aneurysms and subarachnoid hemorrhage. Neurosurgery 2000;46(4):825–30.

20. Lee KC, Joo JY, Kee KS. False localization of rupture by computed tomography in bilateral internal carotid artery aneurysms. Surg Neurol 1996;45:435–41.

21. Nehls DG, Flom RA, Carter LP, et al. Multiple intercerebral aneurysms: determining the site of rupture. J Neurosurg 1985;63:342–8.

22. Karttunen AI, Jartti PH, Ukkola VA, et al. Value of the quantity and distribution of subarachnoid haemorrhage on CT in the localization of a ruptured cerebral aneurysm. Acta Neurochir 2003;145:655–61.

23. van der Jaqt M, Hasan D, Dijvoet HW, et al. Validity of prediction of the site of ruptured intracranial aneurysms with CT. Neurology 1999;152(1):34–9.

24. Kassell NF, Sasaki T, Colohan AR, et al. Cerebral vasospasm following aneurysmal subarachnoid hemorrhage. Stroke 1985;16(4):562–72.

25. Schwartz TH, Solomon RA. Perimesencephalic nonaneurysmal SAH: review of the literature. Neurosurgery 1996;39:433–40.

26. Rinkel GJ, Wijdicks EF, Vermeulen M, et al. Nonaneurysmal perimesencephalic subarachnoid hemorrhage: CT and MR patterns that differ from aneurysmal rupture. AJNR Am J Neuroradiol 1991;12:829–34.

27. Raftopoulos C, Mathurin P, Boscherini D, et al. Prospective analysis of aneurysm treatment in a series of 103 consecutive patients when endovascular embolisation is considered the first option. J Neurosurg 2000;93:175–82.

28. Sleight MJ, Goddard AJP. The impact of multislice CT angiography on the diagnosis and treatment of aneurysmal subarachnoid haemorrhage. BIR Congress Series, Proceedings of the UK Radiological Congress, Manchester, UK, 2004. p. 15.

29. Matsumoto M, Sato M, Nakano M, et al. Three-dimensional computerized tomography angiography-guided surgery of acutely ruptured cerebral aneurysms. J Neurosurg 2001;94:718–27.

30. González-Darder JM, Pesudo-Martínez JV, Feliu-Tatay JV. Microsurgical management of cerebral aneurysms based in CT angiography with three-dimensional reconstruction (3D-CTA) and without preoperative cerebral angiography. Acta Neurochir (Wien) 2001;143:673–9.

31. Wintermark M, Uske A, Chararon M, et al. Multislice computerized tomography angiography in the evaluation of intracranial aneurysms: a comparison with intraarterial digital subtraction angiography. J Neurosurg 2003;98(4):828–36.

32. Dehdashti AR, Binaghi S, Uske A, et al. Comparison of multislice computerized tomography angiography and digital subtraction angiography in the postoperative evaluation of patients with clipped aneurysms. J Neurosurg 2006;104(3):395–403.

33. van der Schaaf IC, Velthuis BK, Wermer MJ, et al. Multislice computed tomography angiography screening for new aneurysms in patients with previously clip-treated intracranial aneurysms: feasibility, positive predictive value, and interobserver agreement. J Neurosurg 2006;105(5):682–8.

34. International Subarachnoid Haemorrhage Collaborative Group. International Subarachnoid Aneurysm Trial (ISAT) of neurosurgical clipping versus endovascular coiling in 2143 patients with ruptured intracranial aneurysms: a randomized trial. Lancet 2002;360:1267–74.

35. Dammert S, Krings T, Moller-Hartmann W, et al. Detection of intracranial aneurysms with multislice CT: comparison with conventional angiography. Neuroradiology 2004;46:427–34.

36. Smith AB, Dillon WP, Gould R, et al. Radiation dose-reduction strategies for neuroradiology CT protocols. AJNR Am J Neuroradiol 2007;28:1628–32.

37. Hirata M, Sugawara Y, Fukutomi Y, et al. Measurement of radiation dose in cerebral CT perfusion study. Radiat Med 2005;23:97–103.

38. Imanishi Y, Fukui A, Niimi H, et al. Radiation-induced temporary hair loss as a radiation damage only occurring in patients who had the combination of MDCT and DSA. Eur Radiol 2005;15:41–6.

39. Dehdashti AR, Rufenacht DA, Delavelle J, et al. Therapeutic decision and management of aneurysmal subarachnoid hemorrhage based on computed tomographic angiography. Br J Neurosurg 2003;17:46–53.

40. Miyamoto S, Yamada K, Kikuta K, et al. Strategy for the proper and safe treatment of cerebral aneurysm. Jpn J Neurosurg (Tokyo) 2003;12:412–8.

41. Hashimoto Y, Kin S, Haraguchi K, et al. Pitfalls in the preoperative evaluation of subarachnoid hemorrhage without digital subtraction angiography: report on 2 cases. Surg Neurol 2007;68:344–8.

42. Walsh M, Adams WM, Mukonoweshuro W. CT angiography of intracranial aneurysms related to arteriovenous malformations: a cautionary tale. Neuroradiology 2006;48:255–8.

43. Gauvrit JY, Leclerc X, Ferre JC, et al. [Imaging of subarachnoid hemorrhage]. J Neuroradiol 2009; 36(2):65–73 [in French].

44. Fiebach JB, Schellinger PD, Geletneky K, et al. MRI in acute subarachnoid haemorrhage: findings with a standardized stroke protocol. Neuroradiology 2004;46(1):44–8.

45. Mitchell P, Wilkinson ID, Hoggard N, et al. Detection of subarachnoid haemorrhage with magnetic resonance imaging. J Neurol Neurosurg Psychiatry 2001;70:205–11.

46. Kidwell CS, Chalela JA, Saver JL, et al. Comparison of MRI and CT for detection of acute intracerebral hemorrhage. JAMA 2004;292:1823–30.

47. Wiesmann M, Mayer TE, Yousry I, et al. Detection of hyperacute subarachnoid hemorrhage of the brain by using magnetic resonance imaging. J Neurosurg 2002;96:684–9.

48. Heiserman JE. MR angiography for the diagnosis of vasospasm after subarachnoid hemorrhage. Is it accurate? Is it safe? AJNR Am J Neuroradiol 2000;21(9):1571–2.

49. Grandin CB, Cosnard G, Hammer F, et al. Vasospasm after subarachnoid hemorrhage: diagnosis with MR angiography. AJNR Am J Neuroradiol 2000;21(9):1611–7.

50. Westerlaan HE, van der Vliet AM, Hew JM, et al. Magnetic resonance angiography in the selection of patients suitable for neurosurgical intervention of ruptured intracranial aneurysms. Neuroradiology 2004;46:867–75.

51. Sato M, Nakano M, Sasanuma J, et al. Preoperative cerebral aneurysm assessment by three-dimensional magnetic resonance angiography: feasibility of surgery without conventional catheter angiography. Neurosurgery 2005;56:903–12.

52. White PM, Wardlaw J, Easton V. Can non-invasive imaging accurately depict intracranial aneurysms? A systematic review. Radiology 2000;217:361–70.

53. Rigamonti A, Ackery A, Baker AJ. Transcranial Doppler monitoring in subarachnoid hemorrhage: a critical tool in critical care. Can J Anesth 2008; 55:112–23.

54. Armonda RA, Bell RS, Vo AH, et al. Wartime traumatic cerebral vasospasm: recent review of combat casualties. Neurosurgery 2006;59: 1215–25.

55. Ecker A, Riewmanschneider PA. Arteriographic demonstration of spasm of the intracranial arteries. With special reference to saccular arterial aneurisms. J Neurosurg 1951;8:600–67.

56. Saqqur M, Aygun D, Demchuck A. Role of transcranial Doppler in neurocritical care. Crit Care Med 2007;35(Suppl 5):s216–23.

57. Kincaid MS. Transcranial Doppler ultrasonography: a diagnostic tool of increasing utility. Curr Opin Anaesthesiol 2008;21:552–9.

58. Sarrafzadeh AS, Haux D, Ludemann L, et al. Cerebral ischemia in aneurysmal subarachnoid hemorrhage: a correlative microdialysis—PET study. Stroke 2004;35:638–43.

59. Vajkoczy P, Horn P, Thome C, et al. Regional cerebral blood flow monitoring in the diagnosis of delayed ischemia following aneurysmal subarachnoid hemorrhage. J Neurosurg 2003;98:1227–34.

60. Zubkov AY, Rabinstien AA. Medical management of cerebral vasospasm: present and future. Neurol Res 2009;31(6):626–31.

61. Smith M. Intensive care management of patients with subarachnoid hemorrhage. Curr opin Anaesthesiol 2007;20:400–7.

62. Keyrouz SG, Diringer MN. Prevention and therapy of vasospasm in subarachnoid hemorrhage. Critical Care 2007;11:220.

63. Vermeulen MJ, Schull MJ. Missed diagnosis of sub-arachnoid hemorrhage in the emergency department. Stroke 2007;38:1216–21.

64. Dorsh NW, King MT. A review of cerebral vasospasm in aneurysmal subarachnoid hemorrhage. Part I: incidence and effects. J Clin Neurosci 1994;1:19–26.

65. Bleck TP. Rebleeding and vasospasm after SAH: new strategies for improving outcome. J Crit Illn 1997;12:572–82.

66. Aaslid R, Markwalder TM, Nornes H. Noninvasive transcranial Doppler ultrasound recording of flow velocity in basal cerebral arteries. J Neurosurg 1982;57:769–74.

67. Aaslid R, Huber R, Nornes H. Evaluation of cerebrovascular spasm with transcranial Doppler ultrasound. J Neurosurg 1984;60:37–41.

68. Daffertshofer M, Gass A, Ringleb P, et al. Transcranial low-frequency ultrasound-mediated thrombolysis in brain ischemia: increased risk of hemorrhage with combined ultrasound and tissue plasminogen activator: results of a phase II clinical trial. Stroke 2005;36(7):1441–6.

69. Mascia L, Fedorko L, terBrugge K, et al. The accuracy of transcranial Doppler to detect vasospasm in patients with aneurysmal subarachnoid hemorrhage. Intensive Care Med 2003;29:1088–94.

70. Sloan MA, Alexandrov AV, Tegeler CH, et al. Assessment: transcranial Doppler ultrasonography: report of the Therapeutics and Technology Assessment Subcommittee of the American Academy of Neurology. Neurology 2004;62(9): 1469–81.

71. Bederson JB, Connolly ES, Batjer HH, et al. Guidelines for the management of aneurysmal subarachnoid hemorrhage: a statement for healthcare professionals from a special writing group of the Stroke Council, American Heart Association. Stroke 2009;40(3):994–1025.

72. Romner B, Brandt L, Berntman L, et al. Simultaneous transcranial Doppler sonography and cerebral blood flow measurements of cerebrovascular CO2-reactivity in patients with aneurysmal subarachnoid haemorrhage. Br J Neurosurg 1991;5(1):31–7.

73. Wozniak MA, Sloan MA, Rothman MI, et al. Detection of vasospasm by transcranial Doppler sonography: the challenges of the anterior and posterior cerebral arteries. J Neuroimaging 1996;6:87–93.

74. Creissard P, Proust F, Langois O. Vasospasm diagnosis: theoretical and real transcranial Doppler sensitivity. Acta Neurochir (Wien) 1995;136(3–4): 181–5.

75. Creissard P, Proust F. Vasospasm diagnosis: theoretical sensitivity of transcranial Doppler evaluated using 135 angiograms demonstrating vasospasm. Practical consequences. Acta Neurochir (Wien) 1994;131(1–2):12–8.

76. Soustiel JF, Bruk B, Shik B, et al. Transcranial Doppler in vertebrobasilar vasospasm after subarachnoid hemorrhage. Neurosurgery 1998; 43:282–91.

77. Lysakowski C, Walder B, Costanza MC, et al. Transcranial Doppler versus angiography in patients with vasospasm due to a ruptured cerebral aneurysm: a systematic review. Stroke 2001; 32:2292–8.

78. Pham M, Johnson A, Bartsch AJ, et al. CT perfusion predicts secondary cerebral infarction after aneurysmal subarachnoid hemorrhage. Neurology 2007;69(8):762–5.

79. Anderson GB, Ashforth R, Steinke DE, et al. CT angiography for the detection of cerebral vasospasm in patients with acute subarachnoid hemorrhage. AJNR Am J Neuroradiol 2000;21: 1011–5.

80. Sanelli PC, Ougorets I, Johnson CE, et al. Using CT in the diagnosis and management of patients with cerebral vasospasm. Semin Ultrasound CT MR 2006;27(3):194–206.

81. Ionita CC, Graffagnino C, Alexander MJ, et al. The value of CT angiography and transcranial Doppler sonography in triaging suspected cerebral vasospasm in SAH prior to endovascular therapy. Neurocrit Care 2008;9:8–12.

82. Ochi RP, Vieco PT, Gross CE. CT angiography of cerebral vasospasm with conventional angiography comparison. AJNR Am J Neuroradiol 1997; 18:265–9.

83. Takagi R, Hayashi H, Kobayashi H, et al. Three-dimensional CT angiography of intracranial vasospasm following subarachnoid haemorrhage. Neuroradiology 1998;40:631–5.

84. Yoon DY, Choi CS, Kim KH, et al. Multidetector-row CT angiography of cerebral vasospasm after aneurysmal subarachnoid hemorrhage: comparison of volume-rendered images and digital subtraction angiography. AJNR Am J Neuroradiol 2006;27: 370–7.

85. Joo SP, Kim TS, Kim YS, et al. Clinical utility of multislice computed tomographic angiography for detection of cerebral vasospasm in acute subarachnoid hemorrhage. Minim Invasive Neurosurg 2006;49:286–90.

86. Chaudhary SR, Ko N, Dillon WP, et al. Prospective evaluation of multidetector-row CT angiography for the diagnosis of vasospasm following subarachnoid hemorrhage: a comparison with digital subtraction angiography. Cerebrovasc Dis 2008; 25:144–50.

87. Konstas AA, Goldmakher GV, Lee TY, et al. Theoretic basis and technical implementations of CT perfusion in acute ischemic stroke, part 1: theoretic basis. AJNR Am J Neuroradiol 2009;30(4): 662–8.

88. Binaghi S, Colleoni ML, Maeder P, et al. CT angiography and perfusion CT in cerebral vasospasm after subarachnoid hemorrhage. AJNR Am J Neuroradiol 2007;28(4):750–8.

89. Wintermark M, Fischbein NJ, Smith WS, et al. Accuracy of dynamic perfusion CT with deconvolution in detecting acute hemispheric stroke. AJNR Am J Neuroradiol 2005;26(1):104–12.

90. Laslo AM, Eastwood JD, Pakkiri P, et al. Perfusion-derived mean transit time predicts early mortality and delayed vasospasm after experimental subarachnoid hemorrhage. AJNR Am J Neuroradiol 2008;29:79–85.

91. Kanazawa R, Kato M, Ishikawa K, et al. Convenience of the computed tomography perfusion

method for cerebral vasospasm detection after subarachnoid hemorrhage. Surg Neurol 2007;67: 604–11.

92. Wintermark M, Ko NU, Smith WS, et al. Vasospasm after subarachnoid hemorrhage: utility of perfusion CT and CT angiography on diagnosis and management. AJNR Am J Neuroradiol 2006;27:26–34.

93. Novak L, Emri M, Molnar P, et al. Regional cerebral (18)FDG uptake during subarachnoid hemorrhage induced vasospasm. Neurol Res 2006;28(8): 864–70.

94. Frykholm P, Andersson JL, Langstrom B, et al. Haemodynamic and metabolic disturbances in the acute states of subarachnoid haemorrhage demonstrated by PET. Acta Neurol Scand 2004; 109(1):25–32.

95. Minhas PS, Menon DK, Smielewski P, et al. Positron emission tomographic cerebral perfusion disturbances and transcranial Doppler findings among patients with neurological deterioration after subarachnoid hemorrhage. Neurosurgery 2003; 52(5):1017–22.

96. Egge A, Sjoholm H, Waterloo K, et al. Serial single-photon emission computed tomographic and transcranial Doppler measurements for evaluation of vasospasm after aneurysmal subarachnoid hemorrhage. Neurosurgery 2005;57:237–42.

97. Leclerc X, Fichten A, Gauvrit JY, et al. Symptomatic vasospasm after subarachnoid haemorrhage: assessment of brain damage by diffusion and perfusion-weighted MRI and single-photon emission computed tomography. Neuroradiology 2002;44(7):610–6.

98. Tranquart F, Ades PE, Groussin P, et al. Postoperative assessment of cerebral blood flow in subarachnoid hemorrhage by means of 99mTc-HMPAO tomography. Eur J Nucl Med 1993;20: 53–8.

99. Ohkuma H, Suzuki S, Kudo K, et al. Cortical blood flow during cerebral vasospasm after aneurysmal subarachnoid hemorrhage: three-dimensional N-isopropyl-p-[(123)I]iodoamphetamine single photon emission CT findings. AJNR Am J Neuroradiol 2003;24(3):444–50.

100. Rajendran JG, Lewis DH, Newell DW, et al. Brain SPECT used to evaluate vasospasm after subarachnoid hemorrhage: correlation with angiography and transcranial Doppler. Clin Nucl Med 2001;26:125–30.

101. Kincaid MS, Souter MJ, Treggiari MM, et al. Accuracy of transcranial Doppler ultrasonography and single-photon emission computed tomography in the diagnosis of angiographically demonstrated cerebral vasospasm. J Neurosurg 2009;110:67–72.

102. Powsner RA, O'Tuama LA, Jabre A, et al. SPECT imaging in cerebral vasospasm following subarachnoid hemorrhage. J Nucl Med 1998;39: 765–9.

103. Koopman K, Teune LK, ter Laan M. An often unrecognized cause of thunderclap headache: reversible cerebral vasoconstriction syndrome. J Headache Pain 2008;9(6):389–91.

104. Johmura Y, Takahashi T, Kuroiwa Y. Acute mountain sickness with reversible vasospasm. J Neurol Sci 2007;263(1–2):174–6.

105. Marshall N, Maclaurin WA, Koulouris G. MRA captures vasospasm in fatal migrainous infarction. Headache 2007;47(2):280–3.

106. Tamatani S, Sasaki O, Takeuchi S, et al. Detection of delayed cerebral vasospasm, after rupture of intracranial aneurysms, by magnetic resonance angiography. Neurosurgery 1997;40(4):748–53.

107. Grieve JP, Stacey R, Moore E, et al. Artefact on MRA following aneurysm clipping: an in vitro study and prospective comparison with conventional angiography. Neuroradiology 1999;41(9):680–6.

108. Weidauer S, Lanfermann H, Raabe A, et al. Impairment of cerebral perfusion and infarct patterns attributable to vasospasm after aneurysmal subarachnoid hemorrhage: a prospective MRI and DSA study. Stroke 2007;38:1831–6.

109. Hertel F, Walter C, Bettag M, et al. Perfusion-weighted magnetic resonance imaging in patients with vasospasm: a useful new tool in the management of patients with subarachnoid hemorrhage. Neurosurgery 2005;56(1):28–35.

110. Ohtonari T, Kakinuma K, Kito T, et al. Diffusion-perfusion mismatch in symptomatic vasospasm after subarachnoid hemorrhage. Neurol Med Chir (Tokyo) 2008;48(8):331–6.

111. Hattingen E, Blasel S, Dettmann E, et al. Perfusion-weighted MRI to evaluate cerebral autoregulation in aneurysmal subarachnoid haemorrhage. Neuroradiology 2008;50(11):929–38.

Medical Complications After Subarachnoid Hemorrhage

Katja E. Wartenberg, MD, PhD[a],
Stephan A. Mayer, MD, FCCM[b],*

KEYWORDS

- Medical complications • Subarachnoid hemorrhage
- Fever • Anemia • Blood transfusion • Hyperglycemia

SCOPE OF THE PROBLEM

Aneurysmal subarachnoid hemorrhage (SAH) is a devastating disease with high disability and mortality rates.[1–3] Poor clinical grade on admission,[1,4–10] age,[1,4–9] large aneurysm size (>10 mm),[1,4,8] and aneurysm rebleeding[1,6,11] have the strongest impact on outcome after SAH. Delayed cerebral ischemia (DCI) from vasospasm, which affects 20% to 45% of patients, is also associated with poor neurologic outcome and mortality[12,13] and has traditionally been the primary focus of postoperative management.

In addition to the direct effects of the initial hemorrhage and secondary neurologic complications, SAH predisposes to medical complications that can have an impact on outcome[14] and increase hospital length of stay.[15] In the placebo arm of the Cooperative Aneurysm Study investigating the effects of nicardipine, the five most frequent non-neurologic complications were anemia, hypertension, cardiac arrhythmia, fever, and electrolyte abnormalities. The proportion of deaths directly attributable to medical complications (23%) was comparable to that of vasospasm (23%) and rebleeding (22%).[16] Advances in aneurysm treatment and neurologic intensive care, with increasing emphasis on aggressive treatment of poor-grade patients, have in all likelihood increased the relative importance of medical complications after SAH.

PHYSIOLOGIC DERANGEMENTS AFTER SUBARACHNOID HEMORRHAGE

Abnormalities of oxygenation, glucose metabolism, and hemodynamic instability within 24 hours of onset can potentially exacerbate the initial brain injury caused by SAH. Claassen and colleagues created a SAH–Physiologic Derangement Score (SAH-PDS), range 0–8, from the most abnormal measurements of physiologic variables (listed in **Table 1**) within 24 hours of admission after SAH. The SAH-PDS was independently associated with death or moderate-to-severe disability (**Fig. 1**) and was found superior to the Acute Physiology and Chronic Health Evaluation-2 (APACHE-2) score and the systemic inflammatory response syndrome (SIRS) score for quantifying the immediate impact of physiologic derangements on outcome after SAH.[1] Interventions to correct these abnormalities, such as tight blood pressure control, brain tissue oxygen tension–directed therapy, or continuous insulin infusion, are reasonable therapeutic options given the current state of knowledge and are promising targets for future safety and feasibility trials.

a Department of Neurology, Neurologic Intensive Care Unit, Martin-Luther University, Halle-Wittenberg, Leipzig, Germany
b Neurological Intensive Care Unit, Division of Neurocritical Care, Neurological Institute, Columbia-Presbyterian Medical Center, 710 West 168th Street, Box 39, New York, NY 10032, USA
* Corresponding author.
E-mail address: sam14@columbia.edu

Neurosurg Clin N Am 21 (2010) 325–338
doi:10.1016/j.nec.2009.10.012

Table 1
Components of the subarachnoid hemorrhage physiologic derangement score

Physiologic Derangement	Pathophysiology	Points
Arterioalveolar gradient >125 mm Hg	Oxygen deficits from neurogenic pulmonary edema, aspiration pneumonia, or neurogenic stunned myocardium with pump failure	3
Serum bicarbonate <20 mm Hg	Lactic acidosis due to acute severe peripheral vasoconstriction and skeletal muscle glycolsysis	2
Serum glucose >180 mg/dL	Elevated blood glucose exacerbates ischemic brain injury, increases the risk of infection and critical illness myopathy, or may be a marker of severe brain injury	2
Mean arterial pressure of <70 or >130 mm Hg	Hypotension may be related to neurogenic stunned myocardium or vasodilatory shock triggered by brainstem compression, and can aggravate ischemic injury when autoregulation is impaired. Hypertension reflects the initial severity of brain injury and may provoke autoregulatory breakthrough and aggravate intracranial hypertension	1
Maximum score		8

Data from Claassen J, Vu A, Kreiter KT, et al. Effect of acute physiologic derangements on outcome after subarachnoid hemorrhage. Crit Care Med 2004;32:832.

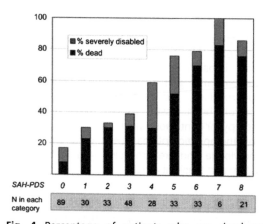

Fig. 1. Percentage of patients who are dead or severely disabled at 3 month by physiologic derangement score (SAH-PDS). (*Modified from* Claassen J, Vu A, Kreiter KT, et al. Effect of acute physiologic derangements on outcome after subarachnoid hemorrhage. Crit Care Med 2004;32:832; with permission.)

FEVER

Fever ($\geq$38.3°C) is a frequent event in patients with SAH (41%–54% [**Fig. 2**])[14,17–21] and in neuro-critical care patients in general.[22] In patients with acute brain injury, fever leads to worsening of cerebral edema and intracranial pressure (ICP),[23,24] exacerbation of ischemic injury,[25] increased oxygen consumption,[24] and depressed level of consciousness.[18] Fever after SAH is associated with an increased risk of symptomatic vasospasm,[18–20] an increased length of intensive care unit (ICU) and hospital stay,[15] and death and poor functional outcome at 3 months (**Fig. 3**).[8,14,18–21] Fever after SAH has been shown to have adverse effects on the outcome of good- and poor-grade patients.[18,19] Infection (pneumonia, urinary tract infection, catheter-related bacteremia, upper respiratory tract infection, or meningitis) can be identified in approximately 34% to 75% of febrile SAH patients,[17,20,21] meaning that in the remainder, the cause of fever may be central or neurogenic in etiology. In the Columbia University SAH Outcomes Project, only pneumonia was significantly associated with fever

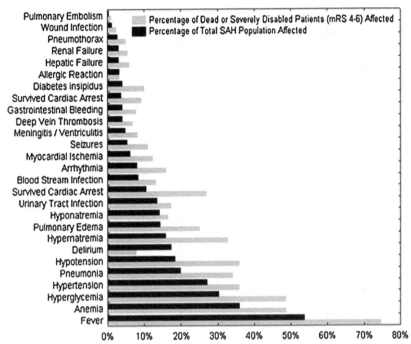

Fig. 2. Frequency of medical complications in the total SAH population (576 patients) and among patients with poor outcome (220 patients, mRS 4–6) at 4 months. (*From* Wartenberg KE, Schmidt JM, Claassen J, et al. Impact of medical complications on outcome after subarachnoid hemorrhage. Crit Care Med 2006;34:617; with permission.)

burden.[18] In a cohort of SAH patients, fever was classified as noninfectious in 48% and infectious in only 18% based on rigorous review of cultures and diagnostic studies. Noninfectious fever tended to present earlier in the hospital course (<72 hours after NICU admission).[26] It has been

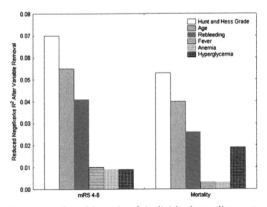

Fig. 3. Attributable risk of individual predictors to poor outcome (mRS 4–6) and mortality (based on Nagelkerke R^2 values). (*From* Wartenberg KE, Schmidt JM, Claassen J, et al. Impact of medical complications on outcome after subarachnoid hemorrhage. Crit Care Med 200634:617; with permission.)

hypothesized that altered rhythmic daily temperature variability may help differentiate central from infectious in SAH patients.[27]

Risk factors for fever burden in the Columbia University SAH Outcomes Project patient group included poor Hunt-Hess scale grade at admission, loss of consciousness at ictus, thick cisternal clot, intraventricular hemorrhage, and aneurysm size greater than or equal to 10 mm.[18] Fever is also a common component of the SIRS, which has been shown to predict poor outcome in SAH patients.[28] Brain stem herniation, hydrocephalus treated with external ventricular drainage, cerebral infarction, respiratory failure, anemia requiring transfusion, and hyperglycemia are neurologic and medical complications with a significant association with fever burden.[18,19] In one study, coiling as method of aneurysm repair was related to a higher fever burden than clipping or no repair, for reasons that are unclear.[19]

Fever control can now be achieved by means of core temperature–controlled surface or endovascular cooling devices. Feasibility studies have demonstrated safe and effective fever control in febrile SAH patients refractory to acetaminophen treatment using the Celsius Control System (Innercool, San Diego, California),[29] and a single-center randomized trial showed a 75% reduction in fever burden with the systemic surface cooling system Artic Sun temperature management system (Medivance, Louisville, Colorado) compared with regular water-circulating cooling blankets.[30] This confirms the results of a previous multicenter fever control trial comparing a catheter-based heat exchange system, the CoolGard/CoolLine system (Alsius, Irvine, California) plus standard fever management (using acetaminophen, ibuprofen, and cooling blankets) to standard therapy alone, in which a 64% reduction in fever burden was shown.[31] Induction of normothermia with ice packs and external surface cooling devices in poor-grade SAH patients significantly reduced episodes of metabolic crisis in the brain assessed by microdialysis markers of metabolic stress (lactate/pyruvate ratio) and ICP.[32]

With all forms of cooling, the main barrier to achieving target temperature is insufficient control of shivering, which increases the systemic rate of metabolism and resting energy expenditure and may potentially adversely affect cerebral oxygenation and ICP.[29,33] Shivering is a natural mechanism that allows the body to create heat if the body temperature falls below the hypothalamic set point. Potentially effective antishivering interventions are listed in **Table 2**. Treatment guidelines almost universally advocate maintenance normothermia for all febrile patients with SAH, despite little evidence to support this practice in the form of randomized controlled trials. Prospective clinical trials are needed to assess the impact of fever control with systemic surface or intravascular cooling devices on development of vasospasm and outcome after SAH.

ANEMIA

Anemia after SAH most likely results from the combined effects of an SAH-related reduction in red blood cell mass,[34] combined with blood losses due to phlebotomy and invasive procedures[35] and hemodilution from fluid administration. In the Columbia University SAH Outcomes Project,

---

Table 2
Interventions to relieve shivering during active cooling to achieve normothermia with systemic surface or intravascular cooling devices

Method	Dosage	Mechanism
Basic management		
Acetaminophen	650–1000 mg orally every 6 h	Inhibits prostaglandin synthesis
Buspirone	30–60 mg orally every 8 h	5HT-1A partial agonist
Skin counterwarming	Bair Hugger polar air cooling system (Arizant Healthcare, Eden Prairie, Minnesota)	Vasodilatation
Advanced management for persistent shivering		
Magnesium sulfate	0.5–1.0 g/h for target serum magnesium of 1–2 mmol/L (3–4 g/dL)	Vasodilatation, muscle relaxant
Clonidine	15–60 µg/h (1.5–3 µg/kg/h)	α2-Receptor agonist
Dexmedetomidine	0.2–1.5 mcg/kg/h	α2-Receptor agonist
Meperidine (Pethidine)	25–100 mg IV every 4 h (or 0.5–1.0 mg/kg/h)	Opioid receptor agonist
Fentanyl	50–200 µg/h	Opioid receptor agonist
Advanced management for refractory shivering		
Propofol	75–300 mg/h	Impairs vasoconstriction and shivering threshold
Rocuronium/Vecuronium	Usually not needed and should be avoided because of increased incidence of critical illness polyneuropathy	Paralysis

Data from Wartenberg KE, Mayer SA. Use of induced hypothermia for neuroprotection: indications and application. Future Neurology 2008;3:325.

anemia (defined as hemoglobin <9 g/dL requiring blood transfusion) occurred in 36% of 580 patients and was the second most common medical complication (see **Fig. 2**).[14] Anemia treated with blood transfusion is associated with an increased risk of mortality and poor functional outcome after SAH (see **Fig. 3**).[14,36] Administration of blood during the hospital course after aneurysm surgery has also been associated with an increased risk of asymptomatic and symptomatic angiographically-confirmed vasospasm.[36] In another study, blood transfusions were significantly related to poor outcome among SAH patients with vasospasm.[37] Multimodality monitoring in SAH patients demonstrated local brain tissue hypoxia (partial pressure of brain tissue oxygen [PbtO$_2$] <20 mm Hg) and cell energy dysfunction (lactate/pyruvate ratio >40) when hemoglobin values were less than 9 g/dL; however, the relationship to functional outcome was not investigated.[38]

It is unclear whether anemia after SAH reflects general illness severity[39] or whether the treatment for anemia—blood transfusion—directly contributes to poor outcome. History of blood transfusion was an independent risk factor for intracerebral hemorrhage and mortality after SAH in the Japan Collaborative Cohort Study and Miyako Study.[40–42] Higher hemoglobin values have been associated with a lower risk of cerebral infarction and poor outcome 3 months after SAH in two different SAH cohorts.[43,44] Blood transfusions were related to poor functional outcome but not to mortality in one of these studies[43] and were not considered in the other.[44] Kramer and colleagues investigated the effect of anemia as opposed to blood transfusion on secondary complications and outcome after SAH. Blood transfusion, but not anemia, was an independent risk factor for poor functional outcome and was associated with the development of nosocomial infections but not symptomatic vasospasm.[45] The extent of hemoglobin decline during the first 2 weeks after SAH predicted unfavorable outcome (severe disability or death) and was more pronounced in patients with poor-grade SAH, thick cisternal clot, and intraventricular hemorrhage.[46]

In the Columbia University SAH Outcomes Project, blood transfusions were related to symptomatic vasospasm and were a significant predictor of mortality and poor functional outcome at 3 months; anemia alone did not influence long-term functional outcome in this model.[47] Packed red blood cells (PRBCs) may be depleted of nitric oxide,[48] an endogenous vasodilator that can reverse vasoconstriction of cerebral arteries and arterioles during vasospasm. Thus, transfusion may result in dilution of this active vasodilatory substance and may subsequently worsen microcirculatory flow or predispose to intraoperative cerebral vasoconstriction.[36] Transfusion of PRBCs increases local PbtO$_2$ in the majority of patients with SAH and other severe brain injuries independent of cerebral perfusion pressure and peripheral oxygen saturation.[49] Stored PRBCs, however, have proinflammatory effects and may induce immunodysfunction and neutrophilic and polymorphonuclear cytotoxicity,[50] which may exacerbate the inflammatory component of vasospasm[36] and increase the risk of nosocomial infections.[45] The deformability of stored and transfused erythrocytes is reduced, which may lead to microvascular sludging,[51] and adenosine triphosphate and 2,3 diphosphoglycerate are depleted,[51] resulting in altered oxygen binding and release.[36] Transfused erythrocytes also contain free iron, which can increase oxidative processes in its ferrous form[52] and aggravate ischemia.[36] Storage of PRBCs has been found to generate interleukin 1,-6, and -8 and tumor necrosis factor α,[53] which may augment ischemia and edema formation.[36]

Given the potential detrimental effects of PRBC transfusion, efforts directed at more physiologic transfusion triggers derived from brain multimodality monitoring (**Table 3**)[54] and prevention of anemia after SAH with erythropoietin should be investigated,[55] particularly given its potential neuroprotective properties.[56]

HYPERGLYCEMIA

Hyperglycemia is known to have an adverse effect on outcome in patients with acute ischemic stroke and to increase the likelihood of intracranial hemorrhage after thrombolytic therapy.[57–59] In the authors' SAH population, hyperglycemia exceeding 11.1 mmol/L (200 mg/dL) occurred in 30% (see **Fig. 2**) and was a significant predictor of poor functional outcome and mortality 3 months after SAH[14] (see **Fig. 3**). Depending on the definition, hyperglycemia can be found in 30% to 100% of SAH patients.[14,60–62] When mean daily glucose burden between day 0 and 10 after SAH (defined as the area under the curve above 5.8 mmol/L or 105 mg/dL) was analyzed, hyperglycemia was found to have a stronger association with moderate-to-severe disability (modified Rankin scale [mRS] 4–6) and loss of high-level functional independence than with mortality, suggesting that hyperglycemia may contribute to physical deconditioning.[63] The relationship of admission or sustained hyperglycemia with poor outcome up to 1 year after SAH has also been confirmed in many other studies.[9,60,62,64–67] In the Intraoperative Hypothermia for Aneurysm

Table 3
Suggestion for transfusion practices in neurocritical care patients

Hemoglobin (g/dL)	Packed Red Blood Cell Transfusion
>10	No
≤7	Yes
7–10	Yes, if PbtO$_2$ <20 mm Hg or rSo$_2$ <60% or cardiopulmonary reserve decreased

Abbreviations: PbtO$_2$, partial pressure of brain tissue oxygen; rSo$_2$, regional oxygen saturation measured by near-infrared spectroscopy.

Data from Leal-Noval SR, Munoz-Gomez M, Murillo-Cabezas F. Optimal hemoglobin concentration in patients with subarachnoid hemorrhage, acute ischemic stroke and traumatic brain injury. Curr Opin Crit Care 2008;14:156.

Surgery Trial population, glucose concentration at the time of aneurysm clipping did not have an impact on mortality at 3 months but influenced physical impairment measured with the National Institute of Health Stroke Scale, neuropsychologic outcome, and intensive care unit (ICU) length-of-stay.[68] In a smaller study of poor-grade SAH patients, early clinical improvement was seen in patients with an admission glucose level less than 180 mg/dL (10.0 mmol/L).[69,70] Elevated blood glucose concentrations on arrival at the hospital were associated with aneurysm rebleeding in another SAH patient cohort.[71] Increased glucose levels, however, have not always been found to be significant predictors of poor functional status after SAH.[66,72,73]

A retrospective study of 352 SAH patients at Massachusetts General Hospital identified hyperglycemia (mean inpatient blood glucose value ≥140 mg/dL) in 73% of patients and found an association with symptomatic vasospasm and increased ICU length of stay.[74] The risk of symptomatic vasospasm was also increased with hyperglycemia in a cohort of 244 SAH patients.[75] These findings are in contrast to an analysis of 175 patients in which elevated admission glucose was not predictive of DCI, despite an association with poor outcome at 3 months.[76]

Acute brain injury may lead to a transient generalized stress response, which may explain the high frequency of hyperglycemia after SAH in patients who do not have a history of diabetes mellitus.[62–64,72,75,77] Hyperglycemia was significantly linked to a history of diabetes mellitus, older age, poor clinical grade, brainstem compression from herniation, higher APACHE-2 physiologic derangement scores, and pulmonary decompensation (congestive heart failure, respiratory failure, and pneumonia) in the authors' study.[63] Hyperglycemia is thus just one aspect of a generalized stress response after SAH which can be triggered by a variety of different perturbations.[78] Activation of the sympathetic nervous system increases glucagon, corticosteroids, and somatotropin secretion and decreases insulin release, all of which cause stress-related hyperglycemia.[60,62,79] When this acute metabolic response is persistent, hyperglycemia predicts the occurrence of symptomatic vasospasm, DCI, and poor long-term functional outcome.[64,66,74,75]

The proportion of SAH patients with known diabetes mellitus is relatively low (<10%).[63,80–82] Although hyperglycemia after SAH could simply reflect pre-existing impaired glucose tolerance, previous multivariate analyses have shown that the relationship between hyperglycemia and poor outcome is independent of other known predictors.[1,9,14,60,62–64,66,76] In a study utilizing monitoring of cerebral metabolism with microdialysis, SAH patients with an acute focal neurologic deficit from the initial hemorrhage or procedural complications had systemic hyperglycemia associated with low cerebral glucose levels and elevated lactate/pyruvate ratios (indicating cerebral metabolic crisis) and worse functional outcome at 6 months.[83] In another microdialysis study, episodes of hyperglycemia were frequent in patients with an acute neurologic deficit or DCI and were accompanied by elevated cerebral glycerol levels (a marker of cellular membrane degradation).[84] Blood glucose elevations have also been related to increased lactate/pyruvate ratios, which argues for increased anaerobic glycolysis with saturation of normal aerobic glucose metabolism.[67] This process may exacerbate tissue injury from ischemia.[60,62,76,79]

Strict glucose control has been associated with reduced ICP, duration of mechanical ventilation, hospital length of stay, use of vasopressors, frequency of seizures, and diabetes insipidus in critically ill neurologic patients.[85] Intensive insulin therapy has also been shown to reduce mortality in critically ill surgical ICU patients[86] and in medical ICU patients admitted for more than 2 days.[87] The first randomized trial of management of poststroke hyperglycemia with 24-hour glucose-potassium-insulin infusions failed to demonstrate a benefit on mortality or disability 90 days after stroke.[88] Glycemic control in this study, however, was poor and the duration of treatment to short. A small trial of 55 patients with SAH demonstrated the feasibility and safety of continuous insulin infusion for glucose values exceeding 7 mmol/L with glucose assessments performed every 2 hours.[89] Retrospective analyses of changes in clinical practice through introduction of insulin protocols in SAH patients showed that achievement of tight glycemic control significantly reduced the likelihood of poor outcome at 6 months[73] and have identified hypoglycemia (<60 mg/dL) as an independent predictor of mortality at discharge.[90]

Balanced against the potential benefits of tight glycemic control is evidence that normalization of hyperglycemia can lead to critical brain tissue hypoglycemia after severe grain injury. Intravenous (IV) insulin therapy for a target glucose of 140 mg/dL (7.8 mmol/L) resulted in critical decreases of cerebral glucose measured with microdialysis at 3 hours after initiation of treatment in 79% of SAH patients, predominantly in men and in the elderly.[91] At 8 hours after start of insulin infusion, cerebral glycerol increased reflecting tissue damage or cellular distress.[91] Another microdialysis study of patients with SAH and other form of brain injury demonstrated a link between high insulin dosages, brain tissue hypoglycemia, elevated lactate/pyruvate ratios, and increased mortality at discharge.[92] Reductions of cerebral glucose has been found related to peri-ischemic cortical depolarizations.[93]

Bilotta and colleagues conducted the first randomized trial of intensive insulin therapy (target glucose 80–120 mg/dL) versus standard insulin therapy (target glucose 80–220 mg/dL) in 78 SAH patients. Rate of infection was the primary outcome measure and was significantly reduced from 42% to 27% in the intensive insulin group. Mortality at 6 months and the frequency of vasospasm were comparable in the two groups.[94] More safety trials of intensive insulin therapy in SAH with cerebral glucose monitoring and efficacy studies exploring long-term outcomes are needed.

CARDIAC COMPLICATIONS

Hypertension treated with continuous IV medication (27%) and hypotension requiring pressors (18%) are common medical complications after SAH, whereas life-threatening arrhythmia (8%), myocardial ischemia (6%), and successful resuscitation from cardiac arrest (4%) rarely occur (see **Fig. 2**).[14,95] The development of clinically relevant arrhythmias, mostly atrial fibrillation or flutter, is associated with older age, a prior history of arrhythmia, hyperglycemia, brainstem herniation, myocardial infarction, a longer NICU length of stay, and poor functional outcome.[95] Electrocardiographic (ECG) abnormalities are found frequently in SAH patients (92%) and encompass ST segment alterations (15%–67%), T-wave changes (12%–92%), prominent U waves (4%–52%), QT prolongation (11%–66%), conduction abnormalities (7.5%), sinus bradycardia (16%) and sinus tachycardia (8.5%).[95–99] Although the majority of these abnormalities do not directly contribute to morbidity or mortality,[97] ST-segment depression has been linked to DCI and poor 3-month outcome.[98]

Neurogenic stunned myocardium is the most severe form of cardiac injury after SAH. It is caused by excessive release of catecholamines from the cardiac sympathetic nerves triggered by the bleeding event and is characterized histologically by myocardial contraction band necrosis.[100] The clinical syndrome of severe acute stunned myocardium is characterized by transient lactic acidosis, cardiogenic shock, pulmonary edema, widespread T-wave inversions with a prolonged QT interval, and reversible left ventricular wall motion abnormalities.[100] Echocardiography and myocardial scintigraphy were performed in 42 SAH patients with stunned myocardium and demonstrated normal myocardial perfusion in all patients, with functional sympathetic denervation and myocardial necrosis in those with regional wall motion abnormalities.[101] In a prospective study of 300 SAH patients undergoing echocardiography and troponin I monitoring, 26% had evidence of regional wall motion abnormalities which persisted through day 9 after SAH. Catecholamine levels obtained on admission were not significantly related to left ventricular dysfunction[102] but might not have been obtained early enough.

The most important risk factor for neurogenic stunned myocardium is poor clinical grade.[102–104] Other predictors of cardiac dysfunction after SAH include older age,[103,105] adrenoreceptor polymorphisms,[106] and prior cocaine or amphetamine use.[102] Tachycardia[102] and troponin I elevation[102,103,105] are almost universally found at in conjunction with neurogenic myocardial stunning. A recent meta-analysis suggested that cardiac abnormalities on ECG, echocardiography, and troponin measurements are related to DCI, poor outcome, and death up to 6 months after SAH.[107,108]

Minor cardiac enzyme elevations occur frequently after SAH, but their significance has been unclear. An analysis of 253 SAH patients deemed at risk for myocardial injury on the basis of acute ECG changes revealed admission cardiac troponin I elevation in 68%. Troponin levels peaked at 1.7 days, and left ventricular wall motion abnormalities were identified by echocardiography in 22%. Higher Hunt-Hess scale grade on admission, intraventricular hemorrhage or global cerebral edema on admission CT, loss of consciousness at ictus, and more severe admission physiologic derangements were predictive of increased cardiac troponin I levels.[109] The association with intracranial pathology underlines a neurogenic mechanism of cardiac injury. Troponin I elevation was associated with a significantly increased risk of abnormal left ventricular wall motion abnormalities on echocardiography, pulmonary edema, hypotension requiring vasopressors, DCI, and cerebral infarction from any cause. Troponin I elevation also independently predicted severe disability and death at hospital discharge.[109]

Another prospective study found peak troponin I levels of greater than 1.0 μg/L in 20% of 223 SAH patients. In this study, female gender, larger body surface area, Hunt-Hess scale grade greater than or equal to 3, higher heart rate, lower systolic blood pressure, higher doses of phenylephrine, higher left ventricular mass index (increased oxygen demand), and shorter time from SAH symptom onset were independently associated with troponin I elevations within 2 days after symptom onset.[104] This again emphasizes the importance of the initial brain injury as a cause of cardiovascular dysfunction and demonstrates the adverse effects of myocardial injury on cardiac performance. Further research is required to test cardio- and neuroprotective intensive care management strategies, which may improve outcome after SAH.

PULMONARY COMPLICATIONS

Pulmonary dysfunction with a disturbance of gas exchange (increased alveolar-arterial oxygen gradient) occurs in up to 80% of SAH patients.[110] Pulmonary complications did not have an independent impact on neurologic outcome at 3 months in the authors' study but remained common and troubling. The most frequent pulmonary complications included pneumonia (20%), pulmonary edema (14%), pneumothorax (3%), and pulmonary embolism (0.3%) (see **Fig. 2**).[14] A previous analysis linked pulmonary events to an increased frequency of symptomatic vasospasm after SAH, but this may reflect fluid overload related to more aggressive hypertensive-hypervolemic therapy.[111]

Pulmonary complications have been independently linked to prolonged ICU and hospital length of stay and poor functional outcome and mortality in several studies.[1,16,110,112,113] A recent study found that bilateral pulmonary infiltrates developed in 27% of 245 SAH patients, mostly due to neurogenic pulmonary edema, aspiration pneumonia, and pulmonary edema complicating neurogenic stunned myocardium. Only pulmonary infiltrates developing later than 72 hours after ictus were predictive of death or poor functional outcome. Pulmonary infiltrates were also associated with poor neurologic grade on admission, symptomatic vasospasm, and prolonged length of hospital stay. Adult respiratory distress syndrome was present in 11% of patients but was not found to be an independent predictor of poor outcome.[113]

Other investigators have linked the delayed onset of pulmonary edema with cardiac dysfunction,[114] presumably reflecting the effects of aggressive volume resuscitation over time. The relationship of pulmonary edema and cardiac dysfunction with ischemic ECG changes, myocardial enzyme elevation, and the requirement of catecholamines for blood pressure stabilization was also confirmed by another group.[115] Adult respiratory distress syndrome and acute lung injury after SAH has been associated with troponin I elevations, length of ICU and hospital stay, and poor short-term (2-week) but not long-term outcome.[15,116] Acute lung injury in SAH patients has also been associated with poor Hunt-Hess scale grade, PRBC transfusion, and severe sepsis.[112]

A review suggested that use of a pulmonary artery catheter during the vasospasm period in SAH targeting an optimal pulmonary artery wedge pressure (10–14 mm Hg) may decrease the incidence of pulmonary edema and sepsis and decrease mortality.[117] The role of newer noninvasive hemodynamic monitoring systems that can provide measurements of stroke volume variability, extravascular lung water, global end-diastolic volume, and other novel measures deserves further study.

ELECTROLYTE ABNORMALITIES

Hyponatremia occurs in 20% to 40% of SAH patients. It may be the result of the syndrome of inappropriate excretion of antidiuretic hormone (SIADH), cerebral salt wasting, or both. Hypomagnesemia (40%), hypokalemia (25%), and hypernatremia (20%) are also common after SAH.[118–120] In the authors' study, hyponatremia (<130 mEq/L) occurred in only 14% (see **Fig. 2**), which might be explained by the standard administration of isotonic saline solutions and strict avoidance of free water in te management protocol.[14] Hyponatremia did not have any prognostic significance in the authors' study[14] nor has it in others.[120,121]

Although SIADH and cerebral salt wasting are often conceptualized as mutually exclusive, it is most likely that SAH patients experience a physiologic shift that favors both of these derangements simultaneously. In a prospective study investigating hyponatremia and volume status in poor-grade SAH patients, hypovolemia and increased natriuresis were identified as the underlying cause consistent with cerebral salt wasting syndrome.[122] Atrial and brain natriuretic peptide levels were initially increased as a consequence of the bleeding event, and renin and aldosterone levels tend to be suppressed by the acute sympathetic response. This can result in excessive sodium excretion and hyponatremia unless these losses are replaced by with isotonic crystalloid fluid resuscitation. Adrenomedullin, a vasorelaxant peptide, can also induce natriuresis, is elevated in the cerebrospinal fluid of SAH patients, and has been correlated with the occurrence of hyponatremia and delayed ischemic deficits.[123]

A surge in arginine vasopressin levels also occurs as a direct consequence of the initial bleeding event, resulting in SIADH physiology. As a result, free water tends to be retained if it is given, resulting in dilutional hyponatremia. In one SAH cohort treated with hypotonic fluids, hyponatremia presented in 57% of patients.[121] A Japanese group conducted a randomized, placebo-controlled trial of IV hydrocortisone (300 mg every 6 hours for 10 days) to maintain serum sodium greater than 140 mmol/L and central venous pressure of 8 to 12 cm H_2O. Sodium excretion and urine volume were significantly decreased, and plasma osmolarity was more often in the normal range in the hydrocortisone compared with the placebo group. This treatment had no impact on symptomatic vasospasm or functional outcome at 30 days, however. In addition, hyperglycemia, hypokalemia, and hypoproteinemia complicated the use of hydrocortisone.[124] Conivaptan is an arginine vasopressin receptor antagonist (V_{1A}/V_2) approved for the treatment of euvolemic and hypervolemic hyponatremia.[125] Initial reports of it use in neurocritical care patients with hyponatremia have yielded promising results.[126]

The 22% frequency of hypernatremia in the authors' study almost certainly reflects treatment for cerebral edema with mannitol or hypertonic saline solutions and, therefore, was mostly iatrogenic. Only 4% of the authors' patients experienced diabetes insipidus.[14] The incidence of hypernatremia was 22% in another SAH patient population and had strong associations with left ventricular dysfunction and troponin I elevation,[118] suggesting a contribution to cardiorespiratory compromise. Hypernatremia may be a marker for extracerebral organ dysfunction and treatment of intracranial hypertension.

INFECTIONS

The most common infections during the course of SAH include pneumonia (20%), urinary tract infection (13%), blood stream infection (8%), and bacterial meningitis/ventriculitis (5%) (see **Fig. 2**).[14,127] After adjusting for length of ICU stay, older age, poor clinical grade, and mechanical ventilation are risk factors for pneumonia.[14] Blood stream infections were associated with mechanical ventilation, urinary tract infections with female gender and central line use, and meningitis/ventriculitis with the presence of intraventricular hemorrhage and extraventricular drainage.[127] In the Columbia University SAH Outcomes Project, none of these infections was independently predictive of poor functional outcome and mortality at 3 months.[14] Pneumonia and urinary tract infection, however, were significantly related to the occurrence of DCI[127] and all infectious complications were associated with prolonged ICU and hospital length of stay.[15,127]

SIRS was diagnosed on at least one ICU day in 87% of 276 SAH patients, and was linked to higher clinical grade, higher Fisher grade, elevated admission mean arterial pressure, aneurysm size, and clipping of the aneurysm. The SIRS burden on the first 4 days after SAH was a strong predictor for the development of symptomatic vasospasm and of poor outcome (death or discharge to nursing facility).[128] The extent to which SIRS physiology after SAH results from nosocomial infection is unclear, but it is an important contributing factor. Hospital-acquired infections should be prevented and treated aggressively, and further studies of the associations of infections with neurologic complications are needed.

OTHER RARE COMPLICATIONS

Renal failure, hepatic failure, deep vein thrombosis, and gastrointestinal bleeding occurred at a frequency of less than 5% in the authors' SAH population and had no impact on neurologic outcome (see **Fig. 2**).[14]

A study of 100 SAH patients found that a low ratio between the lowest platelet during the hospitalization and the admission platelet count (<0.7) an independent predictor of symptomatic vasospasm.[129] This may be explained by increased platelet aggregation and substance release from the platelets resulting in microcirculatory dysfunction.[129] The role of platelet dysfunction in the pathophysiology of vasospasm requires additional studies.

SUMMARY

For years, efforts to improve the outcome of SAH have focused on treatment and prevention of neurologic complications, such as acute hydrocephalus, aneurysm rebleeding, and delayed ischemia from vasospasm. As survival has improved, however, it is increasingly recognized that medical complications also contribute substantially to many of the poor outcomes that result from this disease. Fever, anemia requiring transfusion, hyperglycemia, and neurogenic stunned myocardium seem to have the strongest association with poor outcome after SAH, thus seem to be the most promising candidates for novel treatment strategies.

Given the available evidence, the authors recommend the practice of maintaining normothermia with systemic cooling devices and normoglycemia with continuous insulin infusion monitoring for hypoglycemia, with care to avoid critical brain tissue hypoglycemia in comatose patients undergoing microdialysis monitoring. Phlebotomy should be minimized to prevent severe anemia, and the authors recommend a restrictive blood transfusion policy (a trigger of <7.0 mg/dL) unless active cerebral or myocardial ischemia is present, in which case a transfusion trigger of less than 10.0 mg/dL is reasonable. Measurement of troponin I levels on admission is a sensitive means of identifying neurogenic cardiac injury and identifies patients at risk for cardiopulmonary complications, DCI, and poor outcome. Cardiovascular hemodynamic monitoring may help optimize hypertensive-hemodynamic therapy in patients with neurogenic cardiopulmonary dysfunction. Prevention and treatment of nosocomial infections should be a focus of all neurointensivists. Vasopressin receptor antagonists may aid in combating hyponatremia in SAH patients in the future. Multimodal monitoring pf brain tissue oxygen, microdialysis, cerebral blood flow, and intracortical electroencephalography may become helpful in the assessment, diagnosis, and treatment of medical complications once more experience is gained.

REFERENCES

1. Claassen J, Vu A, Kreiter KT, et al. Effect of acute physiologic derangements on outcome after subarachnoid hemorrhage. Crit Care Med 2004; 32:832.
2. Juvela S. Prehemorrhage risk factors for fatal intracranial aneurysm rupture. Stroke 2003;34:1852.
3. Qureshi AI, Suarez JI, Bhardwaj A, et al. Early predictors of outcome in patients receiving hypervolemic and hypertensive therapy for symptomatic vasospasm after subarachnoid hemorrhage. Crit Care Med 2000;28:824.
4. Claassen J, Carhuapoma JR, Kreiter KT, et al. Global cerebral edema after subarachnoid hemorrhage: frequency, predictors, and impact on outcome. Stroke 2002;33:1225.
5. Kassell NF, Torner JC, Haley EC Jr, et al. The international cooperative study on the timing of aneurysm surgery. Part 1: overall management results. J Neurosurg 1990;73:18.
6. Niskanen MM, Hernesniemi JA, Vapalahti MP, et al. One-year outcome in early aneurysm surgery: prediction of outcome. Acta Neurochir (Wien) 1993;123:25.
7. Rabinstein AA, Friedman JA, Nichols DA, et al. Predictors of outcome after endovascular treatment of cerebral vasospasm. AJNR Am J Neuroradiol 2004;25:1778.
8. Rosengart AJ, Schultheiss KE, Tolentino J, et al. Prognostic factors for outcome in patients with aneurysmal subarachnoid hemorrhage. Stroke 2007;38:2315.
9. Sarrafzadeh A, Haux D, Kuchler I, et al. Poor-grade aneurysmal subarachnoid hemorrhage: relationship of cerebral metabolism to outcome. J Neurosurg 2004;100:400.
10. Torner JC, Kassell NF, Wallace RB, et al. Preoperative prognostic factors for rebleeding and survival in aneurysm patients receiving antifibrinolytic therapy: report of the Cooperative Aneurysm Study. Neurosurgery 1981;9:506.
11. Naidech AM, Janjua N, Kreiter KT, et al. Predictors and impact of aneurysm rebleeding after subarachnoid hemorrhage. Arch Neurol 2005;62:410.
12. Baldwin ME, Macdonald RL, Huo D, et al. Early vasospasm on admission angiography in patients with aneurysmal subarachnoid hemorrhage is a predictor for in-hospital complications and poor outcome. Stroke 2004;35:2506.
13. Claassen J, Bernardini GL, Kreiter K, et al. Effect of cisternal and ventricular blood on risk of delayed cerebral ischemia after subarachnoid hemorrhage: the Fisher scale revisited. Stroke 2001;32:2012.
14. Wartenberg KE, Schmidt JM, Claassen J, et al. Impact of medical complications on outcome after subarachnoid hemorrhage. Crit Care Med 2006; 34:617.
15. Naidech AM, Bendok BR, Tamul P, et al. Medical complications drive length of stay after brain

hemorrhage: a cohort study. Neurocrit Care 2009; 10:11.

16. Solenski NJ, Haley EC Jr, Kassell NF, et al. Medical complications of aneurysmal subarachnoid hemorrhage: a report of the multicenter, cooperative aneurysm study. Participants of the Multicenter Cooperative Aneurysm Study. Crit Care Med 1995;23:1007.

17. Dorhout Mees SM, Luitse MJ, van den Bergh WM, et al. Fever after aneurysmal subarachnoid hemorrhage: relation with extent of hydrocephalus and amount of extravasated blood. Stroke 2008;39: 2141.

18. Fernandez A, Schmidt JM, Claassen J, et al. Fever after subarachnoid hemorrhage: risk factors and impact on outcome. Neurology 2007;68:1013.

19. Naidech AM, Bendok BR, Bernstein RA, et al. Fever burden and functional recovery after subarachnoid hemorrhage. Neurosurgery 2008;63:212.

20. Oliveira-Filho J, Ezzeddine MA, Segal AZ, et al. Fever in subarachnoid hemorrhage: relationship to vasospasm and outcome. Neurology 2001;56: 1299.

21. Todd MM, Hindman BJ, Clarke WR, et al. Perioperative fever and outcome in surgical patients with aneurysmal subarachnoid hemorrhage. Neurosurgery 2009;64:897.

22. Commichau C, Scarmeas N, Mayer SA. Risk factors for fever in the neurologic intensive care unit. Neurology 2003;60:837.

23. Rossi S, Zanier ER, Mauri I, et al. Brain temperature, body core temperature, and intracranial pressure in acute cerebral damage. J Neurol Neurosurg Psychiatr 2001;71:448.

24. Stocchetti N, Protti A, Lattuada M, et al. Impact of pyrexia on neurochemistry and cerebral oxygenation after acute brain injury. J Neurol Neurosurg Psychiatr 2005;76:1135.

25. Ginsberg MD, Busto R. Combating hyperthermia in acute stroke: a significant clinical concern. Stroke 1998;29:529.

26. Rabinstein AA, Sandhu K. Non-infectious fever in the neurological intensive care unit: incidence, causes and predictors. J Neurol Neurosurg Psychiatr 2007;78:1278.

27. Kirkness CJ, Burr RL, Thompson HJ, et al. Temperature rhythm in aneurysmal subarachnoid hemorrhage. Neurocrit Care 2008;8:380.

28. Yoshimoto Y, Tanaka Y, Hoya K. Acute systemic inflammatory response syndrome in subarachnoid hemorrhage. Stroke 2001;32:1989.

29. Badjatia N, O'Donnell J, Baker JR, et al. Achieving normothermia in patients with febrile subarachnoid hemorrhage: feasibility and safety of a novel intravascular cooling catheter. Neurocrit Care 2004;1:145.

30. Mayer SA, Kowalski RG, Presciutti M, et al. Clinical trial of a novel surface cooling system for fever control in neurocritical care patients. Crit Care Med 2004;32:2508.

31. Diringer MN. Treatment of fever in the neurologic intensive care unit with a catheter-based heat exchange system. Crit Care Med 2004;32:559.

32. Oddo M, Frangos S, Milby A, et al. Induced normothermia attenuates cerebral metabolic distress in patients with aneurysmal subarachnoid hemorrhage and refractory Fever. Stroke 2009;40:1913.

33. Badjatia N, Strongilis E, Gordon E, et al. Metabolic impact of shivering during therapeutic temperature modulation: the Bedside Shivering Assessment Scale. Stroke 2008;39:3242.

34. Solomon RA, Post KD, McMurtry JG 3rd. Depression of circulating blood volume in patients after subarachnoid hemorrhage: implications for the management of symptomatic vasospasm. Neurosurgery 1984;15:354.

35. Burnum JF. Medical vampires. N Engl J Med 1986; 314:1250.

36. Smith MJ, Le Roux PD, Elliott JP, et al. Blood transfusion and increased risk for vasospasm and poor outcome after subarachnoid hemorrhage. J Neurosurg 2004;101:1.

37. Di Georgia MA, Deogaonkar A, Ondrejka J, et al. Blood transfusion following subarachnoid hemorrhage worsens outcome [abstract]. Stroke 2005; 36:506.

38. Oddo M, Milby A, Chen I, et al. Hemoglobin concentration and cerebral metabolism in patients with aneurysmal subarachnoid hemorrhage. Stroke 2009;40:1275.

39. Nguyen BV, Bota DP, Melot C, et al. Time course of hemoglobin concentrations in nonbleeding intensive care unit patients. Crit Care Med 2003;31:406.

40. Pham TM, Fujino Y, Tokui N, et al. Mortality and risk factors for stroke and its subtypes in a cohort study in Japan. Prev Med 2007;44:526.

41. Yamada S, Koizumi A, Iso H, et al. History of blood transfusion before 1990 is a risk factor for stroke and cardiovascular diseases: the Japan collaborative cohort study (JACC study). Cerebrovasc Dis 2005;20:164.

42. Yamada S, Koizumi A, Iso H, et al. Risk factors for fatal subarachnoid hemorrhage: the Japan Collaborative Cohort Study. Stroke 2003;34:2781.

43. Naidech AM, Drescher J, Ault ML, et al. Higher hemoglobin is associated with less cerebral infarction, poor outcome, and death after subarachnoid hemorrhage. Neurosurgery 2006; 59:775.

44. Naidech AM, Jovanovic B, Wartenberg KE, et al. Higher hemoglobin is associated with improved outcome after subarachnoid hemorrhage. Crit Care Med 2007;35:2383.

45. Kramer AH, Gurka MJ, Nathan B, et al. Complications associated with anemia and blood transfusion

in patients with aneurysmal subarachnoid hemorrhage. Crit Care Med 2008;36:2070.

46. Kramer AH, Zygun DA, Bleck TP, et al. Relationship between hemoglobin concentrations and outcomes across subgroups of patients with aneurysmal subarachnoid hemorrhage. Neurocrit Care 2009;10:157.

47. Wartenberg KE, Fernandez A, Frontera JA, et al. Impact of red blood cell transfusion on outcome after subarachnoid hemorrhage [abstract]. Crit Care Med 2007;34:A124.

48. McMahon TJ, Moon RE, Luschinger BP, et al. Nitric oxide in the human respiratory cycle. Nat Med 2002;8:711.

49. Smith MJ, Stiefel MF, Magge S, et al. Packed red blood cell transfusion increases local cerebral oxygenation. Crit Care Med 2005;33:1104.

50. Moore EE. Blood substitutes: the future is now. J Am Coll Surg 2003;196:1.

51. Berezina TL, Zaets SB, Morgan C, et al. Influence of storage on red blood cell rheological properties. J Surg Res 2002;102:6.

52. Forceville X, Plouvier E, Claise C. The deleterious effect of heminic iron in transfused intensive care unit patients. Crit Care Med 2002;30:1182.

53. Shanwell A, Kristiansson M, Remberger M, et al. Generation of cytokines in red cell concentrates during storage is prevented by prestorage white cell reduction. Transfusion 1997;37:678.

54. Leal-Noval SR, Munoz-Gomez M, Murillo-Cabezas F. Optimal hemoglobin concentration in patients with subarachnoid hemorrhage, acute ischemic stroke and traumatic brain injury. Curr Opin Crit Care 2008;14:156.

55. Corwin HL, Gettinger A, Pearl RG, et al. Efficacy of recombinant human erythropoietin in critically ill patients: a randomized controlled trial. JAMA 2002;288:2827.

56. Siren AL, Fratelli M, Brines M, et al. Erythropoietin prevents neuronal apoptosis after cerebral ischemia and metabolic stress. Proc Natl Acad Sci U S A 2001;98:4044.

57. Bruno A, Biller J, Adams HP Jr, et al. Acute blood glucose level and outcome from ischemic stroke. Trial of ORG 10172 in Acute Stroke Treatment (TOAST) Investigators. Neurology 1999;52:280.

58. Kase CS, Furlan AJ, Wechsler LR, et al. Cerebral hemorrhage after intra-arterial thrombolysis for ischemic stroke: the PROACT II trial. Neurology 2001;57:1603.

59. Leigh R, Zaidat OO, Suri MF, et al. Predictors of hyperacute clinical worsening in ischemic stroke patients receiving thrombolytic therapy. Stroke 2004;35:1903.

60. Alberti O, Becker R, Benes L, et al. Initial hyperglycemia as an indicator of severity of the ictus in poor-grade patients with spontaneous subarachnoid hemorrhage. Clin Neurol Neurosurg 2000;102:78.

61. Lanzino G. Plasma glucose levels and outcome after aneurysmal subarachnoid hemorrhage. J Neurosurg 2005;102:974.

62. Lanzino G, Kassell NF, Germanson T, et al. Plasma glucose levels and outcome after aneurysmal subarachnoid hemorrhage. J Neurosurg 1993;79:885.

63. Frontera JA, Fernandez A, Claassen J, et al. Hyperglycemia after SAH: predictors, associated complications, and impact on outcome. Stroke 2006;37:199.

64. Kruyt ND, Biessels GJ, de Haan RJ, et al. Hyperglycemia and clinical outcome in aneurysmal subarachnoid hemorrhage: a meta-analysis. Stroke 2009;40:e424.

65. Lee SH, Lim JS, Kim N, et al. Effects of admission glucose level on mortality after subarachnoid hemorrhage: a comparison between short-term and long-term mortality. J Neurol Sci 2008;275:18.

66. McGirt MJ, Woodworth GF, Ali M, et al. Persistent perioperative hyperglycemia as an independent predictor of poor outcome after aneurysmal subarachnoid hemorrhage. J Neurosurg 2007;107:1080.

67. Schlenk F, Vajkoczy P, Sarrafzadeh A. Inpatient hyperglycemia following aneurysmal subarachnoid hemorrhage: relation to cerebral metabolism and outcome. Neurocrit Care 2009;11:56.

68. Pasternak JJ, McGregor DG, Schroeder DR, et al. Hyperglycemia in patients undergoing cerebral aneurysm surgery: its association with long-term gross neurologic and neuropsychological function. Mayo Clin Proc 2008;83:406.

69. Sato M, Nakano M, Asari J, et al. Admission blood glucose levels and early change of neurological grade in poor-grade patients with aneurysmal subarachnoid haemorrhage. Acta Neurochir (Wien) 2006;148:623.

70. Schlenk F, Frieler K, Nagel A, et al. Cerebral microdialysis for detection of bacterial meningitis in aneurysmal subarachnoid hemorrhage patients: a cohort study. Crit Care 2009;13:R2.

71. Kitsuta Y, Suzuki N, Sugiyama M, et al. Changes in level of consciousness and association with hyperglycemia as tool for predicting and preventing re-bleeding after spontaneous subarachnoid hemorrhage. Prehosp Disaster Med 2006;21:190.

72. Dorhout Mees SM, van Dijk GW, Algra A, et al. Glucose levels and outcome after subarachnoid hemorrhage. Neurology 2003;61:1132.

73. Latorre JG, Chou SH, Nogueira RG, et al. Effective glycemic control with aggressive hyperglycemia management is associated with improved outcome in aneurysmal subarachnoid hemorrhage. Stroke 2009;40:1644.

74. Badjatia N, Topcuoglu MA, Buonanno FS, et al. Relationship between hyperglycemia and symptomatic vasospasm after subarachnoid hemorrhage. Crit Care Med 2005;33:1603.

75. Charpentier C, Audibert G, Guillemin F, et al. Multivariate analysis of predictors of cerebral vasospasm occurrence after aneurysmal subarachnoid hemorrhage. Stroke 1999;30:1402.

76. Juvela S, Siironen J, Kuhmonen J. Hyperglycemia, excess weight, and history of hypertension as risk factors for poor outcome and cerebral infarction after aneurysmal subarachnoid hemorrhage. J Neurosurg 2005;102:998.

77. Allport LE, Butcher KS, Baird TA, et al. Insular cortical ischemia is independently associated with acute stress hyperglycemia. Stroke 2004;35:1886.

78. Macmillan CS, Grant IS, Andrews PJ. Pulmonary and cardiac sequelae of subarachnoid haemorrhage: time for active management? Intensive Care Med 2002;28:1012.

79. Capes SE, Hunt D, Malmberg K, et al. Stress hyperglycemia and prognosis of stroke in nondiabetic and diabetic patients: a systematic overview. Stroke 2001;32:2426.

80. Adams HP Jr, Putman SF, Kassell NF, et al. Prevalence of diabetes mellitus among patients with subarachnoid hemorrhage. Arch Neurol 1984;41:1033.

81. Feigin VL, Rinkel GJ, Lawes CM, et al. Risk factors for subarachnoid hemorrhage: an updated systematic review of epidemiological studies. Stroke 2005;36:2773.

82. Inagawa T. Risk factors for aneurysmal subarachnoid hemorrhage in patients in Izumo city, Japan. J Neurosurg 2005;102:60.

83. Kerner A, Schlenk F, Sakowitz O, et al. Impact of hyperglycemia on neurological deficits and extracellular glucose levels in aneurysmal subarachnoid hemorrhage patients. Neurol Res 2007;29:647.

84. Schlenk F, Nagel A, Graetz D, et al. Hyperglycemia and cerebral glucose in aneurysmal subarachnoid hemorrhage. Intensive Care Med 2008;34:1200.

85. Van den Berghe G, Schoonheydt K, Becx P, et al. Insulin therapy protects the central and peripheral nervous system of intensive care patients. Neurology 2005;64:1348.

86. van den Berghe G, Wouters P, Weekers F, et al. Intensive insulin therapy in the critically ill patients. N Engl J Med 2001;345:1359.

87. Van den Berghe G, Wilmer A, Hermans G, et al. Intensive insulin therapy in the medical ICU. N Engl J Med 2006;354:449.

88. Gray CS, Hildreth AJ, Sandercock PA, et al. Glucose-potassium-insulin infusions in the management of post-stroke hyperglycaemia: the UK Glucose Insulin in Stroke Trial (GIST-UK). Lancet Neurol 2007;6:397.

89. Bell DA, Strong AJ. Glucose/insulin infusions in the treatment of subarachnoid haemorrhage: a feasibility study. Br J Neurosurg 2005;19:21.

90. Thiele RH, Pouratian N, Zuo Z, et al. Strict glucose control does not affect mortality after aneurysmal subarachnoid hemorrhage. Anesthesiology 2009;110:603.

91. Schlenk F, Graetz D, Nagel A, et al. Insulin-related decrease in cerebral glucose despite normoglycemia in aneurysmal subarachnoid hemorrhage. Crit Care 2008;12:R9.

92. Oddo M, Schmidt JM, Carrera E, et al. Impact of tight glycemic control on cerebral glucose metabolism after severe brain injury: a microdialysis study. Crit Care Med 2008;36:3233.

93. Hopwood SE, Parkin MC, Bezzina EL, et al. Transient changes in cortical glucose and lactate levels associated with peri-infarct depolarisations, studied with rapid-sampling microdialysis. J Cereb Blood Flow Metab 2005;25:391.

94. Bilotta F, Spinelli A, Giovannini F, et al. The effect of intensive insulin therapy on infection rate, vasospasm, neurologic outcome, and mortality in neurointensive care unit after intracranial aneurysm clipping in patients with acute subarachnoid hemorrhage: a randomized prospective pilot trial. J Neurosurg Anesthesiol 2007;19:156.

95. Frontera JA, Parra A, Shimbo D, et al. Cardiac arrhythmias after subarachnoid hemorrhage: risk factors and impact on outcome. Cerebrovasc Dis 2008;26:71.

96. Brouwers PJ, Wijdicks EF, Hasan D, et al. Serial electrocardiographic recording in aneurysmal subarachnoid hemorrhage. Stroke 1989;20:1162.

97. Sakr YL, Lim N, Amaral AC, et al. Relation of ECG changes to neurological outcome in patients with aneurysmal subarachnoid hemorrhage. Int J Cardiol 2004;96:369.

98. Schuiling WJ, Algra A, de Weerd AW, et al. ECG abnormalities in predicting secondary cerebral ischemia after subarachnoid haemorrhage. Acta Neurochir (Wien) 2006;148:853.

99. van den Bergh WM, Algra A, Rinkel GJ. Electrocardiographic abnormalities and serum magnesium in patients with subarachnoid hemorrhage. Stroke 2004;35:644.

100. Mayer SA, Fink ME, Homma S, et al. Cardiac injury associated with neurogenic pulmonary edema following subarachnoid hemorrhage. Neurology 1994;44:815.

101. Banki NM, Kopelnik A, Dae MW, et al. Acute neurocardiogenic injury after subarachnoid hemorrhage. Circulation 2005;112:3314.

102. Kothavale A, Banki NM, Kopelnik A, et al. Predictors of left ventricular regional wall motion

abnormalities after subarachnoid hemorrhage. Neurocrit Care 2006;4:199.

103. Schuiling WJ, Dennesen PJ, Tans JT, et al. Troponin I in predicting cardiac or pulmonary complications and outcome in subarachnoid haemorrhage. J Neurol Neurosurg Psychiatr 2005;76:1565.

104. Tung P, Kopelnik A, Banki N, et al. Predictors of neurocardiogenic injury after subarachnoid hemorrhage. Stroke 2004;35:548.

105. Urbaniak K, Merchant AI, Amin-Hanjani S, et al. Cardiac complications after aneurysmal subarachnoid hemorrhage. Surg Neurol 2007;67:21.

106. Zaroff JG, Pawlikowska L, Miss JC, et al. Adrenoceptor polymorphisms and the risk of cardiac injury and dysfunction after subarachnoid hemorrhage. Stroke 2006;37:1680.

107. van der Bilt IA, Hasan D, Vandertop WP, et al. Impact of cardiac complications on outcome after aneurysmal subarachnoid hemorrhage: a meta-analysis. Neurology 2009;72:635.

108. Wartenberg KE, Mayer SA. Use of induced hypothermia for neuroprotection: indications and application. Future Neurol 2008;3:325.

109. Naidech AM, Kreiter KT, Janjua N, et al. Cardiac troponin elevation, cardiovascular morbidity, and outcome after subarachnoid hemorrhage. Circulation 2005;112:2851.

110. Gruber A, Reinprecht A, Gorzer H, et al. Pulmonary function and radiographic abnormalities related to neurological outcome after aneurysmal subarachnoid hemorrhage. J Neurosurg 1998;88:28.

111. Friedman JA, Pichelmann MA, Piepgras DG, et al. Pulmonary complications of aneurysmal subarachnoid hemorrhage. Neurosurgery 2003;52:1025.

112. Kahn JM, Caldwell EC, Deem S, et al. Acute lung injury in patients with subarachnoid hemorrhage: incidence, risk factors, and outcome. Crit Care Med 2006;34:196.

113. Kramer AH, Bleck TP, Dumont AS, et al. Implications of early versus late bilateral pulmonary infiltrates in patients with aneurysmal subarachnoid hemorrhage. Neurocrit Care 2009;10:20.

114. McLaughlin N, Bojanowski MW, Girard F, et al. Pulmonary edema and cardiac dysfunction following subarachnoid hemorrhage. Can J Neurol Sci 2005;32:178.

115. Muroi C, Keller M, Pangalu A, et al. Neurogenic pulmonary edema in patients with subarachnoid hemorrhage. J Neurosurg Anesthesiol 2008; 20:188.

116. Naidech AM, Bassin SL, Garg RK, et al. Cardiac troponin I and acute lung injury after subarachnoid hemorrhage. Neurocrit Care 2009;11:177.

117. Kim DH, Haney CL, Van Ginhoven G. Reduction of pulmonary edema after SAH with a pulmonary artery catheter-guided hemodynamic management protocol. Neurocrit Care 2005;3:11.

118. Fisher LA, Ko N, Miss J, et al. Hypernatremia predicts adverse cardiovascular and neurological outcomes after SAH. Neurocrit Care 2006;5:180.

119. McGirt MJ, Blessing R, Nimjee SM, et al. Correlation of serum brain natriuretic peptide with hyponatremia and delayed ischemic neurological deficits after subarachnoid hemorrhage. Neurosurgery 2004;54:1369.

120. Qureshi AI, Suri MF, Sung GY, et al. Prognostic significance of hypernatremia and hyponatremia among patients with aneurysmal subarachnoid hemorrhage. Neurosurgery 2002;50:749.

121. Sherlock M, O'Sullivan E, Agha A, et al. The incidence and pathophysiology of hyponatraemia after subarachnoid haemorrhage. Clin Endocrinol (Oxf) 2006;64:250.

122. Audibert G, Steinmann G, de Talance N, et al. Endocrine response after severe subarachnoid hemorrhage related to sodium and blood volume regulation. Anesth Analg 1922;108:2009.

123. Kubo Y, Ogasawara K, Kakino S, et al. Cerebrospinal fluid adrenomedullin concentration correlates with hyponatremia and delayed ischemic neurological deficits after subarachnoid hemorrhage. Cerebrovasc Dis 2008;25:164.

124. Katayama Y, Haraoka J, Hirabayashi H, et al. A randomized controlled trial of hydrocortisone against hyponatremia in patients with aneurysmal subarachnoid hemorrhage. Stroke 2007; 38:2373.

125. Zeltser D, Rosansky S, van Rensburg H, et al. Assessment of the efficacy and safety of intravenous conivaptan in euvolemic and hypervolemic hyponatremia. Am J Nephrol 2007;27:447.

126. Wright WL, Asbury WH, Gilmore JL, et al. Conivaptan for hyponatremia in the neurocritical care unit. Neurocrit Care 2008;11:6.

127. Frontera JA, Fernandez A, Schmidt JM, et al. Impact of nosocomial infectious complications after subarachnoid hemorrhage. Neurosurgery 2008;62:80.

128. Dhar R, Diringer MN. The burden of the systemic inflammatory response predicts vasospasm and outcome after subarachnoid hemorrhage. Neurocrit Care 2008;8:404.

129. Hirashima Y, Hamada H, Kurimoto M, et al. Decrease in platelet count as an independent risk factor for symptomatic vasospasm following aneurysmal subarachnoid hemorrhage. J Neurosurg 2005;102:882.

Cerebral Salt Wasting: Pathophysiology, Diagnosis, and Treatment

Alan H. Yee, DO[a],*, Joseph D. Burns, MD[b], Eelco F.M. Wijdicks, MD, PhD[a]

KEYWORDS

• Natriuresis • Natriuretic factors • Hyponatremia • SIADH

Hyponatremia can be a vexing problem for those who care for critically ill neurologic patients. Although seemingly simple at first glance, the accurate diagnosis and effective treatment of hyponatremia can be complex. The chief difficulty in this setting often lies in determining what is driving the fall in serum sodium concentration. Cerebral salt wasting (CSW) is a disorder of sodium and water handling that occurs as a result of cerebral disease in the setting of normal kidney function. It is characterized by hyponatremia in association with hypovolemia and, as the name implies, is caused by natriuresis. In routine clinical practice, distinguishing this condition from the more familiar syndrome of inappropriate secretion of antidiuretic hormone (SIADH) can be quite difficult. Nonetheless, this task is crucial because treatments for the two conditions are fundamentally different. Accordingly, it is important for physicians caring for critically ill neurologic patients to have a thorough understanding of this disorder. This article reviews the pathophysiology of CSW. Building on these basic concepts, a rational approach to its diagnosis and treatment is outlined.

HISTORICAL ASPECTS

Early studies of hyponatremia in patients with cerebral disease published in the 1950s described the presence of polyuria, elevated urinary sodium levels, and dehydration despite the presence of a low serum sodium concentration and adequate fluid intake. This syndrome was termed "cerebral salt wasting." At the time, CSW was suspected to be the major cause of hyponatremia in patients with central nervous system (CNS) injury. Shortly after its original description, however, a syndrome of euvolemic hyponatremia associated with normal urine output and inappropriately high levels of antidiuretic hormone (ADH) was described in a patient with bronchogenic carcinoma.[1] This was later termed as the "syndrome of inappropriate antidiuretic hormone release." Following this discovery and over the subsequent 30 years, hyponatremia that developed in patients with neurologic diseases, such as subarachnoid hemorrhage (SAH), was generally attributed to SIADH.[2–6] Beginning in the 1980s, several key studies[7–9] challenged this concept by demonstrating in patients with aneurysmal SAH a syndrome of low blood volume, natriuresis with a net negative sodium balance, and high urinary output, which was consistent with CSW and not SIADH. These publications led to the modern acceptance of CSW as an important cause of hyponatremia in patients with brain injury and to important research that followed investigating the pathophysiologic disturbances of salt and water homeostasis in patients with neurologic disease.

CLINICAL RELEVANCE

Hyponatremia is frequently encountered in patients with neurologic disease. A recent analysis

a Department of Neurology, Mayo Clinic, 200 1st Street SW, Rochester, MN 55905, USA
b Department of Neurology, Boston University, School of Medicine, 72 East Concord Street, Neurology C-3, Boston, MA 02118, USA
* Corresponding author.
E-mail address: Yee.Alan@mayo.edu

Neurosurg Clin N Am 21 (2010) 339–352
doi:10.1016/j.nec.2009.10.011
1042-3680/10/$ – see front matter

of 316 patients with aneurysmal SAH detected hyponatremia in 57% of patients.[10] Although previous investigators have reported lower frequencies,[11–13] it is still the most commonly encountered electrolyte disturbance in the neurologic intensive care unit. Adding to its importance are the occasional serious consequences of severe hyponatremia, which include seizures and worsening of cerebral edema. Although hyponatremia is most reliably encountered in patients with aneurysmal SAH,[7,11,14–30] it occurs not infrequently in a variety of other conditions affecting the CNS, such as head trauma,[31–43] malignancy,[44–51] and CNS infections,[14,52–60] and it has been reported in the postoperative neurosurgical setting.[61–64]

The proportion of patients with hyponatremia related to neurologic disease who have CSW, as opposed to SIADH or some other etiology of hyponatremia, is substantial, although the exact frequency is not clear. This issue has been studied most rigorously in patients with aneurysmal SAH.[7,11,14–30] In one study, up to 67% (six of nine) of patients with hyponatremia after rupture of an intracranial aneurysm had CSW as the etiology of low sodium levels[7] and 75% (six of eight) of SAH cases in other reports.[8] A study by Sherlock and colleagues,[10] however, found that only 6.5% (4 of 62) of patients who presented with spontaneous SAH and subsequent hyponatremia had CSW as the cause of abnormally low sodium levels in their unselected cohort.

The discrepancy between reported prevalence rates may be a result of differences in study population size. Much has to do with how CSW and volume depletion are defined, however, when comparing the available data. There is no universally accepted gold standard in defining extracellular volume status or the specific parameters that classify cerebral-induced salt wasting, leading to significant variability between studies in the definition of low intravascular volume. For example, some authors have measured central venous pressure (CVP),[10] whereas others have used isotope-labeled albumin.[65] This difference in method of volume assessment and inclusion criteria could result in varying frequencies of affected subjects among studies, and it is unclear whether direct comparisons can be made between such trials when identifying CSW as an underlying etiology in hypovolemic hyponatremic patients. An additional confounding variable underlying the variability of CSW frequency in the literature is the manner in which sodium depletion is defined. Single versus multiple day cumulative sodium balance measurements often yield significantly different results.[66]

CSW has been associated with a host of other CNS diseases in addition to aneurysmal SAH. Although the precise frequency of CSW in traumatic brain injury is unknown, an association has been described in a number of case reports, small case series, and studies with greater sample size that incorporate several categories of neurologically injured patients of which small numbers of traumatic brain injury patients are included.[8,31–33,67,68] The best estimate can be found in a study by Vespa,[35] in which 5% to 10% of traumatic brain injury patients were found to have salt wasting. The hyponatremia that frequently occurs in patients with infectious meningitis is most often attributed to SIADH. In several studies of this condition, however, a number of patients with moderate to severe volume contraction in association with decreased serum sodium levels, a combination that is most consistent with CSW, were identified. Further proof of an association between CSW and meningitis is provided by the observation of a trend toward more adverse outcomes in children with meningitis-associated hyponatremia who were treated with fluid restriction.[52,59,69,70] Other conditions in which natriuresis with volume contraction and hyponatremia occur include transsphenoidal pituitary surgery and cerebral malignancies, such as primitive neuroectodermal tumors with intraventricular dissemination, carcinomatous meningitis, glioma, and primary CNS lymphoma.[44–51,61,62]

PATHOPHYSIOLOGY OF CSW

Despite the clear association between the presence of CSW and severe neurologic disease, the mechanism underlying this association has not yet been clearly identified. Maintenance of body sodium and water homeostasis is a vital physiologic process. It is largely governed by intricate interactions between the autonomic nervous system and humoral factors that influence the kidney's handling of sodium and water. Disruption of the normal interactions between these systems can generate sodium and water dysregulation at the level of the nephron, thereby leading to more global alterations in sodium and water homeostasis. It has been postulated that interference of sympathetic input to the kidney and the presence of abnormally elevated circulating natriuretic factors noted after cerebral injury can lead to CSW (**Fig. 1**).

Physiology of the Renin-Angiotensin-Aldosterone System

The renin-angiotensin-aldosterone system (RAAS) is a hormonal pathway involving several enzymatic

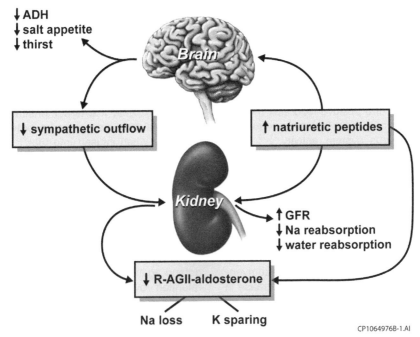

Fig. 1. Proposed mechanisms responsible for the production of CSW syndrome. ADH, antidiuretic hormone; GFR, glomerular filtration rate; K, potassium; Na, sodium; R-AG II, renin-angiotensin II. (*From* Rabinstein A, Wijdicks E. Hyponatremia in critically ill neurologic patients. Neurologist 2003;9:6; with permission.)

steps and humoral factors that serve a central role in maintaining whole-body sodium and water homeostasis. Renin is a circulating enzyme produced and stored within the kidney and released in response to low systemic and renal arterial perfusion. Once released, it initiates a series of intricate sequential enzymatic steps involving the well known angiotensin-converting enzyme, the ultimate product of which is the formation of angiotensin II (AT II). This potent vasopressor agent has immediate effects on blood pressure by influencing the constrictive properties of peripheral vasculature, increasing sympathetic tone, and stimulating the release of ADH.[71] Moreover, AT II augments renal blood flow to maintain an appropriate rate of glomerular filtration and the percentage of sodium to be filtered. AT II activity is not only critical in the immediate phases of hemodynamic control but is also instrumental in maintaining serum sodium homeostasis by stimulating the release of aldosterone, a key mineralocorticoid released from the adrenal gland that regulates extracellular fluid volume and serum potassium concentration (eg, nephrogenic excretion). Aldosterone ultimately causes sodium retention and a subsequent increase in serum sodium concentration by binding to specific intracellular receptors at the distal tubule and collecting ducts, leading to a cascade of protein synthesis of sodium channels, sodium-potassium pumps, and

their regulatory proteins all of which are critical in transepithelial sodium transport.[72]

In large part, effective extracellular fluid volume and sodium concentration are maintained by the degree of RAAS activity and aldosterone bioavailability. These are increased during periods of low circulating fluid volume and decreased when total circulating volume is sufficient or elevated. A cerebrally mediated mechanism for influencing the RAAS system, and renal salt and water handling, may exist.[73–75] Several publications have documented the scientific progress and understanding of a local intrinsic tissue-specific RAAS model within the CNS and its influence on renal physiology.[71,76,77] As detailed in a key review by DiBona,[78] intrinsic cerebral AT II production likely exists and its presence within the CNS conceivably can influence renal sympathetic nerve activity and baroreflex control. More specifically, neuronal synthesis of this hormone within the paraventricular nucleus is released in the rostral ventrolateral medulla, a critical structure in the autonomic neural control of circulation. Tonic excitation of the rostral ventrolateral medulla influenced by endogenous AT II has been postulated to result in increased peripheral sympathetic tone.

Sympathetic Nervous System Hypothesis

The sympathetic nervous system plays an important role in the regulation of sodium and water handling in the kidney.[78–80] In the face of intravascular volume contraction, the autonomic nervous system responds by increasing sympathetic nervous system tone. This in turn induces secretion of renin from the kidneys, subsequently leading to elevations in the bioavailability of AT II and aldosterone, stimulating sodium and water retention. By way of a positive feedback mechanism, AT II itself may have a role in regulating sympathetic nervous system activity.[71,72] Data from animal studies suggest that this circulating hormone can directly affect the sympathetic nervous system by binding to specific receptors located within discrete subcortical brain structures, specifically the subfornical organ and area postrema.[78,81,82] Direct projections from the subfornical organ to the paraventricular nucleus are thought to influence rostral ventrolateral medulla activity indirectly. Activation of these circumventricular regulatory centers leads to an increase in the activity of the sympathetic nervous system by their projections to preganglionic sympathetic neurons within the intermediolateral cell column of the spinal cord[82,83]; the ultimate effect is an increase in mean arterial pressure and retention of sodium and water by the kidney.

Peters and coworkers[14] originally hypothesized that disruption of CNS influence on renal salt and water balance mechanisms could potentially disturb the kidney's ability to maintain proper sodium homeostasis. Specific renal innervation by the sympathetic nervous system, however, was not discovered until nearly 20 years later.[79] Peters' theory was then expanded on to explain more specifically the mechanism underlying CSW.[15,21,22,84] According to this theory, loss of adrenergic tone to the nephron has two important consequences. First, it leads to a decrease in renin secretion by the juxtaglomerular cells, thereby causing decreased levels of aldosterone and decreased sodium reabsorption at the proximal convoluted tubule. Second, it causes dilatation of the afferent arteriole, leading to increased glomerular filtration of plasma and sodium. The failure of renin and aldosterone levels to rise in the setting of CSW-associated volume contraction has been considered to be evidence in favor of this hypothesis. This hypothesis has one crucial flaw: acute CNS injury typically leads to a surge and not a decrease in sympathetic tone during the immediate phases of injury. This is demonstrated by such phenomena as neurogenic pulmonary edema and myocardial dysfunction, which occur because of dramatic sympathetic outflow during periods of severe CNS stress.[85] It has yet to be demonstrated that the changes in the interactions between the autonomic nervous system and the kidneys that are needed to produce a salt-wasting state actually occur in the setting of acute cerebral injury.

Natriuretic Peptide Theory

Natriuretic peptides were initially discovered in the early 1980s after it was demonstrated that atrial myocardial extracts induced a potent natriuretic response when infused into rats.[86] At about the same time, early studies investigating the pathogenesis of sodium and extracellular volume disturbances in patients with SAH led to the hypothesis that a natriuretic factor may be involved.[8,9,17] Subsequently, a number of specific natriuretic substances were identified and their biologic effects have been intensely studied.

Natriuretic peptides are molecules that normally defend against periods of excess water and salt retention by antagonizing the RAAS system, promoting vascular relaxation, and inhibiting excess sympathetic outflow and the generation of vasoconstrictor peptides.[87] Four main natriuretic peptides with purported associations with CSW have been identified: (1) atrial natriuretic peptide (ANP); (2) brain-natriuretic peptide (BNP); (3) C-type natriuretic peptide (CNP); and (4) the more recently discovered dendroaspis natriuretic peptide (DNP).[88,89] Although the former three natriuretic peptides have shown some expressivity within the CNS, each peptide has a unique predominant tissue-specific site of production: ANP and DNP from the myocardial atria; BNP from within the ventricles of the heart; and CNP from the telencephalon, hypothalamus, and endothelium.[90–93]

The natriuretic peptides all have similar, potent effects on the regulation of cardiovascular homeostasis by influencing vascular tone and sodium and water homeostasis. They cause relaxation of vascular smooth muscle thereby leading to dilatation of arteries and veins, most likely by dampening vascular sympathetic tone.[94–96] A similar effect on the nephron's afferent tubule leads to increased filtration of water and sodium through the glomerulus. These molecules also have direct renal tubule natriuretic and diuretic effects by inhibiting angiotensin-induced sodium reabsorption at the proximal convoluted tubule and antagonizing the action of vasopressin at the collecting ducts, respectively.[97,98] Interestingly, local production of natriuretic peptides within the adrenal medulla[99,100] has been demonstrated and might have paracrine inhibitory effects on mineralocorticoid synthesis.[100] This paracrine mechanism might explain why in patients with CSW aldosterone and renin levels fail to rise despite the presence of hypovolemia. Clearance and inactivation of circulating natriuretic peptides occurs by two main mechanisms: endocytosis once bound to a C-type natriuretic receptor (which has equal affinity for the family of peptides),[101,102] and degradation and cleavage by endopeptidases within the vasculature and renal tubular system.[87]

These characteristics of natriuretic peptides make them ideal candidate mediators that may serve as a key link between CNS injury and the development of CSW. Several studies have demonstrated that a rise in serum BNP concentration is evident after SAH.[19–21,103,104] McGirt and colleagues[19] demonstrated the existence of a temporal relationship between elevated BNP levels and the presence of hyponatremia in patients with SAH. Interestingly, in this same study abnormally high levels of BNP correlated well with the presence of cerebral vasospasm, suggesting that BNP may have a direct causal link to the secondary complications often observed in SAH. Besides BNP, other members within this peptide family, ANP in particular, have also been suspected to contribute to the development of CSW.[16,17,28] The caveat to this, however, is that BNP was not measured in these earlier studies, leaving open the possibility that it, rather than ANP, was responsible for the CSW.[28,105] Additionally, more recent evidence has shed light on a new member of the natriuretic peptide family, DNP, as a potential additional causative agent of hyponatremia in patients with aneurysmal SAH.[24] Further investigation is needed to better define the roles played by the different natriuretic peptides in the pathogenesis of CSW.

Several hypotheses have been offered to explain how an intracranial insult could lead to elevations of serum concentrations of these peptides. One plausible hypothesis is that direct damage to cortical and subcortical structures where BNP exists[106] leads to inadvertent release of hormone directly into the circulation.[14] Some investigators have proposed that generation and release of natriuretic peptides from the hypothalamus in disease states, such as SAH, may serve a protective role against elevated intracranial pressure. This cerebral induction of natriuresis could limit further impending rise in intracranial pressure and its subsequent potential unfavorable outcomes.[21,107]

Myocardial tissue has also been proposed to be a source of elevated natriuretic peptide levels in CSW.[104,105] Surges in sympathetic outflow typically occur as a result of acute CNS injury.[85] This increase in sympathetic tone may lead to catecholamine-induced myocardial ventricular strain, thereby causing release of BNP from the atrial myocardium.[85,103] Additionally, the presence of excess catecholamine as a result of acute intracranial disease may be excitotoxic to cardiac myocytes,[85] also potentially causing transient myocardial dysfunction. Related neurohumoral findings have also been demonstrated in other forms of acute cerebral injury, such as ischemic stroke, also implying that like mechanisms are at play.[108] Some authors have speculated that hypervolemic therapy itself, which is frequently administered after SAH, can lead to myocardial chamber stretch with resultant peptide release.[23] Regardless of which individual or combination of molecules is responsible, the mechanistic cause-and-effect link between cerebral damage and natriuretic peptide release with ensuing renal sodium loss has yet to be identified.

Miscellaneous Hypotheses

Kojima and colleagues[26] suggest that a mechanism or mechanisms other than one involving ANP, BNP, or ADH exists that may be responsible for CSW. In an experimental rat model, they measured serum concentrations of these hormones and urinary volume and sodium excretion at several time intervals after induction of SAH while controlling the degree of volume therapy to exclude this as a confounding variable. Findings consistent with CSW occurred in the SAH rats: a significant elevation in urinary volume and sodium excretion, decreased body weight, and an increase in hematocrit. Interestingly, levels of ANP decreased, whereas the BNP and ADH concentrations were unchanged. They concluded that a novel, undefined mechanism, or one that involves DNP, likely underlies the etiology of CSW.

Adrenomedullin (AM) is a more recently discovered endogenous peptide that has been proposed as a mediator of CSW.[30,109,110] Originally discovered in pheochromocytoma tissue[111] and later revealed in human brain matter,[112,113] AM is a potent vasodilator with natriuretic and diuretic properties. Elevation in plasma levels of this peptide has been shown to be high immediately after SAH and may reflect the severity of hemorrhage; however, its levels do not seem to correlate with the presence angiographic vasospasm.[25] Conversely, cerebrospinal fluid concentrations of AM do seem to parallel the development of hyponatremia and delayed ischemic neurologic injury for at least 8 days after the onset of hemorrhage.[27] The release of this hormone in the setting of aneurysmal SAH might serve a protective role against the development or worsening of cerebral vasospasm through its vasoactive properties. The site of CNS production of AM within the hypothalamus extends neuronal projections to regions within the brainstem and spinal cord, which can ultimately effect sympathetic tone.[113] Interestingly, a decrease in renal sympathetic activity with subsequent natriuresis and diuresis has been demonstrated in an animal model after AM was introduced into the cerebral ventricular system.[114] Although new molecules and mechanisms have been described, BNP and ANP continue to be implicated as the main offenders toward the development of CSW, of which the former continues to be of primary suspect.[21]

DIAGNOSIS OF CSW

Differentiating CSW from most other common causes of hyponatremia (diuretic use, adrenal insufficiency, extrarenal-induced volume-deplete states, hypothyroidism, congestive heart failure)[115] is typically not difficult. Obtaining a meticulous history and inventory of recent medications and laboratory studies often reveals the correct diagnosis. The challenge lies in the differentiation of CSW from SIADH, because both disorders cause similar serum and urine laboratory abnormalities and occur in the same neurologic and neurosurgical diseases.[116,117] Accurately distinguishing between these two disorders is crucial, because misdiagnosis can lead to inappropriate therapy, often with serious consequences. Volume restriction instituted for a presumptive diagnosis of SIADH in patients with aneurysmal SAH and CSW, for example, has been shown to increase the risk of delayed ischemic deficits and mortality.[11] Treatment based on an inaccurate diagnosis can also lead to progressive worsening of hyponatremia and its direct neurologic complications.[115] Despite the availability and general ease in obtaining tests for the determination of electrolyte concentrations and osmolality in the serum and urine, only the careful determination of volume status in the hyponatremic patient accurately differentiates CSW from SIADH (**Table 1**).

SIADH is a syndrome of euvolemic hyponatremia. It is characterized by (1) euvolemia and an even fluid balance; (2) hyponatremia (serum sodium <135 mmol/L[115,117]) and hypo-osmolality (serum osmolality <275 mOsm/kg H_2O in an adult); (3) a urine osmolality that is greater than that of maximally dilute urine (>100 mOsm/kg H_2O in an adult); and (4) the presence of an elevated urinary sodium concentration (>40 mmol/L) in an individual with normal salt and water intake.[117] This constellation of findings is a result of excessive ADH-induced water reabsorption from the glomerular filtrate at the distal nephron, which produces inappropriately concentrated urine despite serum hypo-osmolality. CSW, however, is a syndrome of hypovolemic hyponatremia. Its major clinical features are (1) hypovolemia, often with a net

Table 1
Differential diagnosis of CSW and SIADH

Variable	CSW	SIADH
Urine osmolality	↑ (>100 mOsm/kg)	↑ (>100 mOsm/kg)
Urine sodium concentration	↑ (>40 mmol/L)	↑ (>40 mmol/L)
Extracellular fluid volume	↓	↑
Body weight	↓	↔ or ↑
Fluid balance	Negative	Neutral to slightly +
Urine volume	↔ or ↑	↔ or ↓
Heart rate	↔ or ↑	↔
Hematocrit	↑	↔
Albumin	↑	↔
Serum bicarbonate	↑	↔ or ↓
Blood urea nitrogen	↑	↔ or ↓
Serum uric acid	↔ or ↓	↓
Sodium balance	Negative	Neutral or +
Central venous pressure	↓ (< 6 cm H_2O)	↔ or slightly + (6–10 cm H_2O)
Wedge pressure	↓	↔ or slightly ↑

Abbreviations: CSW, cerebral salt wasting; SIADH, syndrome of inappropriate antidiuretic hormone secretion.
Adapted from Rabinstein AA, Wijdicks EF. Hyponatremia in critically ill neurologic patients. Neurologist 2003;9: 290–300; with permission.

negative fluid balance; (2) hyponatremia and serum hypo-osmolality; (3) an elevated urine osmolality (>100 mOsm/kg); and (4) elevated urinary sodium (>40 mEq/L). In contrast to SIADH, the findings in CSW are caused by excessive renal sodium and water excretion. Because sodium excretion is disproportionately higher than that of water, the urine is inappropriately concentrated for the degree of serum hypo-osmolality. Salt wasting typically occurs early following acute cerebral injury and can persist beyond 5 days. Hyponatremia often follows and develops by the first week following the insult.[8,9,11,17]

It is not possible to distinguish CSW from SIADH based on serum and urine laboratory findings alone, because their associated abnormalities are identical. For this reason, accurate determination of the patient's volume status is the key to differentiating these syndromes. Unfortunately, determination of volume status is notoriously difficult to perform accurately in routine clinical practice. Despite the use of complex, labor intensive, and elegant methods of determining intravascular volume status in experimental studies of CSW, no universally accepted standard exists for this purpose.[118] Precisely because of this difficulty in conclusively and consistently differentiating hypovolemic hyponatremia from euvolemic and hypervolemic hyponatremia, Sterns and Silver[118] have recently suggested that differentiating between CSW and SIADH is not currently possible. Rather, they suggest that because hyponatremia from any cause in a brain-injured patient is best treated with hypertonic saline, the two conditions should be considered a single entity called the "cerebral salt wanting syndrome." This idea is intriguing, but needs to be tested to determine its value in clinical practice.

Classical signs and symptoms of hypovolemia including hypotension, orthostatism, lassitude, increased thirst, and muscle cramps all lack specificity, particularly in critically ill patients; however, in the appropriate clinical context (eg, vomiting, diarrhea, diaphoresis, diuretic use, and polyuria), these symptoms can provide clues that the patient is hypovolemic. Weight loss, the absence of jugular venous distention, prolonged capillary refill time or diminished skin turgor, or the presence of dry mucous membranes can be suggestive of diminished extracellular fluid volume. Unfortunately, physical examination provides limited sensitivity in the assessment of hypovolemia.[119,120] Similarly, measurement of serum concentrations of the conventional biochemical markers that normally reflect hypovolemia (renin and aldosterone) is unreliable because these substances are abnormally suppressed in CSW.[22,62,121] Other more common laboratory data used to support a volume-contracted state are the presence of an elevation in serum bicarbonate, blood urea nitrogen concentration, or hematocrit, but none of these is independently diagnostic and all lack specificity. Elevated serum uric acid levels can be seen in the hypovolemic state, but uric acid levels have surprisingly been found to be low in both CSW and SIADH.[122,123]

Measurement of CVP can be useful for estimating intravascular volume status when clinical and laboratory data are nondiagnostic and accurate intravascular volume evaluation is critical. Damaraju and colleagues[124] assessed the intravascular volume status in 25 neurosurgical patients who fulfilled the diagnostic criteria for SIADH by monitoring CVP. Hypovolemia was defined as a CVP less than 5 cm H_2O. Patients with a CVP less than 5 cm H_2O received 50 mL/kg/d of volume replacement and an initial sodium intake of 12 g per day. The main outcome measured was an improvement in serum sodium concentration from two consecutive measurements 12 hours apart or within 72 hours of initiation of therapy. Nineteen of their 25 patients were found to be both hypovolemic and able to achieve normal serum sodium values (defined as >130 mEq/L) within this time frame after therapy. The authors concluded that neurosurgical hyponatremic patients with natriuresis were more likely to be affected by CSW rather than SIADH and that CVP-directed treatment of hyponatremia and volume status in such patients is effective. Although the CVP is a very useful estimate of intravascular volume status, key limitations to its use exist.[125] Placement of a CVP catheter is an invasive procedure associated with rare but important complications.[126] Also, CVP measurements can be inaccurate in the setting of abnormal cardiac function, which is not uncommon in acute cerebral injuries. For example, despite high pulmonary wedge pressures, the CVP can be falsely low-normal in patients with isolated left or right-sided heart failure. Conversely, patients with cor pulmonale can have a falsely elevated CVP.

An accurate and timely diagnosis of CSW relies on several clinical and laboratory features when considered in the appropriate context (eg, SAH). The disorder is characterized by hyponatremia with increased urinary sodium concentration and hypovolemia in the setting of acute intracranial disease. Because other features of CSW are identical to SIADH, the key in distinguishing the two disorders lies in determining the patient's volume status. An estimation of volume status can often be made on the basis of simultaneous consideration of the symptoms, signs, and laboratory parameters discussed previously. Of these, meticulously recorded fluid balance values are probably most informative. In rare patients with hyponatremia in whom precise management of intravascular volume is essential, placement of a central venous catheter for measurement of CVP can be useful.

TREATMENT

The mainstay of therapy for CSW is replacement of the sodium and water that is lost as a result of pathologic natriuresis and diuresis. This is in direct contrast to the treatment of SIADH, the crux of which is free water restriction. Patients with CSW typically have significant extracellular volume depletion and a total-body sodium deficit of at least 2 mmol of sodium/kg body weight.[66] In patients who are hypovolemic, a reasonable initial management strategy is administration of normal saline with the intent of restoring intravascular volume. This is particularly important in patients with aneurysmal SAH, because the risk of vasospasm and its downstream complications is increased in the setting of hypovolemia.[11,17–20,127] Cautiously aggressive administration of intravenous fluids has become the mainstay of initial therapy in patients with SAH and has been shown to prevent volume contraction but not the development of hyponatremia.[128]

Once euvolemia is achieved, attention should be directed to the correction of hyponatremia. One method for augmenting both serum sodium concentration and intravascular volume is the use of mineralocorticoids. One should be mindful that although correction of hyponatremia and hypovolemia can often be achieved,[65,129–132] these medications have not been shown to be beneficial in preventing additional secondary complications of SAH, such as cerebral vasospasm.[131] The authors typically use fludrocortisone, 0.1 to 0.2 mg orally twice a day, starting once the diagnosis of CSW is made and continuing until serum sodium concentrations and intravascular volume remain stably normal, typically 3 to 5 days later. Especially when the serum sodium approaches dangerously low levels (<125 mEq/L) or when large volumes of intravenous fluid are required to maintain euvolemia, intravenous hypertonic saline can also be a useful adjunctive therapy in CSW. A dose of 1.5% sodium chloride can be administered through peripheral veins, and can safely and effectively restore and maintain intravascular volume and serum sodium concentration when administered at rates that are titrated to achieve a normal to slightly positive fluid balance. The authors routinely use 1.5% sodium chloride in patients with CSW at rates between 50 and 150

mL per hour. The use of 3% saline in CSW should be reserved for uncommon patients with CSW who have severe hyponatremia (<120 mEq/L) because it must be administered through a central vein and cannot be given at rates high enough to effectively restore or maintain intravascular volume.

Treatment with hypertonic saline and mineralocorticoids has important side effects. To gage the efficacy of treatment and to avoid osmotic myelinolysis as a consequence of overly rapid correction of hyponatremia, the serum sodium concentration should be carefully and frequently monitored during treatment. In general, the serum sodium concentration should not be increased by more than an average of 0.5 mEq/L/h.[115] Similarly, it is useful to use a serum sodium concentration of 130 mEq/L or greater rather than restoration of a normal concentration of 135 to 145 mEq/L as an end point for treatment. In most patients, this strategy effectively treats the negative consequences of hyponatremia while minimizing the likelihood of causing osmotic myelinolysis. Aggressive fluid and sodium administration and the use of mineralocorticoids can also cause volume overload, hypertension, pulmonary edema, and renal medullary washout,[65] warranting vigilance for these important complications during treatment. Finally, mineralocorticoid-like drugs also frequently cause hypokalemia and, because of their steroid properties, can promote hyperglycemia. Serum glucose and potassium concentration should be carefully monitored during such therapy.[65,129,131,132]

A novel treatment strategy for hyponatremia that has only recently become available highlights the need to differentiate CSW from SIADH. Conivaptan is a nonselective antagonist at the V1a and V2 vasopressin receptor subtypes. By antagonizing the action of vasopressin in the renal collecting duct, it promotes electrolyte-free water excretion (a process termed "aquauresis"), thereby raising serum sodium levels. As its mechanism of action indicates, conivaptan is a highly specific and effective treatment for SIADH caused by a number of conditions.[133] It has recently been approved by the US Food and Drug Administration for the treatment of euvolemic and hypervolemic hyponatremia[133,134] for which it has demonstrated a satisfactory safety profile.[135] Conversely, this medication should not be used to treat hypovolemic hyponatremia, of which CSW is an important cause, because of its tendency to induce a negative fluid balance. The use of this medication in patients with neurologic injury has been examined in only small, uncontrolled retrospective studies.[134] Murphy and colleagues[134] assessed the efficacy of intermittent bolus doses of 20 or 40 mg of intravenous conivaptan to correct acute euvolemic or hypervolemic hyponatremia that developed within 48 hours of admission to the neurologic intensive care unit. The studied patients had a variety of primary neurologic diagnoses, but patients with SAH who were suspected of having CSW were excluded. Patients who received the drug were those who had symptomatic hyponatremia, were at high risk of developing cerebral edema, or had low serum sodium levels refractory to traditional therapy. A 4 to 6 mEq/L rise in serum sodium concentration by 12 hours after a single dose was seen in 59% of patients and there were no adverse effects, including intravenous site reactions or hypotension. Conivaptan clearly shows promise in treating refractory hyponatremia in critically ill neurologic patients. A careful determination of the likely cause of hyponatremia must take place, however, before administering this drug to such patients. Patients with CSW are volume depleted in addition to being hyponatremic, and conivaptan causes volume loss by aquauresis. Because poor outcome has been associated with volume depletion in SAH patients with hypovolemic hyponatremia, conivaptan should not be administered to patients in whom CSW or a high likelihood for cerebral vasospasm is suspected.[11]

SUMMARY

CSW is a syndrome of hypovolemic hyponatremia caused by natriuresis and diuresis. Once thought of as a rare novelty, recent clinical and basic science research has shown that CSW exists, is not uncommon in patients with certain types of brain injury, and can have significant negative consequences if not properly diagnosed and treated. The mechanisms underlying this syndrome have yet to be precisely delineated, although existing evidence strongly implicates abnormal elevations in circulating natriuretic peptides as the key pathophysiologic event. Nonetheless, several fundamental questions have yet to be answered, the most important of which are how cerebral injury leads to the release of excessive amounts of natriuretic peptides and why this occurs in only a small subset of cerebral injury types. The key in diagnosis of CSW lies in distinguishing it from the more common SIADH, although the value of this often imprecise process has recently been called into question.[118] Volume status, but not serum and urine electrolytes and osmolality, is crucial for making this distinction. Volume and sodium repletion are the goals of treatment of patients with CSW, and this can be performed using some combination of isotonic saline, hypertonic saline, and mineralocorticoids.

REFERENCES

1. Schwartz WB, Bennett W, Curelop S, et al. A syndrome of renal sodium loss and hyponatremia probably resulting from inappropriate secretion of antidiuretic hormone. Am J Med 1957;23(4):529–42.
2. Doczi T, Bende J, Huszka E, et al. Syndrome of inappropriate secretion of antidiuretic hormone after subarachnoid hemorrhage. Neurosurgery 1981;9(4):394–7.
3. Doczi T, Tarjanyi J, Huszka E, et al. Syndrome of inappropriate secretion of antidiuretic hormone (SIADH) after head injury. Neurosurgery 1982;10(6 Pt 1):685–8.
4. Wise BL. Syndrome of inappropriate antidiuretic hormone secretion after spontaneous subarachnoid hemorrhage: a reversible cause of clinical deterioration. Neurosurgery 1978;3(3):412–4.
5. Afifi A, Joynt R, Harbison J. Inappropriate antidiuretic hormone secretion in subarachnoid hemorrhage. Trans Am Neurol Assoc 1965;90:217–8.
6. Joynt RJ, Afifi A, Harrison J. Hyponatremia in subarachnoid hemorrhage. Arch Neurol 1965;13(6):633–8.
7. Wijdicks EF, Vermeulen M, ten Haaf JA, et al. Volume depletion and natriuresis in patients with a ruptured intracranial aneurysm. Ann Neurol 1985;18(2):211–6.
8. Nelson PB, Seif SM, Maroon JC, et al. Hyponatremia in intracranial disease: perhaps not the syndrome of inappropriate secretion of antidiuretic hormone (SIADH). J Neurosurg 1981;55(6):938–41.
9. Nelson PB, Seif S, Gutai J, et al. Hyponatremia and natriuresis following subarachnoid hemorrhage in a monkey model. J Neurosurg 1984;60(2):233–7.
10. Sherlock M, O'Sullivan E, Agha A, et al. The incidence and pathophysiology of hyponatraemia after subarachnoid haemorrhage. Clin Endocrinol (Oxf) 2006;64(3):250–4.
11. Wijdicks EF, Vermeulen M, Hijdra A, et al. Hyponatremia and cerebral infarction in patients with ruptured intracranial aneurysms: is fluid restriction harmful? Ann Neurol 1985;17(2):137–40.
12. Hasan D, Wijdicks EF, Vermeulen M. Hyponatremia is associated with cerebral ischemia in patients with aneurysmal subarachnoid hemorrhage. Ann Neurol 1990;27(1):106–8.
13. Fox JL, Falik JL, Shalhoub RJ. Neurosurgical hyponatremia: the role of inappropriate antidiuresis. J Neurosurg 1971;34(4):506–14.
14. Peters JP, Welt LG, Sims EA, et al. A salt-wasting syndrome associated with cerebral disease. Trans Assoc Am Physicians 1950;63:57–64.

15. Palmer BF. Hyponatraemia in a neurosurgical patient: syndrome of inappropriate antidiuretic hormone secretion versus cerebral salt wasting. Nephrol Dial Transplant 2000;15(2):262–8.

16. Isotani E, Suzuki R, Tomita K, et al. Alterations in plasma concentrations of natriuretic peptides and antidiuretic hormone after subarachnoid hemorrhage. Stroke 1994;25(11):2198–203.

17. Wijdicks EF, Ropper AH, Hunnicutt EJ, et al. Atrial natriuretic factor and salt wasting after aneurysmal subarachnoid hemorrhage. Stroke 1991;22(12):1519–24.

18. Igarashi T, Moro N, Katayama Y, et al. Prediction of symptomatic cerebral vasospasm in patients with aneurysmal subarachnoid hemorrhage: relationship to cerebral salt wasting syndrome. Neurol Res 2007;29(8):835–41.

19. McGirt MJ, Blessing R, Nimjee SM, et al. Correlation of serum brain natriuretic peptide with hyponatremia and delayed ischemic neurological deficits after subarachnoid hemorrhage. Neurosurgery 2004;54(6):1369–73.

20. Sviri GE, Feinsod M, Soustiel JF. Brain natriuretic peptide and cerebral vasospasm in subarachnoid hemorrhage: clinical and TCD correlations. Stroke 2000;31(1):118–22.

21. Berendes E, Walter M, Cullen P, et al. Secretion of brain natriuretic peptide in patients with aneurysmal subarachnoid haemorrhage. Lancet 1997;349(9047):245–9.

22. Ganong CA, Kappy MS. Cerebral salt wasting in children: the need for recognition and treatment. Am J Dis Child 1993;147(2):167–9.

23. Inoha S, Inamura T, Nakamizo A, et al. Fluid loading in rats increases serum brain natriuretic peptide concentration. Neurol Res 2001;23(1):93–5.

24. Khurana VG, Wijdicks EF, Heublein DM, et al. A pilot study of dendroaspis natriuretic peptide in aneurysmal subarachnoid hemorrhage. Neurosurgery 2004;55(1):69–75.

25. Kikumoto K, Kubo A, Hayashi Y, et al. Increased plasma concentration of adrenomedullin in patients with subarachnoid hemorrhage. Anesth Analg 1998;87(4):859–63.

26. Kojima J, Katayama Y, Moro N, et al. Cerebral salt wasting in subarachnoid hemorrhage rats: model, mechanism, and tool. Life Sci 2005;76(20):2361–70.

27. Kubo Y, Ogasawara K, Kakino S, et al. Cerebrospinal fluid adrenomedullin concentration correlates with hyponatremia and delayed ischemic neurological deficits after subarachnoid hemorrhage. Cerebrovasc Dis 2008;25(1–2):164–9.

28. Kurokawa Y, Uede T, Ishiguro M, et al. Pathogenesis of hyponatremia following subarachnoid hemorrhage due to ruptured cerebral aneurysm. Surg Neurol 1996;46(5):500–7 [discussion: 507–8].

29. Shimoda M, Yamada S, Yamamoto I, et al. Atrial natriuretic polypeptide in patients with subarachnoid haemorrhage due to aneurysmal rupture: correlation to hyponatremia. Acta Neurochir (Wien) 1989;97(1–2):53–61.

30. Wijdicks EF, Heublein DM, Burnett JC Jr. Increase and uncoupling of adrenomedullin from the natriuretic peptide system in aneurysmal subarachnoid hemorrhage. J Neurosurg 2001;94(2):252–6.

31. Vogel JH. Aldosterone in cerebral salt wasting. Circulation 1963;27:44–50.

32. Lu DC, Binder DK, Chien B, et al. Cerebral salt wasting and elevated brain natriuretic peptide levels after traumatic brain injury: 2 case reports. Surg Neurol 2008;69(3):226–9.

33. Chang CH, Liao JJ, Chuang CH, et al. Recurrent hyponatremia after traumatic brain injury. Am J Med Sci 2008;335(5):390–3.

34. Moro N, Katayama Y, Igarashi T, et al. Hyponatremia in patients with traumatic brain injury: incidence, mechanism, and response to sodium supplementation or retention therapy with hydrocortisone. Surg Neurol 2007;68(4):387–93.

35. Vespa P. Cerebral salt wasting after traumatic brain injury: an important critical care treatment issue. Surg Neurol 2008;69(3):230–2.

36. Lee P, Jones GR, Center JR. Successful treatment of adult cerebral salt wasting with fludrocortisone. Arch Intern Med 2008;168(3):325–6.

37. Jimenez R, Casado-Flores J, Nieto M, et al. Cerebral salt wasting syndrome in children with acute central nervous system injury. Pediatr Neurol 2006;35(4):261–3.

38. Steelman R, Corbitt B, Pate MF. Early onset of cerebral salt wasting in a patient with head and facial injuries. J Oral Maxillofac Surg 2006;64(4):746–7.

39. Berkenbosch JW, Lentz CW, Jimenez DF, et al. Cerebral salt wasting syndrome following brain injury in three pediatric patients: suggestions for rapid diagnosis and therapy. Pediatr Neurosurg 2002;36(2):75–9.

40. Powner DJ, Boccalandro C. Adrenal insufficiency following traumatic brain injury in adults. Curr Opin Crit Care 2008;14(2):163–6.

41. Brimioulle S, Orellana-Jimenez C, Aminian A, et al. Hyponatremia in neurological patients: cerebral salt wasting versus inappropriate antidiuretic hormone secretion. Intensive Care Med 2008;34(1):125–31.

42. Powner DJ, Boccalandro C, Alp MS, et al. Endocrine failure after traumatic brain injury in adults. Neurocrit Care 2006;5(1):61–70.

43. Penney MD, Walters G, Wilkins DG. Hyponatraemia in patients with head injury. Intensive Care Med 1979;5(1):23–6.

44. Roca-Ribas F, Ninno JE, Gasperin A, et al. Cerebral salt wasting syndrome as a postoperative

complication after surgical resection of acoustic neuroma. Otol Neurotol 2002;23(6):992–5.

45. Poon WS, Lolin YI, Yeung TF, et al. Water and sodium disorders following surgical excision of pituitary region tumours. Acta Neurochir (Wien) 1996;138(8):921–7.

46. Oster JR, Perez GO, Larios O, et al. Cerebral salt wasting in a man with carcinomatous meningitis. Arch Intern Med 1983;143(11):2187–8.

47. Oruckaptan HH, Ozisik P, Akalan N. Prolonged cerebral salt wasting syndrome associated with the intraventricular dissemination of brain tumors: report of two cases and review of the literature. Pediatr Neurosurg 2000;33(1):16–20.

48. Kim JH, Kang JK, Lee SA. Hydrocephalus and hyponatremia as the presenting manifestations of primary CNS lymphoma. Eur Neurol 2006;55(1): 39–41.

49. Diringer M, Ladenson PW, Borel C, et al. Sodium and water regulation in a patient with cerebral salt wasting. Arch Neurol 1989;46(8):928–30.

50. Atkin SL, Coady AM, White MC, et al. Hyponatraemia secondary to cerebral salt wasting syndrome following routine pituitary surgery. Eur J Endocrinol 1996;135(2):245–7.

51. Cort JH. Cerebral salt wasting. Lancet 1954; 266(6815):752–4.

52. Moller K, Larsen FS, Bie P, et al. The syndrome of inappropriate secretion of antidiuretic hormone and fluid restriction in meningitis: how strong is the evidence? Scand J Infect Dis 2001;33(1):13–26.

53. Narotam PK, Kemp M, Buck R, et al. Hyponatremic natriuretic syndrome in tuberculous meningitis: the probable role of atrial natriuretic peptide. Neurosurgery 1994;34(6):982–8 [discussion: 988].

54. Huang SM, Chen CC, Chiu PC, et al. Tuberculous meningitis complicated with hydrocephalus and cerebral salt wasting syndrome in a three-year-old boy. Pediatr Infect Dis J 2004;23(9):884–6.

55. Brookes MJ, Gould TH. Cerebral salt wasting syndrome in meningoencephalitis: a case report. J Neurol Neurosurg Psychiatr 2003;74(2):277.

56. Ti LK, Kang SC, Cheong KF. Acute hyponatraemia secondary to cerebral salt wasting syndrome in a patient with tuberculous meningitis. Anaesth Intensive Care 1998;26(4):420–3.

57. Erduran E, Mocan H, Aslan Y. Another cause of hyponatraemia in patients with bacterial meningitis: cerebral salt wasting. Acta Paediatr 1997;86(10): 1150–1.

58. Celik US, Alabaz D, Yildizdas D, et al. Cerebral salt wasting in tuberculous meningitis: treatment with fludrocortisone. Ann Trop Paediatr 2005;25(4): 297–302.

59. Singhi SC, Singhi PD, Srinivas B, et al. Fluid restriction does not improve the outcome of acute meningitis. Pediatr Infect Dis J 1995;14(6):495–503.

60. Chao YN, Chiu NC, Huang FY. Clinical features and prognostic factors in childhood pneumococcal meningitis. J Microbiol Immunol Infect 2008;41(1): 48–53.

61. Olson BR, Gumowski J, Rubino D, et al. Pathophysiology of hyponatremia after transsphenoidal pituitary surgery. J Neurosurg 1997;87(4):499–507.

62. Papadimitriou DT, Spiteri A, Pagnier A, et al. Mineralocorticoid deficiency in post-operative cerebral salt wasting. J Pediatr Endocrinol Metab 2007; 20(10):1145–50.

63. Hensen J, Henig A, Fahlbusch R, et al. Prevalence, predictors and patterns of postoperative polyuria and hyponatraemia in the immediate course after transsphenoidal surgery for pituitary adenomas. Clin Endocrinol (Oxf) 1999;50(4):431–9.

64. Arieff AI. Hyponatremia, convulsions, respiratory arrest, and permanent brain damage after elective surgery in healthy women. N Engl J Med 1986; 314(24):1529–35.

65. Wijdicks EF, Vermeulen M, van Brummelen P, et al. The effect of fludrocortisone acetate on plasma volume and natriuresis in patients with aneurysmal subarachnoid hemorrhage. Clin Neurol Neurosurg 1988;90(3):209–14.

66. Carlotti AP, Bohn D, Rutka JT, et al. A method to estimate urinary electrolyte excretion in patients at risk for developing cerebral salt wasting. J Neurosurg 2001;95(3):420–4.

67. Ishikawa SE, Saito T, Kaneko K, et al. Hyponatremia responsive to fludrocortisone acetate in elderly patients after head injury. Ann Intern Med 1987; 106(2):187–91.

68. Donati-Genet PC, Dubuis JM, Girardin E, et al. Acute symptomatic hyponatremia and cerebral salt wasting after head injury: an important clinical entity. J Pediatr Surg 2001;36(7):1094–7.

69. Kanakriyeh M, Carvajal HF, Vallone AM. Initial fluid therapy for children with meningitis with consideration of the syndrome of inappropriate anti-diuretic hormone. Clin Pediatr (Phila) 1987;26(3):126–30.

70. Maconochie I, Baumer H, Stewart ME. Fluid therapy for acute bacterial meningitis. Cochrane Database Syst Rev 2008;(1):CD004786.

71. Lavoie JL, Sigmund CD. Minireview: overview of the renin-angiotensin system–an endocrine and paracrine system. Endocrinology 2003;144(6):2179–83.

72. Williams GH, Dluhy RG. Disorders of the adrenal cortex. In: Braunwald E, Fauci AS, Kasper DL, et al, editors. Harrison's principles of internal medicine. 15th edition. New York: McGraw-Hill Medical Publishing Division; 2001. p. 2087–9.

73. Paul M, Poyan Mehr A, Kreutz R. Physiology of local renin-angiotensin systems. Physiol Rev 2006;86(3):747–803.

74. Bader M, Peters J, Baltatu O, et al. Tissue renin-angiotensin systems: new insights from

experimental animal models in hypertension research. J Mol Med 2001;79(2–3):76–102.

75. Morimoto S, Sigmund CD. Angiotensin mutant mice: a focus on the brain renin-angiotensin system. Neuropeptides 2002;36(2–3):194–200.

76. Steckelings UM, Obermuller N, Bottari SP, et al. Brain angiotensin: receptors, actions and possible role in hypertension. Pharmacol Toxicol 1992;70(6 Pt 2):S23–7.

77. Steckelings U, Lebrun C, Qadri F, et al. Role of brain angiotensin in cardiovascular regulation. J Cardiovasc Pharmacol 1992;19(Suppl 6):S72–9.

78. DiBona GF. Nervous kidney: interaction between renal sympathetic nerves and the renin-angiotensin system in the control of renal function. Hypertension 2000;36(6):1083–8.

79. Muller J, Barajas L. Electron microscopic and histochemical evidence for a tubular innervation in the renal cortex of the monkey. J Ultrastruct Res 1972;41(5):533–49.

80. DiBona GF. Physiology in perspective: the wisdom of the body. Neural control of the kidney. Am J Physiol Regul Integr Comp Physiol 2005; 289(3):R633–41.

81. DiBona GF. Central sympathoexcitatory actions of angiotensin II: role of type 1 angiotensin II receptors. J Am Soc Nephrol 1999;10(Suppl 11):S90–4.

82. Reid IA. Interactions between ANG II, sympathetic nervous system, and baroreceptor reflexes in regulation of blood pressure. Am J Physiol 1992;262(6 Pt 1):E763–78.

83. Benarroch E, Westmoreland B, Daube J, et al. The internal regulation system. Medical neurosciences: an approach to anatomy, pathology, and physiology by systems and levels. 4th edition. Hagerstown (MD): Lippincott Williams & Wilkins; 1998. 264–9.

84. DiBona GF. Neural control of renal function in health and disease. Clin Auton Res 1994;4(1–2):69–74.

85. Samuels MA. The brain-heart connection. Circulation 2007;116(1):77–84.

86. de Bold AJ, Borenstein HB, Veress AT, et al. A rapid and potent natriuretic response to intravenous injection of atrial myocardial extract in rats. Life Sci 1981;28(1):89–94.

87. Levin ER, Gardner DG, Samson WK. Natriuretic peptides. N Engl J Med 1998;339(5):321–8.

88. Lisy O, Lainchbury JG, Leskinen H, et al. Therapeutic actions of a new synthetic vasoactive and natriuretic peptide, dendroaspis natriuretic peptide, in experimental severe congestive heart failure. Hypertension 2001;37(4):1089–94.

89. Lisy O, Jougasaki M, Heublein DM, et al. Renal actions of synthetic dendroaspis natriuretic peptide. Kidney Int 1999;56(2):502–8.

90. Del Ry S, Cabiati M, Lionetti V, et al. Expression of C-type natriuretic peptide and of its receptor

NPR-B in normal and failing heart. Peptides 2008; 29(12):2208–15.

91. Sudoh T, Minamino N, Kangawa K, et al. C-type natriuretic peptide (CNP): a new member of natriuretic peptide family identified in porcine brain. Biochem Biophys Res Commun 1990;168(2): 863–70.

92. Suga S, Nakao K, Hosoda K, et al. Receptor selectivity of natriuretic peptide family, atrial natriuretic peptide, brain natriuretic peptide, and C-type natriuretic peptide. Endocrinology 1992; 130(1):229–39.

93. Cao LH, Yang XL. Natriuretic peptides and their receptors in the central nervous system. Prog Neurobiol 2008;84(3):234–48.

94. Schultz HD, Gardner DG, Deschepper CF, et al. Vagal C-fiber blockade abolishes sympathetic inhibition by atrial natriuretic factor. Am J Physiol 1988; 255(1 Pt 2):R6–13.

95. Schultz HD, Steele MK, Gardner DG. Central administration of atrial peptide decreases sympathetic outflow in rats. Am J Physiol 1990; 258(5 Pt 2):R1250–6.

96. Steele MK, Gardner DG, Xie PL, et al. Interactions between ANP and ANG II in regulating blood pressure and sympathetic outflow. Am J Physiol 1991; 260(6 Pt 2):R1145–51.

97. Harris PJ, Thomas D, Morgan TO. Atrial natriuretic peptide inhibits angiotensin-stimulated proximal tubular sodium and water reabsorption. Nature 1987;326(6114):697–8.

98. Dillingham MA, Anderson RJ. Inhibition of vasopressin action by atrial natriuretic factor. Science 1986;231(4745):1572–3.

99. Saper CB, Hurley KM, Moga MM, et al. Brain natriuretic peptides: differential localization of a new family of neuropeptides. Neurosci Lett 1989;96(1): 29–34.

100. Lee YJ, Lin SR, Shin SJ, et al. Brain natriuretic peptide is synthesized in the human adrenal medulla and its messenger ribonucleic acid expression along with that of atrial natriuretic peptide are enhanced in patients with primary aldosteronism. J Clin Endocrinol Metab 1994;79(5):1476–82.

101. Maack T, Suzuki M, Almeida FA, et al. Physiological role of silent receptors of atrial natriuretic factor. Science 1987;238(4827):675–8.

102. Johns DG, Ao Z, Heidrich BJ, et al. Dendroaspis natriuretic peptide binds to the natriuretic peptide clearance receptor. Biochem Biophys Res Commun 2007;358(1):145–9.

103. Tomida M, Muraki M, Uemura K, et al. Plasma concentrations of brain natriuretic peptide in patients with subarachnoid hemorrhage. Stroke 1998;29(8):1584–7.

104. Espiner EA, Leikis R, Ferch RD, et al. The neurocardio-endocrine response to acute subarachnoid

haemorrhage. Clin Endocrinol (Oxf) 2002;56(5): 629–35.

105. Rosenfeld JV, Barnett GH, Sila CA, et al. The effect of subarachnoid hemorrhage on blood and CSF atrial natriuretic factor. J Neurosurg 1989;71(1): 32–7.

106. Takahashi K, Totsune K, Sone M, et al. Human brain natriuretic peptide-like immunoreactivity in human brain. Peptides 1992;13(1):121–3.

107. Doczi T, Joo F, Vecsernyes M, et al. Increased concentration of atrial natriuretic factor in the cerebrospinal fluid of patients with aneurysmal subarachnoid hemorrhage and raised intracranial pressure. Neurosurgery 1988;23(1):16–9.

108. Iltumur K, Yavavli A, Apak I, et al. Elevated plasma N-terminal pro-brain natriuretic peptide levels in acute ischemic stroke. Am Heart J 2006;151(5): 1115–22.

109. Lang MG, Paterno R, Faraci FM, et al. Mechanisms of adrenomedullin-induced dilatation of cerebral arterioles. Stroke 1997;28(1):181–5.

110. Dogan A, Suzuki Y, Koketsu N, et al. Intravenous infusion of adrenomedullin and increase in regional cerebral blood flow and prevention of ischemic brain injury after middle cerebral artery occlusion in rats. J Cereb Blood Flow Metab 1997;17(1): 19–25.

111. Kitamura K, Kangawa K, Kawamoto M, et al. Adrenomedullin: a novel hypotensive peptide isolated from human pheochromocytoma. Biochem Biophys Res Commun 1993;192(2):553–60.

112. Satoh F, Takahashi K, Murakami O, et al. Adrenomedullin in human brain, adrenal glands and tumor tissues of pheochromocytoma, ganglioneuroblastoma and neuroblastoma. J Clin Endocrinol Metab 1995;80(5):1750–2.

113. Satoh F, Takahashi K, Murakami O, et al. Immunocytochemical localization of adrenomedullin-like immunoreactivity in the human hypothalamus and the adrenal gland. Neurosci Lett 1996;203(3): 207–10.

114. Saita M, Shimokawa A, Kunitake T, et al. Central actions of adrenomedullin on cardiovascular parameters and sympathetic outflow in conscious rats. Am J Physiol 1998;274(4 Pt 2):R979–84.

115. Adrogue HJ, Madias NE. Hyponatremia. N Engl J Med 2000;342(21):1581–9.

116. Smith DM, McKenna K, Thompson CJ. Hyponatraemia. Clin Endocrinol (Oxf) 2000;52(6): 667–78.

117. Janicic N, Verbalis JG. Evaluation and management of hypo-osmolality in hospitalized patients. Endocrinol Metab Clin North Am 2003;32(2): 459–81 vii.

118. Sterns RH, Silver SM. Cerebral salt wasting versus SIADH: what difference? J Am Soc Nephrol 2008; 19(2):194–6.

119. Chung HM, Kluge R, Schrier RW, et al. Clinical assessment of extracellular fluid volume in hyponatremia. Am J Med 1987;83(5):905–8.

120. McGee S, Abernethy WB III, Simel DL. The rational clinical examination. Is this patient hypovolemic? JAMA 1999;281(11):1022–9.

121. von Bismarck P, Ankermann T, Eggert P, et al. Diagnosis and management of cerebral salt wasting (CSW) in children: the role of atrial natriuretic peptide (ANP) and brain natriuretic peptide (BNP). Childs Nerv Syst 2006;22(10):1275–81.

122. Maesaka JK, Miyawaki N, Palaia T, et al. Renal salt wasting without cerebral disease: diagnostic value of urate determinations in hyponatremia. Kidney Int 2007;71(8):822–6.

123. Maesaka JK, Gupta S, Fishbane S. Cerebral salt-wasting syndrome: does it exist? Nephron 1999; 82(2):100–9.

124. Damaraju SC, Rajshekhar V, Chandy MJ. Validation study of a central venous pressure-based protocol for the management of neurosurgical patients with hyponatremia and natriuresis. Neurosurgery 1997; 40(2):312–6 [discussion: 316–7].

125. Kumar A, Anel R, Bunnell E, et al. Pulmonary artery occlusion pressure and central venous pressure fail to predict ventricular filling volume, cardiac performance, or the response to volume infusion in normal subjects. Crit Care Med 2004;32(3): 691–9.

126. McGee DC, Gould MK. Preventing complications of central venous catheterization. N Engl J Med 2003;348(12):1123–33.

127. Solomon RA, Post KD, McMurtry JG III. Depression of circulating blood volume in patients after subarachnoid hemorrhage: implications for the management of symptomatic vasospasm. Neurosurgery 1984;15(3):354–61.

128. Diringer MN, Wu KC, Verbalis JG, et al. Hypervolemic therapy prevents volume contraction but not hyponatremia following subarachnoid hemorrhage. Ann Neurol 1992;31(5):543–50.

129. Mori T, Katayama Y, Kawamata T, et al. Improved efficiency of hypervolemic therapy with inhibition of natriuresis by fludrocortisone in patients with aneurysmal subarachnoid hemorrhage. J Neurosurg 1999;91(6):947–52.

130. Kinik ST, Kandemir N, Baykan A, et al. Fludrocortisone treatment in a child with severe cerebral salt wasting. Pediatr Neurosurg 2001;35(4):216–9.

131. Katayama Y, Haraoka J, Hirabayashi H, et al. A randomized controlled trial of hydrocortisone against hyponatremia in patients with aneurysmal subarachnoid hemorrhage. Stroke 2007;38(8): 2373–5.

132. Hasan D, Lindsay KW, Wijdicks EF, et al. Effect of fludrocortisone acetate in patients with subarachnoid hemorrhage. Stroke 1989;20(9):1156–61.

133. Decaux G, Soupart A, Vassart G. Non-peptide arginine-vasopressin antagonists: the vaptans. Lancet 2008;371(9624):1624–32.

134. Murphy T, Dhar R, Diringer M. Conivaptan bolus dosing for the correction of hyponatremia in the neuro-intensive care unit. Neurocrit Care 2009;11(1):14–9.

135. Annane D, Decaux G, Smith N. Efficacy and safety of oral conivaptan, a vasopressin-receptor antagonist, evaluated in a randomized, controlled trial in patients with euvolemic or hypervolemic hyponatremia. Am J Med Sci 2009; 337(1):28–36.

Risk Factors and Medical Management of Vasospasm After Subarachnoid Hemorrhage

Christos Lazaridis, MD[a,b,*], Neeraj Naval, MD[c,d,e]

KEYWORDS

- Vasospasm • Aneurysmal subarachnoid hemorrhage
- Triple-H therapy • Cerebral blood flow

Aneurysmal subarachnoid hemorrhage (aSAH) comprises 5% of all strokes and affects as many as 30,000 Americans each year.[1,2] Commonly, it involves a younger population. In fact half of the patients are younger than 55 years[3]; as a result, the loss of productive life years approaches that for ischemic stroke and intracerebral hemorrhage.[4] About 10% to 15% of patients die from the initial rupture and never make it to the hospital.[5,6] For the survivors, rebleeding becomes an immediate concern, with an incidence of 4% to 15% in different series in the first 24 hours, carrying very high mortality and morbidity.[7,8] Prevention of rebleeding with prompt exclusion of the ruptured aneurysm from the circulation has become the standard of care for most patients; also, interest in the use of short-term antifibrinolytics has reemerged.[9,10] After this first phase of the disease, patients may deteriorate secondary to hydrocephalus, delayed ischemic neurologic deficits (DIND) (also called delayed cerebral ischemia [DCI]), and multiple medical complications including cardiomyopathy and nosocomial infections. In addition, there is increasing recognition and understanding of the mechanisms of early brain injury (EBI) as a major contributor to poor neurologic outcomes.[11,12] DIND has been classically associated with angiographic vasospasm, especially when manifested with clinical symptoms referable to the vascular territory of the involved vessel. Treatment consists of a combination of interventional procedures, such as mechanical and/or chemical angioplasty for amenable lesions[13] and medical therapy summarized under the term triple-H (hypertension, hypervolemia, hemodilution) therapy. This approach is considered the standard of care by many despite the absence of high-quality evidence on the effectiveness of these interventions.[14] In recent years, several investigators have challenged the traditional presumption linking DIND and DCI exclusively with angiographic vasospasm. Alternative mechanisms have been proposed, including microvascular spasm with cerebral blood flow (CBF) autoregulatory failure, microthrombosis and microembolism, cortical spreading depolarizations and ischemia, and delayed neuronal apoptosis triggered by EBI.[15–18] In this article,

[a] Department of Neurology, Neurosciences Intensive Care Unit, Medical University of South Carolina, 96 Jonathan Lucas Street, Suite 428, Charleston, SC 29425, USA
[b] Department of Neurosurgery, Neurosciences Intensive Care Unit, Medical University of South Carolina, 96 Jonathan Lucas Street, Suite 428, Charleston, SC 29425, USA
[c] Department of Neurology, Johns Hopkins University, 600 North Wolfe Street, Baltimore, MD 21287, USA
[d] Department of Neurosurgery, Johns Hopkins University, 600 North Wolfe Street, Baltimore, MD 21287, USA
[e] Department of Anesthesia–Critical Care, Johns Hopkins University, 600 North Wolfe Street, Baltimore, MD 21287, USA
* Corresponding author. Department of Neurology, Neurosciences Intensive Care Unit, Medical University of South Carolina, 96 Jonathan Lucas Street, Suite 428, Charleston, SC 29425.
E-mail address: lazaridi@musc.edu

Neurosurg Clin N Am 21 (2010) 353–364
doi:10.1016/j.nec.2009.10.006

the known risk factors, prevention, and current medical management of DIND are reviewed.

RISK FACTORS

Angiographic vasospasm is seen in 30% to 70% of patients post aSAH[19,20]; typically it can be expected to start after postbleed day 3, although hyperacute or early vasospasm has been reported.[21,22] Symptoms of cerebral ischemia with high risk for debilitating stroke and mortality are experienced by 20% to 30% of patients. The presence and the amount of oxyhemoglobin in the subarachnoid cisterns is believed to be the major trigger of the phenomena that ultimately cause smooth muscle spasm, narrowing of the arterial lumen, and impaired blood flow autoregulation.[23,24] In their seminal paper, Fisher and colleagues[25] found a strong correlation linking thick cisternal clot with angiographic and clinical vasospasm. The Fisher computed tomographic (CT) rating scale is widely used by neurointensivists and neurosurgeons and has been recently modified to incorporate intraventricular hemorrhage as a significant predictor for vasospasm and also to denote increasing risk as the grade increases.[26,27] Techniques to remove blood or increase clearance of blood from the basal cisterns with either intracisternal[28] or intrathecal lysis, head shaking,[29] and lumbar drainage[30] have been attempted with variable results. Other potential risk factors include poor clinical grade, early angiographic spasm, history of hypertension, and admission mean arterial pressure (MAP).[27] There have been conflicting reports regarding age as a predictor, with one study identifying age less than 35 years as a risk factor,[31] although this finding was not confirmed by others.[32,33] One prospective study of 70 patients demonstrated that apart from thick subarachnoid clot, a history of smoking was independently associated with development of symptomatic spasm.[32] Volume status of the patient with aSAH is considered critical, and a large part of critical care in this disease centers on its regulation. Hypovolemia is believed to be a potentially significant contributor to DCI and can be common if not prevented, especially in the presence of natriuresis secondary to cerebral salt-wasting syndrome (CSWS).[34]

PREVENTION AND VOLUME MANAGEMENT

Current guidelines advise maintenance of normal circulating blood volume instead of prophylactic hyperdynamic, hypervolemic therapy.[35] Lennihan and colleagues randomized patients with aSAH into hypervolemic versus normovolemic regimens based on the measurements of pulmonary artery diastolic pressures (PADPs) for the first 3 days and central venous pressure (CVP) measurements thereafter, and until day 14, they measured CBF using xenon (Xe) washout. There was no difference between the 2 groups in mean global CBF, rate of symptomatic spasm, or functional outcome.[36] Subsequently, Egge and colleagues[37] published similar results in their randomized prospective trial that compared hypervolemic to normovolemic approaches, finding no difference in the occurrence of vasospasm, TCD ultrasonography recordings, or SPECT (single-photon emission computed tomography) CBF measurements. These studies, despite the small number of patients, suggest that euvolemia should be the goal because extra volume translates neither to an increase in CBF nor to improved outcomes. Importantly, fluid management should also take into account the not-uncommon presence of cardiomyopathy[38,39] and neurogenic pulmonary edema.[40] Even moderate volume overload can lead to further lung[41] and cerebral edema in these patients, and positive fluid balance has been associated with increased mortality in neurologic and general critical care populations.[42,43] This discussion raises the question of volume assessment to guide therapy. It is common practice to calculate daily fluid balance (DFB) as a measure of the need for more or less fluid administration, but the correlation of DFB with actual circulating blood volume as measured by integrated pulse spectrophotometry and pulse dye densitometry has been shown to be poor.[44,45] As a consequence, several institutional protocols for the management of aSAH call for insertion of central venous and/or pulmonary artery catheters for the measurement of CVP, PADP, and pulmonary artery occlusion pressures (PAOPs) as measures of right and left heart preload and also for cardiac output (CO) estimations. The major limitation of this approach, apart from its being invasive, relates to the inaccuracy of extrapolating cardiac filling pressures to volumetric assessments. This inaccuracy is accentuated when cardiac compliance is altered, as may be seen with neurogenic stunned myocardium. The failure of these static pressures to predict volume responsiveness has been demonstrated across the spectrum from healthy volunteers to critically ill mechanically ventilated (MV) patients with sepsis; accordingly, dynamic parameters, such as systolic pressure variation and pulse pressure variation for MV patients, are recommended.[46–48] An alternative for advanced hemodynamic monitoring is a device that combines single indicator transpulmonary thermodilution technique and pulse contour continuous CO measurements (PiCCO, PULSION Medical Systems AG, Munich, Germany).[49] This device has been used extensively to guide management of different populations of critically ill patients, including those with conditions such as septic[50] and cardiogenic[51] shock and acute respiratory distress syndrome,[52] and it has been used for management in the operating theater. The potential theoretical benefits are direct volumetric measurements of intrathoracic blood volume (ITBV), global end diastolic volume (GEDV), and extravascular lung water (EVLW) volume and also continuous dynamic volume responsiveness parameter (stroke volume variation [SVV]) and CO monitoring. It does require positive pressure MV and minimal spontaneous breathing efforts. The device has been used in patients with aSAH and was found to be a useful tool for volume and hemodynamic augmentation (HA) management.[53–55] The authors also use PiCCO for selected patients and to target normovolemia goals (GEDV index, 680–800 mL/m^2; ITBV index, 850–1000 mL/m^2; SVV ≤ 10%; and EVLW index ≤ 10 mL/kg). It remains to be seen in a prospective trial if this device proves more useful over traditional measures such as DFB and cardiac filling pressures in patients with aSAH. A last comment on the prevention of hypovolemia concerns the occurrence of CSWS. Despite an incomplete understanding of the pathophysiology of the syndrome, it is considered when large urinary output is accompanied by hyponatremia. A similar clinical picture can be seen secondary to iatrogenic reasons such as overzealous fluid administration and the use of natural diuretics, such as hypertonic saline (HTS).[56] Fludrocortisone is often used as an adjunct to volume and sodium replacement in CSWS. It has been evaluated in 2 randomized controlled trials (RCTs) as a means to prevent hyponatremia and volume contraction, with mixed results.[57,58] An alternative or supplementary fluid management technique is to use colloids, such as 5% albumin, not only as a volume expander but also to potentially prevent sodium and fluid losses associated with CSWS.[59]

NEUROPROTECTION

Nimodipine administration from the time of admission and for 21 days is considered the standard of care and is the only recommendation carrying a class I, level A evidence grade in current guidelines.[35] A recent Cochrane review analyzed a total of 12 studies on calcium antagonists (heavily weighted by a single large trial of nimodipine[60]) and found an outcome improvement with a relative risk reduction of 18% (95% confidence interval [CI], 7%–28%) and an absolute risk reduction of 5.1%.[61] Treatment with nimodipine may prevent 1 poor outcome in every 13 patients with aSAH.[62] However, the medication does not prevent vasospasm[63] and is believed to improve outcome through a neuroprotective mechanism. Alternative explanations have been proposed to explain this beneficial effect, including enhanced fibrinolysis[64] and the observation that nimodipine transforms cortical spreading ischemia back to cortical spreading hyperemia.[65] In recent years, many centers have incorporated the use of HMG-CoA (3-hydroxy-3-methyl-glutaryl-coenzyme A) reductase inhibitors such as "statins" in their standard armamentarium in the treatment of patients with aSAH. A meta-analysis by Sillberg and colleagues[66] included 3 double-blind RCTs of statin versus placebo and found significantly reduced incidence of vasospasm (relative risk [RR] 0.73; 95% CI, 0.54–0.99, number needed to treat [NNT] 6.25), delayed ischemic deficits (RR 0.38; 95% CI, 0.17–0.83, NNT 5), and mortality (RR 0.22; 95% CI, 0.06–0.82, NNT 6.7). All 3 trials have included small numbers of patients, and there is heterogeneity in regards to primary end points. Furthermore, 2 large retrospective studies have reported no benefits from statin use in vasospasm incidence or clinical outcomes.[67,68] The potentially favorable benefit-risk ratio of statins makes them attractive for wide use in aSAH; the authors hope that future large RCTs such as STASH, which is a multicenter placebo-controlled double-blinded phase 3 trial assessing the clinical benefit of SimvaSTatin in Aneurysmal Subarachnoid Hemorrhage, will provide a definitive answer. The hypothesis is that simvastatin 40 mg given within 96 hours of ictus over 3 weeks reduces the incidence and duration of DCI after aSAH when compared with placebo (Dr Peter Kirkpatrick, chief investigator, University of Cambridge, UK).

As mentioned earlier, DIND seems to be the end result of multiple cooperating mechanisms, and relieving angiographic vessel narrowing does not necessarily translate to clinical improvement. The endothelin receptor-A antagonist (clazosentan) studies may provide another valuable clue in dissociating angiographic vasospasm, clinical outcomes, and DCI. CONSCIOUS-1 was a randomized, double-blind, placebo-controlled phase 2 dose-finding trial of intravenous clazosentan with the aim of preventing vasospasm in patients with aSAH. Clazosentan significantly decreased moderate and severe angiographic vasospasm in a dose-dependent manner; nevertheless, no significant benefit on any morbidity or mortality end points was observed.[69] It is possible that the study was underpowered, and a phase 3 clinical trial (CONSCIOUS-2) is designed to focus on clinical outcomes in patients undergoing aneurysm clipping receiving placebo or 5 mg/h of clazosentan.[70] This lack of a clinical effect has led certain investigators to further challenge conventional notions and question if angiographic vasospasm is no more than an epiphenomenon.[16]

Other medical therapies that have been evaluated for the prevention of vasospasm and poor outcomes include the nonglucocorticoid 21-aminosteroid tirilazad, magnesium, aspirin, low molecular weight heparin, nitroglycerin, and nitric oxide donors. Meta-analysis of the tirilazad mesylate study included 3797 patients and found no effect on clinical outcome despite a decrease in symptomatic vasospasm.[71] Magnesium therapy has been studied in a large placebo-controlled trial of continuous intravenous infusion for 14 days with promising results (Magnesium and Acetylsalicylic acid in Subarachnoid Hemorrhage [MASH]). Van den Bergh and colleagues[72] noticed a reduction in poor outcomes at 3 months by 23%, and the RR of a good outcome was 3.4 (95% CI, 1.3–8.9) for treated patients. A (MASH II) phase 3 clinical trial is currently under way with an aim to include 1200 patients before 2010 to further define the role of intravenous magnesiun infusion in patients with aSAH.[73]

DIAGNOSIS AND MULTIMODALITY NEUROMONITORING

Before the discussion of HA as the mainstay of medical management, the diagnosis and neuromonitoring of vasospasm and DCI are reviewed. The gold standard for detection of angiographic vessel narrowing is conventional digital-subtraction angiography (DSA). When clinical symptoms correlate with an area of narrowing on DSA, the diagnosis of clinical vasospasm is made. It should be noted that the presence of large vessel narrowing is not necessary for DCI to occur; in fact, Rabinstein and colleagues[74] reported that the presence and location of angiographically demonstrated vasospasm failed to correlate with areas of cerebral infarction in as many as one-third of their cases. Transcranial Doppler (TCD) ultrasonography is commonly used on a daily basis in the neurocritical care unit to follow patients with aSAH and with moderate to high risk for DCI.

The American Academy of Neurology expert committee has given a Type A, Class II level of evidence supporting the use of TCD ultrasonography in diagnosis of severe spasm.[75] A meta-analysis of 7 trials out of 26 reports evaluated the accuracy of TCD ultrasonography as compared with DSA. For the middle cerebral artery (MCA), sensitivity of TCD ultrasonography was 67% and specificity was 99%, with a positive predictive value of 97% and negative predictive value of 78%. The accuracy of TCD ultrasonography was considerably less for detecting spasm in vessels other than the MCA.[76] The noninvasiveness, ease, and wide availability have made TCD ultrasonography the most common neuromonitor for patients with aSAH. As cautioned before and in relation to DSA, Minhas and colleagues observed no correlation between positron emission tomography (PET) and TCD ultrasonography among patients who developed delayed neurologic deficits after aSAH. They concluded that TCD ultrasonography–derived indices correlate poorly with cerebral perfusion values.[77]

TCD ultrasonography, apart from measurement of flow velocities, can also be used to characterize the state of pressure autoregulation, which has been shown to be deranged in patients with aSAH.[78,79] Soehle and colleagues calculated and followed the moving correlation coefficient between slow changes of arterial blood pressure (ABP) and mean (Mx) or systolic flow velocity. The investigators demonstrated an increase in Mx during vasospasm reflecting a derangement of cerebral pressure autoregulation.[80] The authors have mentioned earlier the potentially beneficial effect of statins in preventing DCI and improving outcomes. A plausible explanation of this effect was published by the Cambridge group and it relates to an improvement in the state of pressure-flow autoregulation as measured by the transient hyperemic response test (TCD ultrasonography derived).[81]

Using brain tissue oxygen ($PtiO_2$) as a surrogate for CBF, Jaeger and colleagues found deranged CBF-autoregulation that does not improve after aSAH-ictus to be closely associated to the development of DCI. They calculated ORx (oxygen reactivity index), which is the moving linear (Pearson) correlation coefficient between the values of cerebral perfusion pressure (CPP) and $PtiO_2$ and varies between −1 and +1. The more positive, the more it indicates a passive relationship between CBF and MAP/CPP, meaning a pressure-passive nonreactive vascular bed. Of note, $PtiO_2$ alone was not different between the DCI and non-DCI groups.[82] The investigation of vascular reactivity and pressure autoregulation indices in patients with aSAH is fascinating and potentially it may yield an early marker for detection of DCI before clinical symptoms ensue. The investigation also provides alternative mechanisms and therapeutic targets for DCI, placing the focus from the proximal segments of the circle of Willis to the microcirculation responsible for CBF regulation.

Microdialysis (MD) is increasingly used in the neuromonitoring of patients with severe TBI and aSAH. A consensus meeting on MD based on the available literature noted that glutamate was found to be the earliest marker of the onset of vasospasm followed over time by lactate, the lactate/pyruvate (L/P) ratio, and glycerol.[83] Sarrafzadeh and colleagues[84] compared MD with PET in 15 patients with aSAH and found glutamate to have the closest correlation with regional CBF (rCBF). Lactate, L/P ratio, and glycerol were significantly higher in symptomatic patients. It is also of interest to note that in this same study and in most symptomatic patients the measured PET-rCBF values were higher than the accepted critical thresholds of ischemia. In an earlier comparison of MD with TCD ultrasonography and DSA by the same group of investigators, MD was shown to be more specific but less sensitive as a diagnostic tool for DIND.[85] Brain tissue oxygenation is actively being researched, especially in TBI, and several centers use it routinely to prevent, detect, and treat secondary brain insults. Retrospective data from a prospective database of patients with aSAH were reported. The investigators observed an association of lower PtiO$_2$ with mortality. More specifically, low PtiO$_2$ on the first day of monitoring, lower mean daily PtiO$_2$, lower mean minimum PtiO$_2$, and longer cumulative duration of compromised PtiO$_2$ tend to be associated with an increased mortality rate at 1 month after aSAH in this cohort.[86] Finally, perfusion imaging in patients with aSAH using PET, SPECT, MRI, and CT methodologies is actively investigated. CT can provide expediently combined computed tomography angiogram and dynamic computed tomographic perfusion (CTP) scans and is becoming increasingly used for the diagnosis of DCI. CTP is based on the central volume principle, which states that the CBF value is the ratio of the blood volume within all blood vessels in a given volume of tissue (cerebral blood volume [CBV], which is measured in milliliters per gram) to the mean transit time (MTT, measured in seconds) of the contrast agent, from the arterial input to the venous drainage, within the volume being evaluated (CBF = CBV/MTT).[87] Recent articles are finding MTT to be an early predictor for DCI and angiographic vasospasm in animal models and human subjects.[88,89] In addition, relative CBF and MTT values have correlated well with estimated rCBF as measured by SPECT in patients with vasospasm after aSAH.[90]

TREATMENT: HEMODYNAMIC AUGMENTATION

The traditional approach to the medical treatment of cerebral vasospasm after aSAH for the prevention of DCI is summarized under the terms of triple-H therapy. The rationale behind this therapy is the enhancement of CBF by an increase in the circulating blood volume, increase in CPP, and improved rheologic properties via hemodilution. It is interesting that this management is considered as the standard of care despite the paucity of well-conducted RCTs. In the following paragraphs the authors review the available literature and describe current thinking under the term HA. Transluminal balloon angioplasty of affected segments combined with intra-arterial vasodilators may be considered in addition to HA in patients with symptomatic vasospasm refractory to triple-H therapy, whereas other proponents of its use suggest using HA merely as a bridge to the more definitive endovascular intervention; this methodology is the subject of discussion in another article (See the article by McGuinness and Gandhi elsewhere in this issue for further exploration of this topic.).

The first report in relation to triple-H therapy is credited to Kosnik and Hunt[91] (1976) when they described 7 patients post clipping for aSAH who developed delayed neurologic deficits. The investigators treated these patients successfully with phenylephrine for blood pressure augmentation and colloids for volume expansion. Shortly after this first report, Kassell and colleagues[92] published their cohort of 58 patients who developed angiographic and clinical spasm post clipping. Treatment with a hypervolemic-hypertensive regimen was able to reverse clinical symptoms in 47 patients. Most publications that followed consist of case reports, series, retrospective data, and noncontrolled studies. Treggiari and colleagues[93] reviewed the literature on the prophylactic application of triple-H therapy and found only 2 RCTs. The investigators commented on the great variability of study protocols and prophylactic regimens used and concluded that there is insufficient evidence to make any recommendations. The issue of prophylactic euvolemia versus hypervolemia has been discussed earlier, and currently the consensus is against prophylactic hypervolemia.

When a patient develops neurologic deficit, volume status should be quickly optimized. In a study of 6 euvolemic patients who developed

DIND and were imaged via PET scanning, Jost and colleagues were able to demonstrate an enhancement of rCBF after a normal saline bolus. Importantly, areas with ischemic level of CBF increased to nonischemic levels with volume expansion. It is notable that the bolus did not increase ABP, CO, or cardiac filling pressures as measured by central venous and pulmonary artery catheters.[94] The number of patients investigated is small and there are no outcome data; nevertheless, this elegant study shows the beneficial potential of volume loading in enhancement of CBF in ischemic brain regions. Subsequently, the Cambridge group has researched the effect of 23.5% HTS infusion on CBF as measured by Xe-CT and on cerebral autoregulation as measured by TCD ultrasonography and by waveform cross correlation of continuous ABP, intracranial pressure (ICP), and CPP monitoring.[95] Subjects for this study were 35 patients with low-grade aSAH. HTS administration significantly increased ABP and CPP at 30 minutes post infusion followed by a decrease in ICP, and also there was a dose-dependent effect of CBF increments on favorable outcome (mRS [modified Rankin scale] at hospital discharge). In this study, CBF augmentation by HTS was independent of baseline levels. Transient autoregulatory impairment was seen with HTS administration likely secondary to vasodilation with an eventual increase in CPP. A significant contribution to the literature on HA is the article by Muench and colleagues.[55] This is a combined experimental animal and clinical intervention study involving 10 patients with aSAH. For both parts of the study, advanced hemodynamic monitoring with a central venous catheter and the PiCCO device and advanced neuromonitoring with intra-parenchymal ICP monitor, $PtiO_2$ probe, and thermal diffusion rCBF microprobe were used. The aim of the study was to investigate the influence of the 3 components of triple-H therapy on rCBF and brain tissue oxygenation in healthy animals with intact pressure autoregulation and in patients with aSAH with potentially deranged autoregulation. Their findings have important implications. Specifically, in the animal experiment, neither induced hypertension nor hypervolemia altered ICP, $PtiO_2$, or rCBF. In patients, who all had deranged autoregulation from day 1, induced hypertension resulted in significant increase of rCBF and $PtiO_2$. This benefit of ABP augmentation was lost when it was combined with hypervolemic hemodilution, which led to a decrease in $PtiO_2$ likely due to an adverse effect on oxygen delivery. State of autoregulation and oxygen carrying capacity of the blood should be critically considered during HA application.

Hemodilution conceptually leads to decreased blood viscosity and improved rheology. Ekelund and colleagues showed that isovolemic hemodilution to a hematocrit value of 0.28 from 0.36 does increase CBF, but it comes with a pronounced reduction in oxygen delivery capacity, translating to an overall increase in the volume of ischemic brain regions. In addition, hypervolemia conferred no benefit, further suggesting that there may be a hemoglobin (Hgb) threshold that should not be exceeded irrespective of volume status.[96] Kramer and colleagues have published a retrospective cohort study of 245 patients with aSAH. Anemia (Hgb <10 g/dL) and use of transfusions were both associated with worse outcomes; with both variables entered into logistic regression, only transfusion remained significantly predictive. Transfusion-related outcome worsening was stronger among patients without vasospasm.[97] Cause and effect are impossible to decipher from such a retrospective design in which there may be uncontrolled confounders. Other reports have shown an association of higher Hgb levels with improved outcome after correction for other clinical predictors.[98] The authors agree with the investigators of the previously referenced studies that a liberal versus a restrictive transfusion strategy trial is justified in patients with aSAH and that extrapolations from the literature on non–brain injured patients are not appropriate. Further understanding of the optimal Hgb level and transfusion triggers could be guided by advanced neuromonitoring. Recently, the Penn group has reported their findings from monitoring brain tissue oxygenation and MD metabolic parameters in patients with poor-grade aSAH who received blood transfusions. They found the incidence of brain hypoxia and cell energy dysfunction to increase significantly when Hgb level was less than 9 g/dL. This finding was independent of other relevant physiologic variables (such as CPP, CVP, Pao_2/Fio_2 ratio [partial pressure of arterial oxygen to fraction of inspired oxygen ratio]) and from the presence of clinical vasospasm.[99] Significant limitations are again the small sample size and the lack of correlation with clinical outcomes. The optimal Hgb level is currently unknown and most experts maintain a level close to 10 g/dL, especially during the peak vasospasm period and in symptomatic patients.

The previously discussed studies serve as a proof of concept for cautious volume expansion, with attention to Hgb levels and oxygen delivery, in the euvolemic patient with neurologic deterioration during the vasospasm period, and this is the first step that the authors take in the management of such patients. Advanced hemodynamic monitoring often becomes necessary to guide fluid administration. CVP and PADP/PAOP measurements are most commonly used, we have mentioned the possible caveats with their use in the patient with aSAH. It will be interesting to see if ITBV and GEDV prove to be more sensitive indices and if the assistance of knowing EVLW can help optimize volume with avoidance of pulmonary edema.

To directly increase CBF, manipulation of ABP and CO become the major tools. ABP augmentation is achieved with the use of vasopressors such as phenylephrine, dopamine (DA), and norepinephrine (NE). The target blood pressure is titrated according to clinical neurologic examination, direct rCBF measurements, and tissue oxygen and metabolic parameters when available, and to adverse effects related to end-organ damage. Neurogenic stunned myocardium and cardiomyopathy as well as cardiogenic and noncardiogenic pulmonary edema must be taken into account. There are no comparative studies between vasopressor agents in the setting of HA for aSAH. The choice depends on comorbidities such as cardiac function and patient tolerance. Miller and colleagues treated a cohort of 24 patients with aSAH with phenylephrine for the prevention of DCI; two-thirds of them had vascular risk factors but normal cardiac index before augmentation. There were no clinically significant episodes of pulmonary edema or myocardial infarctions and no extracardiac toxicity. Phenylephrine was discontinued in only 1 patient, and 88% of the patients exhibited neurologic improvement.[100] The effect of CPP augmentation with DA as compared with NE on brain tissue oxygenation and MD parameters was studied by Johnston and colleagues in a small number of patients with severe TBI. Although TBI has a potentially different pathophysiology from that of aSAH, the investigators noted no significant differences between the 2 agents on cerebral oxygenation or metabolic parameters. DA leads to a significantly higher cardiac index without a difference in MAP. Overall, there were no large differences observed in terms of CBF or $CMRO_2$ (cerebral metabolic rate of oxygen). CPP augmentation with NE significantly reduced $AVDO_2$ (arteriojugular venous difference of oxygen) and increased $PbtO_2$ (brain tissue partial pressure), and the response was more predictable than with the use of DA.[101] The same group had similar results when DA was compared with NE using TCD ultrasonography FVm (mean flow velocity) as a surrogate for CBF. Their conclusion was that NE may be more reliable and efficient for CPP augmentation in patients with TBI.[102] The authors use NE or phenylephrine as

a first choice in patients with preserved cardiac function. If there is any cardiac compromise, a combination of NE with dobutamine or milrinone is considered, or DA.

Kim and colleagues treated 16 patients with vasospasm post aSAH and assigned them to 3 different groups for HA. One group received hypervolemia only, the second group received MAP augmentation with phenylephrine, and the third one received CO augmentation with dobutamine. CBF was measured with Xe-CT, and all 3 groups had similar baseline values. The important finding of this study is the direct effect of increased CO to an increment of CBF independent of MAP.[103] CO augmentation is an alternative and complementary method for HA, and as the investigators argue, it may be safer than induced hypertension. Of note, hypervolemia alone had no effect on CBF in this study. Milrinone is another potentially useful agent for CO augmentation in the setting of aSAH. Naidech and colleagues[104] suggested that dobutamine and milrinone could be equal choices for patients with moderate MAP and systemic vascular resistance, but dobutamine may be superior in hypotensive patients or patients with low systemic vascular resistance. Apart from CO augmentation in the setting of HA, CO augmentation may be required secondary to a neurogenic stunned myocardium or to a so-called takotsubo cardiomyopathy.[105,106] Patients may develop cardiogenic shock, and a few case reports and case series describe rescue therapy with employment of an intra-aortic balloon pump (IABP) in patients with aSAH.[107,108] In fact, the common use of vasopressors may not be appropriate in the presence of takotsubo cardiomyopathy in view of the proposed pathophysiology of the syndrome, meaning catecholamine excess. Tung and colleagues[109] in a multivariate model examining predictors of neurocardiogenic injury found the use of phenylephrine, a pure alpha agonist, to be independently associated with higher levels of troponin release. This was not a result of the higher systolic blood pressure achieved with phenylephrine, suggesting direct toxicity of this pressor to the myocardium. In this scenario, mechanical circulatory support in the form of an IABP may be the more appropriate therapy instead of increasing doses of vasoactive medications, as suggested for patients with myocardial stunning caused by sudden emotional stress.[110] As a last comment on IABP use, the authors refer to the study by Spann and colleagues because this is the only study administering IABP therapy in a prospective fashion in 6 patients with aSAH who were deemed by them at high risk for DCI but before they developed any vasospasm or cardiac dysfunction. The objective was to measure the effect of IABP on CBF, which is measured after administration of Xe-133. This study provides evidence of the beneficial effect of IABP on CBF even in patients with apparently not severely compromised cardiac function.[111]

SUMMARY

The understanding of DIND pathomechanisms is evolving. Arterial vessel narrowing is neither necessary nor always sufficient to cause DCI. Advanced hemodynamic monitoring and neuro-monitoring hold promise in prevention, early detection, and therapy guidance. Knowledge of the state of pressure autoregulation, vascular reactivity, local CBF, and tissue oxygen and metabolic parameters could potentially lead to targeted interventional and medical manipulations. The aim is to reduce the toll of DIND on patients with aSAH and to minimize complications of applied therapies.

REFERENCES

1. Graf CJ, Nibbelink DW. Cooperative study of intracranial aneurysms and subarachnoid hemorrhage: report on a randomized treatment study, 3: intracranial surgery. Stroke 1974;5:557–601.
2. King JT Jr. Epidemiology of aneurysmal subarachnoid hemorrhage. Neuroimaging Clin N Am 1997;7: 659–68.
3. Anderson C, Anderson N, Bonita R, et al. Epidemiology of aneurysmal subarachnoid hemorrhage in Australia and New Zealand: incidence and case fatality from the Australasian Cooperative Research on Subarachnoid Hemorrhage Study (ACROSS). Stroke 2000;31:1843–50.
4. Johnston SC, Selvin S, Gress DR. The burden, trends, and demographics of mortality from subarachnoid hemorrhage. Neurology 1998;50: 1413–8.
5. Huang J, Van Gelder JM. The probability of sudden death from rupture of intracranial aneurysms: a meta-analysis. Neurosurgery 2002;51: 1101–5.
6. Schievink WI. Intracranial aneurysms. N Engl J Med 1997;336:28–40.
7. Kassell NF, Torner JC. Aneurysmal rebleeding: a preliminary report from the Cooperative Aneurysm Study. Neurosurgery 1983;13:479–81.
8. Ohkuma H, Tsurutani H, Suzuki S. Incidence and significance of early aneurysmal rebleeding before neurosurgical or neurological management. Stroke 2001;32:1176–80.
9. Hillman J, Fridriksson S, Nilsson O, et al. Immediate administration of tranexamic acid and reduced incidence of early rebleeding after aneurysmal subarachnoid hemorrhage: a prospective randomized study. J Neurosurg 2002;97:771–8.
10. Starke RM, Kim GH, Fernandez A, et al. Impact of a protocol for acute antifibrinolytic therapy on aneurysm rebleeding after subarachnoid hemorrhage. Stroke 2008;39:2617–21.
11. Cahill J, Calvert JW, Zhang JH. Mechanisms of early brain injury after subarachnoid hemorrhage. J Cereb Blood Flow Metab 2006;26(11):1341–53.
12. Cahill J, Zhang JH. Subarachnoid hemorrhage: is it time for a new direction? Stroke 2009;40(Suppl 3): S86–7.
13. Eddleman CS, Hurley MC, Naidech AM, et al. Endovascular options in the treatment of delayed ischemic neurological deficits due to cerebral vasospasm. Neurosurg Focus 2009;26(3):E6.
14. Rinkel G, Feigin V, Algra A, et al. Circulatory volume expansion therapy for aneurysmal subarachnoid haemorrhage. Cochrane Database Syst Rev 2004;(4):CD000483.
15. Pluta RM, Hansen-Schwartz J, Dreier J, et al. Cerebral vasospasm following subarachnoid hemorrhage: time for a new world of thought. Neurol Res 2009;31(2):151–8.
16. Vergouwen MD, Vermeulen M, Coert BA, et al. Delayed cerebral ischemia after aneurysmal subarachnoid hemorrhage: is angiographic vasospasm an epiphenomenon? Stroke 2009;40(2): e39.
17. Vergouwen MD, Vermeulen M, Coert BA, et al. Microthrombosis after aneurysmal subarachnoid hemorrhage: an additional explanation for delayed cerebral ischemia. J Cereb Blood Flow Metab 2008;28(11):1761–70.
18. Stein SC, Levine JM, Nagpal S, et al. Vasospasm as the sole cause of cerebral ischemia: how strong is the evidence? [review]. Neurosurg Focus 2006; 21(3):E2.
19. Dorsch NW. Cerebral arterial spasm—a clinical review. Br J Neurosurg 1995;9:403–12.
20. Heros RC, Zervas NT, Varsos V. Cerebral vasospasm after subarachnoid hemorrhage: an update. Ann Neurol 1983;14:599–608.
21. Baldwin ME, Macdonald RL, Huo D, et al. Early vasospasm on admission angiography in patients with aneurysmal subarachnoid hemorrhage is a predictor for in-hospital complications and poor outcome. Stroke 2004;35:2506–11.
22. Qureshi AI, Sung GY, Suri MA, et al. Prognostic value and determinants of ultraearly angiographic vasospasm after aneurysmal subarachnoid hemorrhage. Neurosurgery 1999;44:967–74.
23. Kolias AG, Sen J, Belli AJ. Pathogenesis of cerebral vasospasm following aneurysmal subarachnoid hemorrhage: putative mechanisms and novel approaches. Neurosci Res 2009;87(1):1–11.

24. Macdonald RL, Weir BK. A review of hemoglobin and the pathogenesis of cerebral vasospasm. Stroke 1991;22:971–82.

25. Fisher CM, Kistler JP, Davis JM. Relation of cerebral vasospasm to subarachnoid hemorrhage visualized by computerized tomographic scanning. Neurosurgery 1980;6:1–9.

26. Claassen J, Bernardini GL, Kreiter K, et al. Effect of cisternal and ventricular blood on risk of delayed cerebral ischemia after subarachnoid hemorrhage: the Fisher scale revisited. Stroke 2001;32:2012–20.

27. Frontera JA, Claassen J, Schmidt JM, et al. Prediction of symptomatic vasospasm after subarachnoid hemorrhage: the modified fisher scale. Neurosurgery 2006;59:21–7.

28. Amin-Hanjani S, Ogilvy CS, Barker FG. Does intracisternal thrombolysis prevent vasospasm after aneurysmal subarachnoid hemorrhage? A meta-analysis. Neurosurgery 2004;54:326–34.

29. Kawamoto S, Tsutsumi K, Yoshikawa G, et al. Effectiveness of the head-shaking method combined with cisternal irrigation with urokinase in preventing cerebral vasospasm after subarachnoid hemorrhage. J Neurosurg 2004;100:236–43.

30. Klimo P Jr, Kestle JR, MacDonald JD, et al. Marked reduction of cerebral vasospasm with lumbar drainage of cerebrospinal fluid after subarachnoid hemorrhage. J Neurosurg 2004;100:215–24.

31. Rabb CH, Tang G, Chin LS, et al. A statistical analysis of factors related to symptomatic cerebral vasospasm. Acta Neurochir 1994;127:27–31.

32. Lasner TM, Weil RJ, Riina HA, et al. Cigarette smoking-induced increase in the risk of symptomatic vasospasm after aneurysmal subarachnoid hemorrhage. J Neurosurg 1997;87(3):381–4.

33. Inagawa T. Cerebral vasospasm in elderly patients treated by early operation for ruptured intracranial aneurysms. Acta Neurochir 1992;115:79–85.

34. Wijdicks EFM, Vermeulen M, ten Haaf JA, et al. Volume depletion and natriuresis in patients with a ruptured intracranial aneurysm. Ann Neurol 1985;18:211–6.

35. Bederson JB, Connolly ES Jr, Batjer HH, et al. American Heart Association Guidelines for the management of aneurysmal subarachnoid hemorrhage: a statement for healthcare professionals from a special writing group of the Stroke Council, American Heart Association. Stroke 2009;40(3): 994–1025.

36. Lennihan L, Mayer SA, Fink ME, et al. Effect of hypervolemic therapy on cerebral blood flow after subarachnoid hemorrhage: a randomized controlled trial. Stroke 2000;31:383–91.

37. Egge A, Waterloo K, Sjoholm H, et al. Prophylactic hyperdynamic postoperative fluid therapy after aneurismal subarachnoid hemorrhage: a clinical, prospective, randomized, controlled study. Neurosurgery 2001;49:593–605.

38. van der Bilt IA, Hasan D, Vandertop WP, et al. Impact of cardiac complications on outcome after aneurysmal subarachnoid hemorrhage: a meta-analysis. Neurology 2009;72(7):635–42.

39. Fujita K, Fukuhara T, Munemasa M, et al. Ampulla cardiomyopathy associated with aneurysmal subarachnoid hemorrhage: report of 6 patients. Surg Neurol 2007;68(5):556–61.

40. Muroi C, Keller M, Pangalu A, et al. Neurogenic pulmonary edema in patients with subarachnoid hemorrhage. J Neurosurg Anesthesiol 2008;20(3): 188–92.

41. Corsten L, Raja A, Guppy K, et al. Contemporary management of subarachnoid hemorrhage and vasospasm: the UIC experience. Surg Neurol 2001;56(3):140–8.

42. Mascia L, Sakr Y, Pasero D, et al. Sepsis Occurrence in Acutely Ill Patients (SOAP) Investigators. Extracranial complications in patients with acute brain injury: a post-hoc analysis of the SOAP study. Intensive Care Med 2008;34(4):720–7.

43. Vincent JL, Sakr Y, Sprung CL, et al. Sepsis Occurrence in Acutely Ill Patients Investigators. Sepsis in European intensive care units: results of the SOAP study. Crit Care Med 2006;34(2):344–53.

44. Kasuya H, Onda H, Yoneyama T, et al. Bedside monitoring of circulating blood volume after subarachnoid hemorrhage. Stroke 2003;34(4): 956–60.

45. Hoff RG, van Dijk GW, Algra A, et al. Fluid balance and blood volume measurement after aneurysmal subarachnoid hemorrhage. Neurocrit Care 2008; 8(3):391–7.

46. Kumar A, Anel R, Bunnell E, et al. Pulmonary artery occlusion pressure and central venous pressure fail to predict ventricular filling volume, cardiac performance, or the response to volume infusion in normal subjects. Crit Care Med 2004;32(3): 691–9.

47. Osman D, Ridel C, Ray P, et al. Cardiac filling pressures are not appropriate to predict hemodynamic response to volume challenge. Crit Care Med 2007; 35(1):64–8.

48. Michard F, Boussat S, Chemla D, et al. Relation between respiratory changes in arterial pulse pressure and fluid responsiveness in septic patients with acute circulatory failure. Am J Respir Crit Care Med 2000;162(1):134–8.

49. Gödje O, Höke K, Goetz AE, et al. Reliability of a new algorithm for continuous cardiac output determination by pulse-contour analysis during hemodynamic instability. Crit Care Med 2002; 30(1):52–8.

50. Spöhr F, Hettrich P, Bauer H, et al. Comparison of two methods for enhanced continuous circulatory

monitoring in patients with septic shock. Intensive Care Med 2007;33(10):1805–10.

51. Friesecke S, Heinrich A, Abel P, et al. Comparison of pulmonary artery and aortic transpulmonary thermodilution for monitoring of cardiac output in patients with severe heart failure: validation of a novel method. Crit Care Med 2009;37(1): 119–23.

52. Berkowitz DM, Danai PA, Eaton S, et al. Accurate characterization of extravascular lung water in acute respiratory distress syndrome. Crit Care Med 2008;36(6):1803–9.

53. Segal E, Greenlee JD, Hata SJ, et al. Monitoring intravascular volumes to direct hypertensive, hypervolemic therapy in a patient with vasospasm. J Neurosurg Anesthesiol 2004;16:296–8.

54. Mutoh T, Kazumata K, Ajiki M, et al. Goal-directed fluid management by bedside transpulmonary hemodynamic monitoring after subarachnoid hemorrhage. Stroke 2007;38(12):3218–24.

55. Muench E, Horn P, Bauhuf C, et al. Effects of hypervolemia and hypertension on regional cerebral blood flow, intracranial pressure, and brain tissue oxygenation after subarachnoid hemorrhage. Crit Care Med 2007;35(8):1844–51.

56. Naval NS, Stevens RD, Mirski MA, et al. Controversies in the management of aneurysmal subarachnoid hemorrhage [review]. Crit Care Med 2006; 34(2):511–24.

57. Hasan D, Lindsay KW, Wijdicks EF, et al. Effect of fludrocortisone acetate in patients with subarachnoid hemorrhage. Stroke 1989;20:1156–61.

58. Mori T, Katayama Y, Kawamata T, et al. Improved efficiency of hypervolemic therapy with inhibition of natriuresis by fludrocortisone in patients with aneurysmal subarachnoid hemorrhage. J Neurosurg 1999;91:947–52.

59. Mayer SA, Solomon RA, Fink ME, et al. Effect of 5% albumin solution on sodium balance and blood volume after subarachnoid hemorrhage. Neurosurgery 1998;42:759–67.

60. Pickard JD, Murray GD, Illingworth R, et al. Effect of oral nimodipine on cerebral infarction and outcome after subarachnoid haemorrhage: British aneurysm nimodipine trial. BMJ 1989;298:636–42.

61. Rinkel GJE, Feigin VL, Algra A, et al. Calcium antagonists for aneurysmal subarachnoid haemorrhage. Cochrane Database Syst Rev 2005;(1):CD000277.

62. Zubkov AY, Rabinstein AA. Medical management of cerebral vasospasm: present and future. Neurol Res 2009;31(6):626–31.

63. Feigin VL, Rinkel GJ, Algra A, et al. Calcium antagonists in patients with aneurismal subarachnoid hemorrhage: a systematic review. Neurology 1998;50:876–83.

64. Roos YB, Levi M, Carroll TA, et al. Nimodipine increases fibrinolytic activity in patients with aneurysmal subarachnoid hemorrhage. Stroke 2001;32:1860–2.

65. Dreier JP, Körner K, Ebert N, et al. Nitric oxide scavenging by hemoglobin or nitric oxide synthase inhibition by N-nitro-L-arginine induces cortical spreading ischemia when K+ is increased in the subarachnoid space. J Cereb Blood Flow Metab 1998;18:978–90.

66. Sillberg VA, Wells GA, Perry JJ. Do statins improve outcomes and reduce the incidence of vasospasm after aneurysmal subarachnoid hemorrhage: a meta-analysis. Stroke 2008;39(9):2622–6.

67. Kramer AH, Gurka MJ, Nathan B, et al. Statin use was not associated with less vasospasm or improved outcome after subarachnoid hemorrhage. Neurosurgery 2008;62(2):422–7 [discussion: 427–30].

68. McGirt MJ, Garces Ambrossi GL, Huang J, et al. Simvastatin for the prevention of symptomatic cerebral vasospasm following aneurysmal subarachnoid hemorrhage: a single-institution prospective cohort study. J Neurosurg 2009;110(5):968–74.

69. Macdonald RL, Kassell NF, Mayer S, et al. CONSCIOUS-1 Investigators. Clazosentan to overcome neurological ischemia and infarction occurring after subarachnoid hemorrhage (CONSCIOUS-1): randomized, double-blind, placebo-controlled phase 2 dose-finding trial. Stroke 2008;39(11): 3015–21.

70. Pearl JD, Macdonald RL. Vasospasm after aneurysmal subarachnoid hemorrhage: need for further study. Acta Neurochir Suppl 2008;105: 207–10.

71. Jang YG, Ilodigwe D, Macdonald RL. Metaanalysis of tirilazad mesylate in patients with aneurysmal subarachnoid hemorrhage. Neurocrit Care 2009; 10(1):141–7.

72. van den Bergh WM, Algra A, van Kooten F, et al. MASH Study Group. Magnesium sulfate in aneurysmal subarachnoid hemorrhage: a randomized controlled trial. Stroke 2005;36(5):1011–5.

73. Dorhout Mees SM, MASH-II Study Group. Magnesium in aneurysmal subarachnoid hemorrhage (MASH II) phase III clinical trial MASH-II study group. Int J Stroke 2008;3(1):63–5.

74. Rabinstein AA, Friedman JA, Weigand SD, et al. Predictors of cerebral infarction in aneurysmal subarachnoid hemorrhage. Stroke 2004;35: 1862–6.

75. Sloan MA, Alexandrov AV, Tegeler CH, et al. Therapeutics and Technology Assessment Subcommittee of the American Academy of Neurology. Assessment: transcranial Doppler ultrasonography: report of the Therapeutics and Technology Assessment Subcommittee of the American Academy of Neurology. Neurology 2004;62: 1468–81.

76. Lysakowski C, Walder B, Costanza MC, et al. Transcranial Doppler versus angiography in patients with vasospasm due to a ruptured cerebral aneurysm: a systematic review. Stroke 2001;32:2292–8.

77. Minhas PS, Menon DK, Smielewski P, et al. Positron emission tomographic cerebral perfusion disturbances and transcranial Doppler findings among patients with neurological deterioration after subarachnoid hemorrhage. Neurosurgery 2003; 52(5):1017–22.

78. Lam JM, Smielewski P, Czosnyka M, et al. Predicting delayed ischemic deficits after aneurysmal subarachnoid hemorrhage using a transient hyperemic response test of cerebral autoregulation. Neurosurgery 2000;47:819–26.

79. Rätsep T, Asser T. Cerebral hemodynamic impairment after aneurysmal subarachnoid hemorrhage as evaluated using transcranial Doppler ultrasonography: relationship to delayed cerebral ischemia and clinical outcome. J Neurosurg 2001; 95:393–401.

80. Soehle M, Czosnyka M, Pickard JD, et al. Continuous assessment of cerebral autoregulation in subarachnoid hemorrhage. Anesth Analg 2004; 98(4):1133–9.

81. Tseng MY, Czosnyka M, Richards H, et al. Effects of acute treatment with statins on cerebral autoregulation in patients after aneurysmal subarachnoid hemorrhage. Neurosurg Focus 2006;21(3): E10.

82. Jaeger M, Schuhmann MU, Soehle M, et al. Continuous monitoring of cerebrovascular autoregulation after subarachnoid hemorrhage by brain tissue oxygen pressure reactivity and its relation to delayed cerebral infarction. Stroke 2007;38(3): 981–6.

83. Bellander BM, Cantais E, Enblad P, et al. Consensus meeting on microdialysis in neurointensive care. Intensive Care Med 2004;30(12):2166–9.

84. Sarrafzadeh A, Haux D, Plotkin M, et al. Bedside microdialysis reflects dysfunction of cerebral energy metabolism in patients with aneurysmal subarachnoid hemorrhage as confirmed by 15 O-H2 O-PET and 18 F-FDG-PET. J Neuroradiol 2005;32(5):348–51.

85. Unterberg AW, Sakowitz OW, Sarrafzadeh AS, et al. Role of bedside microdialysis in the diagnosis of cerebral vasospasm following aneurysmal subarachnoid hemorrhage. J Neurosurg 2001;94: 740–9.

86. Ramakrishna R, Stiefel M, Udoetuk J, et al. Brain oxygen tension and outcome in patients with aneurysmal subarachnoid hemorrhage. J Neurosurg 2008;109(6):1075–82.

87. Lad SP, Guzman R, Kelly ME, et al. Cerebral perfusion imaging in vasospasm [review]. Neurosurg Focus 2006;21(3):E7.

88. Laslo AM, Eastwood JD, Pakkiri P, et al. CT perfusion-derived mean transit time predicts early mortality and delayed vasospasm after experimental subarachnoid hemorrhage. AJNR Am J Neuroradiol 2008;29(1):79–85.

89. Pham M, Johnson A, Bartsch AJ, et al. CT perfusion predicts secondary cerebral infarction after aneurysmal subarachnoid hemorrhage. Neurology 2007;69(8):762–5.

90. Sviri GE, Mesiwala AH, Lewis DH, et al. Dynamic perfusion computerized tomography in cerebral vasospasm following aneurysmal subarachnoid hemorrhage: a comparison with technetium-99m-labeled ethyl cysteinate dimer-single-photon emission computerized tomography. J Neurosurg 2006;104(3):404–10.

91. Kosnik EJ, Hunt WE. Postoperative hypertension in the management of patients with intracranial arterial aneurysms. J Neurosurg 1976;45(2):148–54.

92. Kassell NF, Peerless SJ, Durward QJ, et al. Treatment of ischemic deficits from vasospasm with intravascular volume expansion and induced arterial hypertension. Neurosurgery 1982;11(3): 337–43.

93. Treggiari MM, Walder B, Suter PM, et al. Systematic review of the prevention of delayed ischemic neurological deficits with hypertension, hypervolemia, and hemodilution therapy following subarachnoid hemorrhage [review]. J Neurosurg 2003;98(5): 978–84.

94. Jost SC, Diringer MN, Zazulia AR, et al. Effect of normal saline bolus on cerebral blood flow in regions with low baseline flow in patients with vasospasm following subarachnoid hemorrhage. J Neurosurg 2005;103(1):25–30.

95. Tseng MY, Al-Rawi PG, Czosnyka M, et al. Enhancement of cerebral blood flow using systemic hypertonic saline therapy improves outcome in patients with poor-grade spontaneous subarachnoid hemorrhage. J Neurosurg 2007; 107(2):274–82.

96. Ekelund A, Reinstrup P, Ryding E, et al. Effects of iso- and hypervolemic hemodilution on regional cerebral blood flow and oxygendelivery for patients with vasospasm after aneurysmal subarachnoid hemorrhage. Acta Neurochir (Wien) 2002;144: 703–12.

97. Kramer AH, Gurka MJ, Nathan B, et al. Complications associated with anemia and blood transfusion in patients with aneurysmal subarachnoid hemorrhage. Crit Care Med 2008;36(7):2070–5.

98. Naidech AM, Jovanovic B, Wartenberg KE, et al. Higher hemoglobin is associated with improved outcome after subarachnoid hemorrhage. Crit Care Med 2007;35(10):2383–9.

99. Oddo M, Milby A, Chen I, et al. Hemoglobin concentration and cerebral metabolism in patients

with aneurysmal subarachnoid hemorrhage. Stroke 2009;40(4):1275–81.

100. Miller JA, Dacey RG Jr, Diringer MN. Safety of hypertensive hypervolemic therapy with phenylephrine in the treatment of delayed ischemic deficits after subarachnoid hemorrhage. Stroke 1995; 26(12):2260–6.

101. Johnston AJ, Steiner LA, Chatfield DA, et al. Effect of cerebral perfusion pressure augmentation with dopamine and norepinephrine on global and focal brain oxygenation after traumatic brain injury. Intensive Care Med 2004;30(5):791–7.

102. Steiner LA, Johnston AJ, Czosnyka M, et al. Direct comparison of cerebrovascular effects of norepinephrine and dopamine in head-injured patients. Crit Care Med 2004;32(4):1049–54.

103. Kim HD, Joseph M, Ziadi S, et al. Increases in cardiac output can reverse flow deficits from vasospasm independent of blood pressure: a study using xenon computed tomographic measurement of cerebral blood flow. Neurosurgery 2003;53(5): 1044–51.

104. Naidech A, Du Y, Kreiter KT, et al. Dobutamine versus milrinone after subarachnoid hemorrhage. Neurosurgery 2005;56(1):21–6.

105. Lee VH, Connolly HM, Fulgham JR, et al. Tako-tsubo cardiomyopathy in aneurysmal subarachnoid hemorrhage: an underappreciated ventricular dysfunction. J Neurosurg 2006;105(2):264–70.

106. Kawai S, Kitabatake A, Tomoike H, Takotsubo Cardiomyopathy Group. Guidelines for diagnosis of takotsubo (ampulla) cardiomyopathy. Circ J 2007;71(6):990–2.

107. Apostolides PJ, Greene KA, Zabramski JM, et al. Intra-aortic balloon pump counterpulsation in the management of concomitant cerebral vasospasm and cardiac failure after subarachnoid hemorrhage: technical case report. Neurosurgery 1996; 38(5):1056–9 [discussion: 1059–60].

108. Rosen CL, Sekhar LN, Duong DH. Use of intra-aortic balloon pump counterpulsation for refractory symptomatic vasospasm. Acta Neurochir (Wien) 2000;142(1):25–32.

109. Tung P, Kopelnik A, Banki N, et al. Predictors of neurocardiogenic injury after subarachnoid hemorrhage. Stroke 2004;35(2):548–51.

110. Wittstein IS, Thiemann DR, Lima JA, et al. Neurohumoral features of myocardial stunning due to sudden emotional stress. N Engl J Med 2005; 352(6):539–48.

111. Spann RG, Lang DA, Birch AA, et al. Intra-aortic balloon counterpulsation: augmentation of cerebral blood flow after aneurysmal subarachnoid haemorrhage. Acta Neurochir (Wien) 2001;143(2):115–23.

Inflammation and Cerebral Vasospasm After Subarachnoid Hemorrhage

Gustavo Pradilla, MD[a], Kaisorn L. Chaichana, MD[a],
Stanley Hoang, BS[b], Judy Huang, MD[a],
Rafael J. Tamargo, MD[a],*

KEYWORDS

- Cerebral vasospasm • Subarachnoid hemorrhage
- Inflammation • Leukocytes • Endothelial cells
- Hemoglobin • Haptoglobin • Nitric oxide

Aneurysmal subarachnoid hemorrhage (aSAH) remains a leading cause of morbidity and mortality in patients who survive the initial ictus, primarily as a result of the development of delayed or chronic vasospasm.[1–4] Vasospasm after aSAH in humans is a biphasic phenomenon[5] in which an acute phase that typically occurs 3 to 4 hours after an aSAH and generally resolves rapidly, is followed by a chronic phase that occurs 3 to 14 days later.[5] This chronic or delayed phase is characterized by sustained arterial narrowing that can lead to permanent deficits and death in 20% to 40% of patients.[1–3,6] Cerebral vasospasm has also been observed in other conditions, including traumatic brain injury,[7–15] after craniotomies,[16–18] and in meningitis.[19–23] Interactions between leukocytes and endothelial cells are fundamental factors in the inflammatory response to injury, and seem to be critical components in the pathophysiology of posthemorrhagic cerebral vasospasm.[24] This review summarizes the growing body of evidence that supports the prominent role of inflammation in this condition, and discusses its potential implications in the development of diagnostic and therapeutic strategies for this condition.

THE INFLAMMATORY HYPOTHESIS OF VASOSPASM AFTER SUBARACHNOID HEMORRHAGE

During SAH, blood deposition into the subarachnoid space results in release of free hemoglobin (Hgb), which is extremely toxic.[25] To counteract free Hgb toxicity, the immune system stimulates rapid expression of specific cell adhesion molecules (CAMs) on the luminal surface of the endothelial cells.[24] This allows macrophages and neutrophils to bind to the endothelial cells and enter the subarachnoid space, where they phagocytose extravasated red blood cells (RBCs) and remove free Hgb. The binding and clearance of extracorpuscular Hgb relies on the identification of Hgb only when it is conjugated with haptoglobin (Hp),[25] a serum protein that binds to free Hgb with high affinity.[25]

After RBC phagocytosis and Hgb clearance, however, macrophages and neutrophils remain trapped in the subarachnoid space because of the absence of lymphatics in the central nervous system (CNS) and impaired cerebrospinal fluid (CSF) flow caused by the SAH,[24] and within 2 to

[a] Division of Cerebrovascular Neurosurgery, Department of Neurosurgery, The Johns Hopkins University School of Medicine, Meyer Building 8-181, 600 North Wolfe Street, Baltimore, MD 21287, USA
[b] Stanford University, School of Medicine, Palo Alto, CA 94305, USA
* Corresponding author
E-mail address: rtamarg@jhmi.edu

Neurosurg Clin N Am 21 (2010) 365–379
doi:10.1016/j.nec.2009.10.008
1042-3680/10/$ – see front matter © 2010 Elsevier Inc. All rights reserved.

4 days after their entry into the subarachnoid space, macrophages and neutrophils die and degranulate.[26–31] This results in a release of intracellular endothelins (ET) and oxygen-free radicals into the interstitial and subarachnoid spaces that ultimately cause an inflammation-induced arteriopathy and arterial vasoconstriction.[26,28–32] Arterial narrowing, however, is only 1 manifestation of the inflammatory response that follows SAH; the clinical deterioration of patients with arterial narrowing by imaging or ultrasonography is the result of a more complex and robust inflammatory response that results in meningitis and cerebritis. This hypothesis explains why the meningitic syndrome and arterial spasm seen after aSAH, which results in delayed ischemic deficits and

stroke, is also present in other pathophysiologic entities such as bacterial meningitis and traumatic brain injury (TBI), among others.[19] This hypothesis is illustrated in **Fig. 1**.

HEMATOLOGICAL COMPONENTS OF VASOSPASM
Hgb and Hp

Hgb is the iron-carrying oxygen transport metalloprotein that constitutes most of the structure of the RBCs. Although intracorpuscular Hgb is usually degraded by macrophages in the reticuloendothelial system, extracorpuscular Hgb is a proinflammatory molecule[33] that requires complex interactions for proper recycling. Free Hgb also

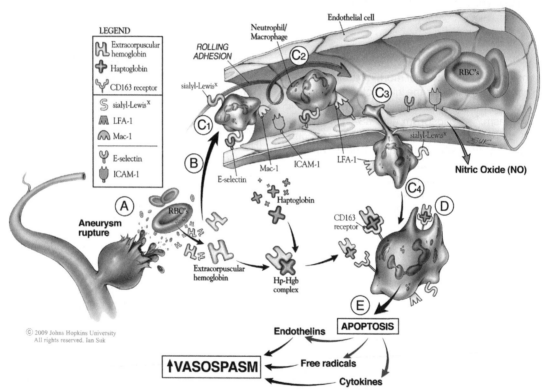

Fig. 1. Cascade of events resulting in posthemorrhagic cerebral vasospasm. (A) Rupture of a cerebral aneurysm results in subarachnoid hemorrhage. (B) Extravasated RBCs are lysed and release Hgb into the subarachnoid space that induces upregulation of CAMs on leukocytes and endothelial cells. (C1) Circulating granulocytes and neutrophils transiently bind with selectins on endothelial cells (E-selectins) through their sialyl-Lewis moieties and roll along the intraluminal surface. (C2) Leukocyte rolling is arrested by tethering to the endothelial surface through strong bonds between leukocyte integrins (LFA-1 and Mac-1) and endothelial immunoglobulin superfamily proteins (ICAM1). (C3) Transendothelial leukocyte migration into the subarachnoid space occurs. (C4) Intrathecal leukocytes migrate toward senescent RBCs and phagocytose free Hgb molecules. (D) Extracorpuscular Hgb binds to Hp and forms an Hp-Hgb complex. The CD163 scavenger receptor on the macrophage surface binds with variable affinity to the Hp-Hgb complex depending on the Hp genotype (weaker in Hp 2-2 genotypes than in Hp 1-1) and internalizes it for phagocytosis, thereby degrading Hgb into bilirubin. (E) Trapped intrathecal leukocytes undergo apoptosis within days, and release ET, free radicals, and proinflammatory cytokines, which in turn enhance leukocyte migration, decrease NO-mediated vasodilation, and result in delayed chronic cerebral vasospasm. (*Courtesy of* Johns Hopkins University, Baltimore, MD.)

reduces vasodilation induced by nitric oxide (NO), and the synergistic proinflammatory and vasospastic effects of extravascular Hgb seem to be critical in the development of vasospasm.[27,30]

Hepatocytes synthesize large quantities of Hp in serum.[34] This protein couples with Hb through a stable, high affinity bond[35–38] and ameliorates the toxicity of free extracorpuscular Hgb. Although in humans the Hp gene has 2 alleles, designated Hp 1 and Hp 2, other mammalian species have only a single Hp1 allele.[39–41] The dimeric protein coded by Hp 1-1 more efficiently binds and promotes the clearance of Hgb molecules when compared with the cyclical Hp 2-2 protein,[42] and seems to have superior antiinflammatory, immunomodulatory, antioxidant, and vasodilatory effects in vitro and in animal studies.[42–46] Hp 2-2, however, provides protection against some infectious disease, a characteristic that has promoted its dissemination in the human gene pool.

The Inflammatory Response

Inflammation constitutes a biphasic response with an acute and a chronic period. Although the acute period constitutes a short event that occurs immediately after the initial injury and uses polymorphonuclear neutrophils, macrophages, and monocytes as its primary effector cells,[47,48] the chronic period occurs in a delayed manner in days or weeks, and has lymphocytes and plasma cells as the main effector cells.[49,50] Acute inflammation results from the combination of a vascular response that includes arteriolar relaxation (increasing blood flow) and local endothelial cell contraction (increasing vascular permeability)[47,48] and a cellular response that involves neutrophils, macrophages, and monocytes, which migrate to the inflamed site and phagocytose the particles that stimulated the inflammatory response. These inflammatory effector cells eventually degranulate, and release enzymes and other toxic intermediates into the extravascular space that precede and subsequently promote chronic inflammation.[51] Continuous proinflammatory stimulation primarily mediated by lymphocytes and monocytes/macrophages that invade the affected tissue and release cytokines (eg, interferon-γ), reactive oxygen species, and hydrolytic enzymes result in chronic inflammation.[49,50] This chronic component develops in days or weeks, and can persist for many months or years.[49,50]

INFLAMMATION AND CHRONIC VASOSPASM

Although Ecker and Riemenschneider[52] first described angiographic cerebral vasospasm in 6 patients with aSAH in 1951, William Gull[53] had already reported a case consistent with vasospasm in England in 1859. Cerebral arterial vasospasm was experimentally recreated in laboratory models in the early twentieth century,[54–57] and the clinicopathologic correlation of cerebral infarction in the presence of a patent cerebral vasculature was provided by Robertson[56] in 1949, who studied a series of patients with ruptured aneurysms and concomitant cerebral infarction, and hypothesized that the infarctions resulted from transient spasm of the supplying arteries and not from mechanical compression from the aneurysms. The first correlation of angiographic vasospasm and focal neurologic deficits, however, was not reported until Fisher and colleagues' study in 1977.[58] Despite increasing clinical and experimental evidence, the pathophysiology of vasospasm continues to be elusive and modest therapeutic progress has been made to date.

Clinical Correlates of Inflammation and Vasospasm

Hyperthermia

Hyperthermia or fever was the first clinical sign that indicated a subjacent inflammatory response in these patients,[59] and its appearance correlated with the onset of chronic vasospasm.[60] These observations were later confirmed by Weir and colleagues,[61] who found that of all patients with aSAH who developed clinical vasospasm, 60% had a temperature greater than 37.5°C in the 6 days before vasospasm onset, which represented nearly twice the incidence of patients with lower temperatures. These findings were replicated in other studies that also correlated persistent fever after aSAH with less favorable outcomes.[62]

Leukocytosis

Increased white blood cell (WBC) counts have been shown to correlate with an increased risk of clinically significant vasospasm and worst outcomes.[61,63–67] Although the impact of leukocytosis on clinical outcomes was first reported in 1974 by Neil-Dwyer and Cruikshank,[65] a link between increased WBCs and vasospasm was not confirmed until 1987, when Spallone and colleagues[67] correlated leukocytosis with the development of ischemia after aSAH. Detailed chronologic correlation between leukocytosis and the time course of chronic vasospasm was later provided by Niikawa and colleagues,[66] and an independent association between peak leukocyte counts and the development of cerebral vasospasm was then reported in a multivariate analysis by McGirt and colleagues.[64]

Serologic markers of inflammation in vasospasm

Immune complexes are seen in patients with post-hemorrhagic vasospasm,[68–70] along with activated complement cascade proteins,[68,71] and C-reactive protein (CRP).[72] In fact, Rothoerl and colleagues[72] have shown that CRP is significantly increased in patients who developed symptomatic vasospasm and that it correlates with the worst neurologic outcomes.

Histopathologic changes in vasospastic cerebral vessels

Evidence of a significant inflammatory arteriopathy has been described on histopathologic examination of cerebral arteries from patients with clinical and angiographic vasospasm and is consistently replicated in multiple experimental models of the disease.[73–77] For instance, increased endothelial penetration of monocytes within arteries in proximity to ruptured-aneurysm sites,[73] macrophage invasion of the tunica media and adventitia of vessels in angiographic vasospasm,[75] and positive immunofluorescence for IgM and C3 in the endothelium of spastic arteries in patients with aSAH[74,76] have been reported.

Experimental Evidence of Inflammation in Vasospasm

Induction of vasospasm with proinflammatory agents

A clear pathophysiologic link between inflammation and cerebral vasospasm has been difficult to demonstrate despite numerous clinical studies that correlated a robust inflammatory response with the progression of vasospasm.[60–67,69,70,78] To elucidate the nature and causality of this relationship, researchers have replicated arterial vasospasm in the absence of blood products and other conditions associated with SAH by administering several proinflammatory agents in experimental models.[79–83] Vasospasm has been successfully induced by injected latex and dextran beads into the cistern magna of dogs,[81] administration of polystyrene latex beads[83] and talc (crystallized hydrous magnesium sulfate),[79,80] and locally delivered lipopolysaccharide (LPS) into the subarachnoid space of rabbits.[82] Controlled release of LPS in particular resulted in chronic vasospasm in a dose-dependent fashion, which replicated the basilar artery vasospasm induced by SAH in the same model.[82] These studies demonstrated that significant arterial vasospasm could be induced despite the absence of RBCs or Hgb in the subarachnoid space and provide further confirmation of the role of inflammation in the development of chronic vasospasm.

Prevention of vasospasm with immunosuppressive or antiinflammatory agents

Immunosuppressive or antiinflammatory agents have been postulated as potential treatments for chronic cerebral vasospasm in various animal models[84–92] and in a few human clinical trials[93–97] with varied results. Among the proposed agents, corticosteroids,[84–86,93,94] cyclosporine,[81,87,95–97] tacrolimus (FK-506),[88–90] and nonsteroidal antiinflammatory drugs (NSAIDs)[85–92] have been most extensively studied.

Corticosteroids are steroidal hormones with antiinflammatory and immunosuppressive properties[98] that primarily affect lymphocyte proliferation and function, and tend to suppress chronic rather than acute inflammation.[99] Experimental administration of high dose methylprednisolone decreased cerebral vasospasm, ameliorated arterial wall abnormalities, and suppressed prostaglandin E2 synthesis in animal models.[84–96] Human clinical studies by Chyatte and colleagues[93] in 21 patients at high risk for vasospasm by clinical criteria showed that methylprednisolone therapy improved neurologic outcomes, decreased mortality, and reduced delayed cerebral ischemia. A multicenter study by Hashi and colleagues[94] then followed that included 52 centers with 140 enrolled patients and evaluated the effects of hydrocortisone administration after vasospasm onset. Results showed improved mental status, speech, and motor function in hydrocortisone treated patients 1 month after treatment.

Cyclosporine causes T-cell dysfunction by inhibiting interleukin-2 (IL-2) transcription,[100] and its use in animal models of experimental SAH has produced conflicting results.[91,95,101] Clinical studies with cyclosporine have also had mixed results. Although in a study by Manno and colleagues[95] cyclosporine failed to prevent chronic vasospasm in patients with Fisher grade 3 SAH, a study by Ryba and colleagues[76,97] showed that a combination of cyclosporine with nimodipine significantly improved outcomes in patients who underwent early clipping (<72 hours) after a SAH.

In addition to their antipyretic and analgesic effects, NSAIDs also have potent antiinflammatory properties, mediated in part by a nonselective inhibition of cyclooxygenase expression, which reduces prostaglandin synthesis.[102] Furthermore, certain NSAIDs such as ibuprofen have been shown to prevent leukocyte migration into the periadventitial space[103–105] by inhibition of endothelial intercellular adhesion molecule 1 (ICAM1; CD54) expression. White and colleagues[92] have also shown that intravenous NSAID administration in a canine model of SAH significantly reduced the severity of vasospasm. In this study, however, NSAIDs were injected 30 minutes before and 3 hours after induction of SAH, and despite their positive findings these time points would limit therapeutic replication in human trials.[92]

Decreased levels of activated complement proteins in serum have been shown to ameliorate cerebral vasospasm in experimental models[83,106,107] and in human subjects.[108,109] Nafamostat mesilate is a serine protease inhibitor that prevents complement activation and experimentally reduced angiographic vasospasm in rabbits with hemorrhagic[109] and latex bead-induced vasospasm.[83] These findings were replicated in a small clinical trial in which Nafamostat reduced the incidence of vasospasm alone[109] and in combination with a thromboxane synthetase inhibitor.[108]

Current Molecular Evidence of Inflammation in Vasospasm

CAMs and leukocyte migration

The development of monoclonal antibodies led to the discovery of cell-adhesion molecules (CAMs), which facilitated a detailed understanding of leukocyte-endothelial cell interactions during inflammation. The 3 classes of CAMs that regulate leukocyte-endothelial cell interactions are selectins, integrins, and immunoglobulin superfamily proteins. Identification of the location and variable expression of CAMs elucidated and clarified the complex process that results in leukocyte adhesion, diapedesis, and migration, which is now known to involve 3 primary steps: selectin-facilitated rolling, chemokine-induced activation, and integrin-dependent arrest.[51] The initial tethering of leukocytes to the vessel walls results from the interaction between sialylated carbohydrates on the leukocyte membrane and endothelial selectins.[110] This interaction is followed by binding of leukocyte receptors to chemoattractants released from the injured tissue and integrin activation.[111] Integrins in turn bind to immunoglobulin superfamily members expressed on the endothelium, which increases leukocyte adhesiveness and causes rolling leukocytes to arrest.[112] Arrested leukocytes then diapedese and migrate to sites of inflammation.[113]

Selectins

Selectin expression facilitates the formation of adhesions between leukocytes and endothelial cells and reflects an evolving inflammatory response.[114,115] E-selectin has been found to be elevated in SAH patients, with higher concentrations seen in patients who develop moderate or severe vasospasm.[116] Although P-selectin levels

appeared to be higher in patients with low-grade SAH who developed ischemia, L-selectins were higher in patients who did not develop delayed cerebral ischemia.[117,118] Selectin inhibition in a mouse model of SAH resulted in improved lumen patency and decreased peripheral WBC counts when compared with SAH controls.[119]

Integrins

The main integrins involved in leukocyte adhesion and migration are LFA-1 and Mac-1.[120,121] The authors have analyzed the effects of systemically administered anti-LFA-1 and Mac-1 monoclonal antibodies on morphometric arterial vasospasm in rats,[122] rabbits,[123] and monkeys after experimental SAH[124] and found a significant decrease in posthemorrhagic vasospasm in all models, which correlated with fewer periadventitial infiltration of neutrophils and macrophages.[122] Intracisternal monoclonal antibody administration in a rabbit model by Bavbek and colleagues[125] produced similar results.

Statins are 3-hydroxy-3-methylglutaryl coenzyme A reductase inhibitors clinically used as cholesterol-reducing agents. Their ability to reduce the expression of proinflammatory cytokines and inhibit leukocyte integrins confers them potent antiinflammatory activity also.[126,127] In a randomized controlled trial by Tseng and colleagues,[128] patients with aSAH (n = 80) were randomized to receive either oral pravastatin or placebo within 72 hours of their initial hemorrhage. Patients treated with pravastatin had a 32% reduction in vasospasm incidence, vasospasm-related neurologic deficits decreased by 83%, and mortality decreased by 75% when compared with patients treated with placebo.[128] A subsequent study by the same group found that pravastatin also improved neurologic outcomes at 6 months.[129] In addition, a case-control series by Parra and colleagues[130] showed decreased incidences of clinical vasospasm and improved 14-day functional outcomes in patients receiving statins before developing aSAH compared with patients who did not use statins. Kramer and colleagues and McGirt and colleagues,[131,132] however, in recent retrospective studies did not find significant differences in the severity of angiographic or clinical vasospasm, or in the neurologic outcomes of patients receiving statins after aSAH.

Immunoglobulin superfamily proteins

Immunoglobulin superfamily proteins, such as ICAM1, have been found to be upregulated in patients who develop clinical vasospasm[116] and increased expression correlates with poor neurologic outcomes following aSAH.[133–135] The authors have shown that anti-ICAM1 monoclonal antibodies can decrease the extent of femoral artery vasospasm and inhibit periadventitial infiltration of macrophages and neutrophils in a rat model.[136] This antibody produced a similar effect in basilar artery vasospasm and inflammatory cell infiltration as an anti-LFA-1 monoclonal antibody in animal models.[122]

The use of drugs like statins and ibuprofen, which downregulate immunoglobulin superfamily expression, also decreases vasospasm in experimental studies. Several clinical studies have shown that statins decrease serum ICAM1 levels in hypercholesterolemic patients,[126,127,137–139] and may contribute to the beneficial effects of statins in reducing the incidence of vasospasm in clinical trials.[128–131,140] Ibuprofen is another antiinflammatory with anti-ICAM1 and antivascular cell adhesion molecule 1 (VCAM1) activity.[103,141] Local sustained delivery of ibuprofen via controlled-release polymers significantly inhibited femoral artery vasospasm and decreased the number of periadventitial monocytes and macrophages when administered at 0 and 6 hours after hemorrhage in a rat model.[105] These results were replicated in rabbit[142] and monkey SAH models.[104] Chyatte and colleagues[85] also demonstrated that ibuprofen prevented ultrastructural changes in the cerebral vessel walls of dogs after blood injection. Clinical use of ibuprofen, however, is limited because its efficacy at preventing vasospasm has been shown only if it is administered within 6 hours of hemorrhage.[104,105,142]

The critical role of leukocytes and inflammation in the pathophysiology of chronic vasospasm is widely supported by the experimental findings described earlier and by the efficacy of monoclonal antibodies against integrins and immunoglobulin superfamily CAMs in animal models. In the rabbit and primate SAH models, treatment with monoclonal antibodies against CAMs prevents leukocyte migration and vasospasm despite the presence of RBCs and Hgb in the subarachnoid space, which shows that chronic vasospasm does not occur in the absence of leukocytes or attenuated inflammation.

Other proinflammatory proteins

Cytokines and other proinflammatory proteins such as c-Jun N-terminal kinase (JNK) and poly (ADP-ribose) polymerase (PARP) have also been implicated in vasospasm. The main proinflammatory cytokines that have been shown to be elevated in patients with vasospasm include IL-1, IL-6, IL-8, and tumor necrosis factor α.[143–149] Administration of drugs that inhibit cytokine production has resulted in attenuation of vasospasm in animal models.[150,151] JNK is a mitogen-activated kinase involved in the inflammatory response.[152] The use of a JNK inhibitor has been found to decrease angiographic vasospasm, improve neurologic function, reduce leukocyte infiltration, and decrease IL-6 production following blood injection in a canine model.[153] PARP is a nuclear enzyme that regulates CAM expression and neutrophil recruitment during inflammation.[154] In a rabbit model of SAH Satoh and colleagues[155] showed that PARP activation occurred in the smooth muscles and adventitia of blood-exposed vessels, and that a PARP inhibitor decreased the severity of vasospasm.

NO Depletion and ET Elevation

Endothelium-derived relaxing factor or NO is synthesized in the blood vessel wall in response to shear stress or metabolic dysfunction, and results in significant arterial vasodilation.[156] After hemorrhage, however, free Hgb disrupts several components of NO-mediated vasodilation. Besides inflammation, NO dysfunction is believed to play a contributory role in the development of posthemorrhagic vasospasm and has been a target in several experimental studies.[156] Following aSAH, CSF levels of nitrites, a major source of endogenous NO,[157,158] have been found to be significantly decreased in patients who develop vasospasm.[159,160] The authors have shown that intrathecal NO supplementation via controlled-released polymers prevented vasospasm in rat and rabbit models of SAH,[161,162] and that delayed polymer implantation 24 or 48 hours after SAH also ameliorated vasospasm.[162] Several studies have also shown that selective intracerebral NO injection,[163] intraventricular NO injection,[164] and systemic nitrite infusions improved the severity or decreased the incidence of vasospasm experimental and clinical studies.[160]

ET are powerful vasoconstrictors commonly expressed by vascular endothelial cells.[165,166] Although several studies have documented significant intrathecal ET-1 level increases in aSAH patients that develop vasospasm,[167,168] others have not.[169] Anti-ET-1 monoclonal antibodies,[170] anti-ET receptors antibodies,[171,172] and ET activation enzyme inhibitors[173] have been shown to decrease vasospasm in some,[171,172] but not all studies[174]; therefore, additional studies are needed to clarify its role in the pathophysiology of chronic vasospasm.

NONHEMORRHAGIC VASOSPASM

Cerebral vasospasm seems to develop in other pathologic conditions that affect the CNS in the absence of aSAH, such as TBI,[9,10,15] infectious meningitis,[19–23] and after craniotomies.[16–18] Inflammation also seems to contribute significantly to the development of vasospasm in these other conditions.

Reported incidences of vasospasm in patients after TBI have ranged from 25% to 40%,[9] regardless of intracranial penetration.[10,175] The incidence[176] and the pathophysiology[15,175] of post-TBI vasospasm closely resemble those of posthemorrhagic vasospasm. Post-TBI vasospasm is also biphasic; it has an acute and a chronic period,[15] and its time course parallels posthemorrhagic vasospasm.[175] Despite the limited experimental and clinical studies on post-TBI, these observations suggest that trauma or trauma-related hemorrhage triggers a perivascular inflammatory response that results in cerebral vasospasm.

In addition to posttraumatic vasospasm, it has been reported that vasospasm can develop in patients who have undergone craniotomies for nonvascular causes.[16–18] Bejjani and colleagues[16] reported a case of a 6-year-old girl who underwent a craniotomy for an intracranial schwannoma who later developed angiographically confirmed vasospasm. El Hendawy and colleagues[17] reported 14 cases of vasospasm following craniotomies for intraaxial and extraaxial brain tumors, including gliomas and meningiomas. As with posttraumatic vasospasm, it is believed that the same mechanisms underlying post-aSAH vasospasm may explain postcraniotomy vasospasm.

Several cases of meningitis-associated cerebral vasospasm have been reported.[19–23] The authors have shown that meningitis-associated vasospasm follows a time course similar to aSAH-associated vasospasm,[19] and that its pathophysiology could also be explained by the inflammatory hypothesis. Following bacterial meningeal colonization and infection, endothelial activation signaling is triggered, leukocyte infiltration into the subarachnoid space occurs, and cytokines and other proinflammatory agents are released,[177–182] which upregulate CAM expression,[179–183] and enhance the inflammatory response that results in cerebral vasospasm.[179–183]

FUTURE DIRECTIONS

Despite numerous studies with promising experimental therapies for aSAH-induced vasospasm,[184–186] hypertensive-hypervolemic-hemodilutional ("triple H") therapy[187] still remains as the mainstay of clinical vasospasm treatment. Large prospective controlled trials, however, have failed to show that prophylactic triple H therapy significantly reduces the incidence of clinical or angiographic vasospasm or that it improves neurologic outcomes.[184–188] Additional treatments including transluminal balloon angioplasty,[189,190] lumbar drainage of CSF,[191,192] and intracisternal thrombolysis[193] have been used as salvage therapies but they typically result in minimal benefits and increased complications. Pharmacologic therapies involving systemic calcium channel blockers (nimodipine),[185,194] a nonglucocorticoid free radical scavenger (tirilazad mesilate),[195,196] and intraarterial[197,198] have suffered from these same limitations. Arterial narrowing was prevented effectively by nicardipine[199] and clazosentan[200] in clinical trials, but neurologic outcomes remained unchanged.

Limited progress has been made in the development of techniques to identify prospectively aSAH patients at risk for chronic cerebral vasospasm that would enable early and selective application of targeted therapies to prevent or ameliorate the inflammatory response and restore NO-mediated vasodilation. Among the potential molecular markers for predicting which patients will develop clinical vasospasm following aSAH, the Hp genotype has gained recent interest.[201] Of all aSAH patients, 30% develop symptomatic vasospasm, 50% develop asymptomatic angiographic vasospasm, and 20% do not show signs of angiographic or clinical vasospasm. This distribution follows the prevalence of Hp genotypes in humans,[202] and the Hp 2-2 genotype in particular seems to be present in 30% of humans, which correlates with the incidence of clinical vasospasm in aSAH patients. The authors have genetically engineered mice to express the Hp 2-2 genotype,[39–41] and showed that Hp 2-2 mice developed more severe morphometric and clinical vasospasm after experimental SAH than wild-type Hp 1-1 mice.[201] Vasospasm in these animals correlated with increased periadventitial neutrophils and macrophages, which strongly suggests a relationship between the Hp 2-2 genotype, inflammation, and cerebral vasospasm.[201] Further studies are needed to clarify the relationship between the Hp genotype and inflammation, and only prospective clinical studies will define the effect of an Hp genotype in the development of chronic cerebral vasospasm.

Based on the substantial evidence on the contribution of inflammation to the pathophysiology of vasospasm presented, a hypothesis that links the various pathophysiologic events described in this review and elsewhere in the literature with the development of chronic vasospasm has been formulated: after aSAH, erythrocyte extravasation into the subarachnoid space induces endothelial upregulation of CAMs, primarily of ICAM1, which can also be upregulated by bacterial meningitis and traumatic SAH. ICAM1 upregulation enables endothelial cells to bind to LFA-1 or Mac-1 proteins on the leukocyte surface and mediate transendothelial leukocyte migration into the peri-adventitial space. Once in the subarachnoid space, extravasated leukocytes phagocytose subarachnoid erythrocytes in SAH or bacteria in bacterial meningitis. The absence of a lymphatic intrathecal system prevents leukocyte recirculation and trapped leukocytes die and degranulate in the subarachnoid space 2 to 4 days after the triggering event, which corresponds to the onset and time course of chronic vasospasm in humans. Leukocyte degranulation results in ET and oxygen free radicals release, and NO dysfunction. Although these molecular mechanisms are strongly amplified in Hp 2-2, they are moderately present in Hp 2-1 patients and lead to clinical vasospasm in Hp 2-2 patients, angiographic vaso-spasm in Hp 2-1 patients, and do not result in vasospasm in Hp 1-1 patients. Validation of this hypothesis will require extensive future testing in experimental models and clinical settings.

SUMMARY

Delayed or chronic cerebral vasospasm results in major morbidity and mortality for patients after aSAH. Despite extensive clinical and experimental analysis of this phenomenon its pathophysiology remains poorly understood and the biologic and genetic principles behind the variability in the development of clinical vasospasm have not been elucidated. The cumulative evidence presented strongly supports the role that inflammation and leukocyte-endothelial cell interactions play in the pathophysiology of vasospasm, but translation of these findings into clinically effective therapies will require further molecular and genetic understanding of this inflammatory arteriopathy.

REFERENCES

1. Kassell NF, Torner JC, Haley EC Jr, et al. The International Cooperative Study on the timing of aneurysm surgery. Part 1: overall management results. J Neurosurg 1990;73:18.
2. Kassell NF, Torner JC, Jane JA, et al. The International Cooperative Study on the timing of aneurysm surgery. Part 2: surgical results. J Neurosurg 1990;73:37.
3. Solenski NJ, Haley EC Jr, Kassell NF, et al. Medical complications of aneurysmal subarachnoid hemorrhage: a report of the multicenter, cooperative aneurysm study. Participants of the Multicenter Cooperative Aneurysm Study. Crit Care Med 1995;23:1007.
4. Suarez JI, Tarr RW, Selman WR. Aneurysmal subarachnoid hemorrhage. N Engl J Med 2006;354:387.
5. Weir B, Grace M, Hansen J, et al. Time course of vasospasm in man. J Neurosurg 1978;48:173.
6. Haley EC Jr, Kassell NF, Torner JC, et al. A randomized trial of two doses of nicardipine in aneurysmal subarachnoid hemorrhage. A report of the Cooperative Aneurysm Study. J Neurosurg 1994;80:788.
7. Armin SS, Colohan AR, Zhang JH. Traumatic subarachnoid hemorrhage: our current understanding and its evolution over the past half century. Neurol Res 2006;28:445.
8. Hamer J, Krastel A. Cerebral vasospasm after brain injury. Neurochirurgia (Stuttg) 1976;19:185.
9. Martin NA, Doberstein C, Alexander M, et al. Post-traumatic cerebral arterial spasm. J Neurotrauma 1995;12:897.
10. Martin NA, Doberstein C, Zane C, et al. Posttrau-matic cerebral arterial spasm: transcranial Doppler ultrasound, cerebral blood flow, and angiographic findings. J Neurosurg 1992;77:575.
11. Pasqualin A, Vivenza C, Rosta L, et al. Cerebral vasospasm after head injury. Neurosurgery 1984;15:855.
12. Sander D, Klingelhofer J. Cerebral vasospasm following post-traumatic subarachnoid hemorrhage evaluated by transcranial Doppler ultraso-nography. J Neurol Sci 1993;119:1.
13. Soustiel JF, Shik V. Posttraumatic basilar artery vasospasm. Surg Neurol 2004;62:201.
14. Taneda M, Kataoka K, Akai F, et al. Traumatic subarachnoid hemorrhage as a predictable indicator of delayed ischemic symptoms. J Neurosurg 1996;84:762.
15. Zubkov AY, Lewis AI, Raila FA, et al. Risk factors for the development of post-traumatic cerebral vaso-spasm. Surg Neurol 2000;53:126.
16. Bejjani GK, Duong DH, Kalamarides M, et al. Cerebral vasospasm after tumor resection. A case report. Neurochirurgie 1997;43:164.
17. el Hendawy M, Wronski J, Juniewicz H, et al. Cerebral vasospasm detection by TCD after supratentorial brain tumours surgery. Neurol Neurochir Pol 2000;34:114.
18. Yamashima T, Kida S, Yamamoto S. An electron microscopic study of cerebral vasospasm with resultant myonecrosis in cases of subarachnoid haemorrhage, meningitis and trans-sylvian surgery. J Neurol 1986;233:348.

19. Chaichana K, Riley LH 3rd, Tamargo RJ. Delayed cerebral vasospasm secondary to bacterial meningitis after lumbosacral spinal surgery: case report. Neurosurgery 2007;60:E206.

20. Ferris EJ, Rudikoff JC, Shapiro JH. Cerebral angiography of bacterial infection. Radiology 1968;90:727.

21. Pfister HW, Borasio GD, Dirnagl U, et al. Cerebrovascular complications of bacterial meningitis in adults. Neurology 1992;42:1497.

22. Ries S, Schminke U, Fassbender K, et al. Cerebrovascular involvement in the acute phase of bacterial meningitis. J Neurol 1997;244:51.

23. Yamashima T, Kashihara K, Ikeda K, et al. Three phases of cerebral arteriopathy in meningitis: vasospasm and vasodilatation followed by organic stenosis. Neurosurgery 1985;16:546.

24. Gallia GL, Tamargo RJ. Leukocyte-endothelial cell interactions in chronic vasospasm after subarachnoid hemorrhage. Neurol Res 2006;28:750.

25. Ascenzi P, Bocedi A, Visca P, et al. Hemoglobin and heme scavenging. IUBMB Life 2005;57:749.

26. Claassen J, Bernardini GL, Kreiter K, et al. Effect of cisternal and ventricular blood on risk of delayed cerebral ischemia after subarachnoid hemorrhage: the Fisher scale revisited. Stroke 2001;32:2012.

27. Dietrich HH, Dacey RG Jr. Molecular keys to the problems of cerebral vasospasm. Neurosurgery 2000;46:517.

28. Fisher CM, Kistler JP, Davis JM. Relation of cerebral vasospasm to subarachnoid hemorrhage visualized by computerized tomographic scanning. Neurosurgery 1980;6:1.

29. Hijdra A, van Gijn J, Nagelkerke NJ, et al. Prediction of delayed cerebral ischemia, rebleeding, and outcome after aneurysmal subarachnoid hemorrhage. Stroke 1988;19:1250.

30. Nishizawa S, Laher I. Signaling mechanisms in cerebral vasospasm. Trends Cardiovasc Med 2005;15:24.

31. Qureshi AI, Sung GY, Razumovsky AY, et al. Early identification of patients at risk for symptomatic vasospasm after aneurysmal subarachnoid hemorrhage. Crit Care Med 2000;28:984.

32. Doering TJ, Brix J, Schneider B, et al. Cerebral hemodynamics and cerebral metabolism during cold and warm stress. Am J Phys Med Rehabil 1996;75:408.

33. Rother RP, Bell L, Hillmen P, et al. The clinical sequelae of intravascular hemolysis and extracellular plasma hemoglobin: a novel mechanism of human disease. JAMA 2005;293:1653.

34. Hooper DC, Steer CJ, Dinarello CA, et al. Haptoglobin and albumin synthesis in isolated rat hepatocytes. Response to potential mediators of the acute-phase reaction. Biochim Biophys Acta 1981;653:118.

35. Giblett ER. The haptoglobins of human serum. J Forensic Sci 1963;8:446.

36. McCormick DJ, Atassi MZ. Hemoglobin binding with haptoglobin: delineation of the haptoglobin binding site on the alpha-chain of human hemoglobin. J Protein Chem 1990;9:735.

37. Wejman JC, Hovsepian D, Wall JS, et al. Structure and assembly of haptoglobin polymers by electron microscopy. J Mol Biol 1984;174:343.

38. Wejman JC, Hovsepian D, Wall JS, et al. Structure of haptoglobin and the haptoglobin-hemoglobin complex by electron microscopy. J Mol Biol 1984;174:319.

39. Bowman BH, Kurosky A. Haptoglobin: the evolutionary product of duplication, unequal crossing over, and point mutation. Adv Hum Genet 1982;12:189.

40. Langlois MR, Delanghe JR. Biological and clinical significance of haptoglobin polymorphism in humans. Clin Chem 1996;42:1589.

41. Smithies O. Zone electrophoresis in starch gels: group variations in the serum proteins of normal human adults. Biochem J 1955;61:629.

42. Javid J. The effect of haptoglobin polymer size on hemoglobin binding capacity. Vox Sang 1965;10:320.

43. Asleh R, Guetta J, Kalet-Litman S, et al. Haptoglobin genotype- and diabetes-dependent differences in iron-mediated oxidative stress in vitro and in vivo. Circ Res 2005;96:435.

44. Blum S, Asaf R, Guetta J, et al. Haptoglobin genotype determines myocardial infarct size in diabetic mice. J Am Coll Cardiol 2007;49:82.

45. Lange V. [Haptoglobin polymorphism–not only a genetic marker]. Anthropol Anz 1992;50:281 [in German].

46. Melamed-Frank M, Lache O, Enav BI, et al. Structure-function analysis of the antioxidant properties of haptoglobin. Blood 2001;98:3693.

47. Serhan CN. Resolution phase of inflammation: novel endogenous anti-inflammatory and proresolving lipid mediators and pathways. Annu Rev Immunol 2007;25:101.

48. Serhan CN, Savill J. Resolution of inflammation: the beginning programs the end. Nat Immunol 2005;6:1191.

49. Filer A, Raza K, Salmon M, et al. Targeting stromal cells in chronic inflammation. Discov Med 2007;7:20.

50. O'Shea JJ, Murray PJ. Cytokine signaling modules in inflammatory responses. Immunity 2008;28:477.

51. Springer TA. Traffic signals for lymphocyte recirculation and leukocyte emigration: the multistep paradigm. Cell 1994;76:301.

52. Ecker A, Riemenschneider PA. Arteriographic demonstration of spasm of the intracranial arteries, with special reference to saccular arterial aneurysms. J Neurosurg 1951;8:660.

53. Gull WM. Cases of aneurism of the cerebral vessels. Guys Hosp Rep 1859;5:281.

54. Florey H. Microscopical observations on the circulation of blood in the cerebral cortex. Brain 1925; 48:43.

55. Jackson IJ. Aseptic hemogenic meningitis. An experimental study of aseptic meningeal reactions due to blood and its breakdown products. Arch Neurol Psychiatry 1949;62:572.

56. Robertson EG. Cerebral lesions due to intracranial aneurysms. Brain 1949;72:150.

57. Chou WH, Choi DS, Zhang H, et al. Neutrophil protein kinase Cdelta as a mediator of stroke-reperfusion injury. J Clin Invest 2004;114:49.

58. Fisher CM, Roberson GH, Ojemann RG. Cerebral vasospasm with ruptured saccular aneurysm–the clinical manifestations. Neurosurgery 1977;1:245.

59. Henker R, Carlson KK. Fever: applying research to bedside practice. AACN Adv Crit Care 2007;18:76.

60. Rousseaux P, Scherpereel B, Bernard MH, et al. Fever and cerebral vasospasm in ruptured intracranial aneurysms. Surg Neurol 1980;14:459.

61. Weir B, Disney L, Grace M, et al. Daily trends in white blood cell count and temperature after subarachnoid hemorrhage from aneurysm. Neurosurgery 1989;25:161.

62. Oliveira-Filho J, Ezzeddine MA, Segal AZ, et al. Fever in subarachnoid hemorrhage: relationship to vasospasm and outcome. Neurology 2001;56: 1299.

63. Maiuri F, Gallicchio B, Donati P, et al. The blood leukocyte count and its prognostic significance in subarachnoid hemorrhage. J Neurosurg Sci 1987; 31:45.

64. McGirt MJ, Mavropoulos JC, McGirt LY, et al. Leukocytosis as an independent risk factor for cerebral vasospasm following aneurysmal subarachnoid hemorrhage. J Neurosurg 2003;98: 1222.

65. Neil-Dwyer G, Cruickshank J. The blood leucocyte count and its prognostic significance in subarachnoid haemorrhage. Brain 1974;97:79.

66. Niikawa S, Hara S, Ohe N, et al. Correlation between blood parameters and symptomatic vasospasm in subarachnoid hemorrhage patients. Neurol Med Chir (Tokyo) 1997;37:881.

67. Spallone A, Acqui M, Pastore FS, et al. Relationship between leukocytosis and ischemic complications following aneurysmal subarachnoid hemorrhage. Surg Neurol 1987;27:253.

68. Ostergaard JR, Kristensen BO, Svehag SE, et al. Immune complexes and complement activation following rupture of intracranial saccular aneurysms. J Neurosurg 1987;66:891.

69. Pellettieri L, Carlson CA, Lindholm L. Is the vasospasm following subarachnoidal hemorrhage an immunoreactive disease? Experientia 1981;37: 1170.

70. Pellettieri L, Nilsson B, Carlsson CA, et al. Serum immunocomplexes in patients with subarachnoid hemorrhage. Neurosurgery 1986;19:767.

71. Kasuya H, Shimizu T. Activated complement components C3a and C4a in cerebrospinal fluid and plasma following subarachnoid hemorrhage. J Neurosurg 1989;71:741.

72. Rothoerl RD, Axmann C, Pina AL, et al. Possible role of the C-reactive protein and white blood cell count in the pathogenesis of cerebral vasospasm following aneurysmal subarachnoid hemorrhage. J Neurosurg Anesthesiol 2006;18:68.

73. Crompton MR. The pathogenesis of cerebral infarction following the rupture of cerebral berry aneurysms. Brain 1964;87:491.

74. Hoshi T, Shimizu T, Kito K, et al. [Immunological study of late cerebral vasospasm in subarachnoid hemorrhage. Detection of immunoglobulins, C3, and fibrinogen in cerebral arterial walls by immunofluorescence method]. Neurol Med Chir (Tokyo) 1984;24:647 [in Japanese].

75. Hughes JT, Schianchi PM. Cerebral artery spasm. A histological study at necropsy of the blood vessels in cases of subarachnoid hemorrhage. J Neurosurg 1978;48:515.

76. Ryba M, Jarzabek-Chorzelska M, Chorzelski T, et al. Is vascular angiopathy following intracranial aneurysm rupture immunologically mediated? Acta Neurochir (Wien) 1992;117:34.

77. Shimizu T, Kito K, Hoshi T, et al. [Immunological study of late cerebral vasospasm in subarachnoid hemorrhage]. Neurol Med Chir (Tokyo) 1982;22: 613 [in Japanese].

78. Walton JN. The prognosis and management of subarachnoid haemorrhage. Can Med Assoc J 1955;72:165.

79. Mori T, Nagata K, Ishida T, et al. Sequential morphological changes of the constrictive basilar artery in a canine model of experimental cerebral vasospasm by talc injection. J Vet Med Sci 1994; 56:535.

80. Nagata K, Sasaki T, Mori T, et al. Cisternal talc injection in dog can induce delayed and prolonged arterial constriction resembling cerebral vasospasm morphologically and pharmacologically. Surg Neurol 1996;45:442.

81. Peterson JW, Kwun BD, Hackett JD, et al. The role of inflammation in experimental cerebral vasospasm. J Neurosurg 1990;72:767.

82. Recinos PF, Pradilla G, Thai QA, et al. Controlled release of lipopolysaccharide in the subarachnoid space of rabbits induces chronic vasospasm in the absence of blood. Surg Neurol 2006;66:463.

83. Yanamoto H, Kikuchi H, Okamoto S, et al. Cerebral vasospasm caused by cisternal injection of

polystyrene latex beads in rabbits is inhibited by a serine protease inhibitor. Surg Neurol 1994; 42:374.

84. Chyatte D. Prevention of chronic cerebral vasospasm in dogs with ibuprofen and high-dose methylprednisolone. Stroke 1989;20:1021.

85. Chyatte D, Rusch N, Sundt TM Jr. Prevention of chronic experimental cerebral vasospasm with ibuprofen and high-dose methylprednisolone. J Neurosurg 1983;59:925.

86. Chyatte D, Sundt TM Jr. Response of chronic experimental cerebral vasospasm to methylprednisolone and dexamethasone. J Neurosurg 1984; 60:923.

87. Handa Y, Hayashi M, Takeuchi H, et al. Effect of cyclosporine on the development of cerebral vasospasm in a primate model. Neurosurgery 1991;28:380.

88. Mori T, Nagata K, Ishida T, et al. FK-506: a new immunosuppressive agent, failed to reduce cerebral vasospasm after experimental subarachnoid hemorrhage. J Vet Med Sci 1993;55:581.

89. Nagata K, Sasaki T, Iwama J, et al. Failure of FK-506, a new immunosuppressant, to prevent cerebral vasospasm in a canine two-hemorrhage model. J Neurosurg 1993;79:710.

90. Nishizawa S, Peterson JW, Shimoyama I, et al. Therapeutic effect of a new immunosuppressant, FK-506, on vasospasm after subarachnoid hemorrhage. Neurosurgery 1993;32:986.

91. Peterson JW, Nishizawa S, Hackett JD, et al. Cyclosporine A reduces cerebral vasospasm after subarachnoid hemorrhage in dogs. Stroke 1990; 21:133.

92. White RP, Robertson JT. Comparison of piroxicam, meclofenamate, ibuprofen, aspirin, and prostacyclin efficacy in a chronic model of cerebral vasospasm. Neurosurgery 1983;12:40.

93. Chyatte D, Fode NC, Nichols DA, et al. Preliminary report: effects of high dose methylprednisolone on delayed cerebral ischemia in patients at high risk for vasospasm after aneurysmal subarachnoid hemorrhage. Neurosurgery 1987;21:157.

94. Hashi K, Takakura K, Sano K, et al. [Intravenous hydrocortisone in large doses in the treatment of delayed ischemic neurological deficits following subarachnoid hemorrhage–results of a multi-center controlled double-blind clinical study]. No To Shinkei 1988;40:373 [in Japanese].

95. Manno EM, Gress DR, Ogilvy CS, et al. The safety and efficacy of cyclosporine A in the prevention of vasospasm in patients with Fisher grade 3 subarachnoid hemorrhages: a pilot study. Neurosurgery 1997;40:289.

96. Ryba M, Pastuszko M, Iwanska K, et al. Cyclosporine A prevents neurological deterioration of patients with SAH–a preliminary report. Acta Neurochir (Wien) 1991;112:25.

97. Ryba M, Pastuszko M, Dziewiecki C, et al. A strategy for analyzing multiple parameters with application to aneurysmal SAH patients all of them clipped but treated with and without cyclosporine. Acta Neurochir (Wien) 1993;122:194.

98. Pozzesi N, Gizzi S, Gori F, et al. IL-2 induces and altered CD4/CD8 ratio of splenic T lymphocytes from transgenic mice overexpressing the glucocorticoid-induced protein GILZ. J Chemother 2007; 19:562.

99. Elenkov IJ. Glucocorticoids and the Th1/Th2 balance. Ann N Y Acad Sci 2004;1024:138.

100. Pritchard DI. Sourcing a chemical succession for cyclosporin from parasites and human pathogens. Drug Discov Today 2005;10:688.

101. Ryba M, Grieb P, Bidzinski J, et al. Cyclosporine A for the prevention of neurological deficit following subarachnoid hemorrhage. Stroke 1991;22:531.

102. Green GA. Understanding NSAIDs: from aspirin to COX-2. Clin Cornerstone 2001;3:50.

103. Kapiotis S, Sengoelge G, Sperr WR, et al. Ibuprofen inhibits pyrogen-dependent expression of VCAM-1 and ICAM-1 on human endothelial cells. Life Sci 1996;58:2167.

104. Pradilla G, Thai QA, Legnani FG, et al. Local delivery of ibuprofen via controlled-release polymers prevents angiographic vasospasm in a monkey model of subarachnoid hemorrhage. Neurosurgery 2005;57:184.

105. Thai QA, Oshiro EM, Tamargo RJ. Inhibition of experimental vasospasm in rats with the periadventitial administration of ibuprofen using controlled-release polymers. Stroke 1999;30:140.

106. German JW, Gross CE, Giclas P, et al. Systemic complement depletion inhibits experimental cerebral vasospasm. Neurosurgery 1996;39:141.

107. Yanamoto H, Kikuchi H, Okamoto S, et al. Preventive effect of synthetic serine protease inhibitor, FUT-175, on cerebral vasospasm in rabbits. Neurosurgery 1992;30:351.

108. Kaminogo M, Yonekura M, Onizuka M, et al. Combination of serine protease inhibitor FUT-175 and thromboxane synthetase inhibitor OKY-046 decreases cerebral vasospasm in patients with subarachnoid hemorrhage. Neurol Med Chir (Tokyo) 1998;38:704.

109. Yanamoto H, Kikuchi H, Sato M, et al. Therapeutic trial of cerebral vasospasm with the serine protease inhibitor, FUT-175, administered in the acute stage after subarachnoid hemorrhage. Neurosurgery 1992;30:358.

110. Kansas GS. Selectins and their ligands: current concepts and controversies. Blood 1996;88:3259.

111. Campbell JJ, Qin S, Bacon KB, et al. Biology of chemokine and classical chemoattractant receptors: differential requirements for adhesion-triggering versus chemotactic responses in lymphoid cells. J Cell Biol 1996;134:255.

112. Chan JR, Hyduk SJ, Cybulsky MI. Chemoattractants induce a rapid and transient upregulation of monocyte alpha4 integrin affinity for vascular cell adhesion molecule 1 which mediates arrest: an early step in the process of emigration. J Exp Med 2001;193:1149.

113. Schenkel AR, Mamdouh Z, Muller WA. Locomotion of monocytes on endothelium is a critical step during extravasation. Nat Immunol 2004;5:393.

114. Lasky LA. Selectins: interpreters of cell-specific carbohydrate information during inflammation. Science 1992;258:964.

115. Rosen SD. Cell surface lectins in the immune system. Semin Immunol 1993;5:237.

116. Polin RS, Bavbek M, Shaffrey ME, et al. Detection of soluble E-selectin, ICAM-1, VCAM-1, and L-selectin in the cerebrospinal fluid of patients after subarachnoid hemorrhage. J Neurosurg 1998;89:559.

117. Nissen JJ, Mantle D, Blackburn A, et al. The selectin superfamily: the role of selectin adhesion molecules in delayed cerebral ischaemia after aneurysmal subarachnoid haemorrhage. Acta Neurochir Suppl 2000;76:55.

118. Nissen JJ, Mantle D, Gregson B, et al. Serum concentration of adhesion molecules in patients with delayed ischaemic neurological deficit after aneurysmal subarachnoid haemorrhage: the immunoglobulin and selectin superfamilies. J Neurol Neurosurg Psychiatry 2001;71:329.

119. Lin CL, Dumont AS, Calisaneller T, et al. Monoclonal antibody against E selectin attenuates subarachnoid hemorrhage-induced cerebral vasospasm. Surg Neurol 2005;64:201.

120. de Fougerolles AR, Stacker SA, Schwarting R, et al. Characterization of ICAM-2 and evidence for a third counter-receptor for LFA-1. J Exp Med 1991;174:253.

121. Springer TA. Adhesion receptors of the immune system. Nature 1990;346:425.

122. Clatterbuck RE, Oshiro EM, Hoffman PA, et al. Inhibition of vasospasm with lymphocyte function-associated antigen-1 monoclonal antibody in a femoral artery model in rats. J Neurosurg 2002;97:676.

123. Pradilla G, Wang PP, Legnani FG, et al. Prevention of vasospasm by anti-CD11/CD18 monoclonal antibody therapy following subarachnoid hemorrhage in rabbits. J Neurosurg 2004;101:88.

124. Clatterbuck RE, Gailloud P, Ogata L, et al. Prevention of cerebral vasospasm by a humanized anti-CD11/CD18 monoclonal antibody administered after experimental subarachnoid hemorrhage in nonhuman primates. J Neurosurg 2003;99:376.

125. Bavbek M, Polin R, Kwan AL, et al. Monoclonal antibodies against ICAM-1 and CD18 attenuate cerebral vasospasm after experimental subarachnoid hemorrhage in rabbits. Stroke 1998;29:1930.

126. Ascer E, Bertolami MC, Venturinelli ML, et al. Atorvastatin reduces proinflammatory markers in hypercholesterolemic patients. Atherosclerosis 2004;177:161.

127. Chello M, Carassiti M, Agro F, et al. Simvastatin blunts the increase of circulating adhesion molecules after coronary artery bypass surgery with cardiopulmonary bypass. J Cardiothorac Vasc Anesth 2004;18:605.

128. Tseng MY, Czosnyka M, Richards H, et al. Effects of acute treatment with pravastatin on cerebral vasospasm, autoregulation, and delayed ischemic deficits after aneurysmal subarachnoid hemorrhage: a phase II randomized placebo-controlled trial. Stroke 2005;36:1627.

129. Tseng MY, Hutchinson PJ, Czosnyka M, et al. Effects of acute pravastatin treatment on intensity of rescue therapy, length of inpatient stay, and 6-month outcome in patients after aneurysmal subarachnoid hemorrhage. Stroke 2007;38:1545.

130. Parra A, Kreiter KT, Williams S, et al. Effect of prior statin use on functional outcome and delayed vasospasm after acute aneurysmal subarachnoid hemorrhage: a matched controlled cohort study. Neurosurgery 2005;56:476.

131. Kramer AH, Gurka MJ, Nathan B, et al. Statin use was not associated with less vasospasm or improved outcome after subarachnoid hemorrhage. Neurosurgery 2008;62:422.

132. McGirt MJ, Garces Ambrossi GL, Huang J, et al. Simvastatin for the prevention of symptomatic cerebral vasospasm following aneurysmal subarachnoid hemorrhage: a single-institution prospective cohort study. J Neurosurg 2009;110:968.

133. Cheong JH, Kim JM, Bak KH, et al. Correlation between cerebral vasospasm after subarachnoid hemorrhage and intracellular adhesion molecule-1 levels in serum and cerebrospinal fluid. J Korean Med Sci 2005;38:1.

134. Mack WJ, Mocco J, Hoh DJ, et al. Outcome prediction with serum intercellular adhesion molecule-1 levels after aneurysmal subarachnoid hemorrhage. J Neurosurg 2002;96:71.

135. Mocco J, Mack WJ, Kim GH, et al. Rise in serum soluble intercellular adhesion molecule-1 levels with vasospasm following aneurysmal subarachnoid hemorrhage. J Neurosurg 2002;97:537.

136. Oshiro EM, Hoffman PA, Dietsch GN, et al. Inhibition of experimental vasospasm with anti-intercellular adhesion molecule-1 monoclonal antibody in rats. Stroke 1997;28:2031.

137. Doo YC, Han SJ, Han SW, et al. Effect of preexisting statin use on expression of C-reactive protein, adhesion molecules, interleukin-6, and antioxidized low-density lipoprotein antibody in patients with unstable angina undergoing coronary stenting. Clin Cardiol 2005;28:72.

138. Koh KK, Son JW, Ahn JY, et al. Vascular effects of diet and statin in hypercholesterolemic patients. Int J Cardiol 2004;95:185.

139. Rezaie-Majd A, Prager GW, Bucek RA, et al. Simvastatin reduces the expression of adhesion molecules in circulating monocytes from hypercholesterolemic patients. Arterioscler Thromb Vasc Biol 2003;23:397.

140. Lynch JR, Wang H, McGirt MJ, et al. Simvastatin reduces vasospasm after aneurysmal subarachnoid hemorrhage: results of a pilot randomized clinical trial. Stroke 2005;36:2024.

141. Hofbauer R, Frass M, Gmeiner B, et al. Rapid, fluorescence-based assay for microtiter plates to test drug influences on neutrophil transmigration through endothelial cell monolayers. Life Sci 1999;65:2453.

142. Frazier JL, Pradilla G, Wang PP, et al. Inhibition of cerebral vasospasm by intracranial delivery of ibuprofen from a controlled-release polymer in a rabbit model of subarachnoid hemorrhage. J Neurosurg 2004;101:93.

143. Aihara Y, Kasuya H, Onda H, et al. Quantitative analysis of gene expressions related to inflammation in canine spastic artery after subarachnoid hemorrhage. Stroke 2001;32:212.

144. Fassbender K, Hodapp B, Rossol S, et al. Inflammatory cytokines in subarachnoid haemorrhage: association with abnormal blood flow velocities in basal cerebral arteries. J Neurol Neurosurg Psychiatry 2001;70:534.

145. Gaetani P, Tartara F, Pignatti P, et al. Cisternal CSF levels of cytokines after subarachnoid hemorrhage. Neurol Res 1998;20:337.

146. Hendryk S, Jarzab B, Josko J. Increase of the IL-1 beta and IL-6 levels in CSF in patients with vasospasm following aneurysmal SAH. Neuro Endocrinol Lett 2004;25:141.

147. Nam DH, Kim JS, Hong SC, et al. Expression of interleukin-1 beta in lipopolysaccharide stimulated monocytes derived from patients with aneurysmal subarachnoid hemorrhage is correlated with cerebral vasospasm. Neurosci Lett 2001;312:41.

148. Schoch B, Regel JP, Wichert M, et al. Analysis of intrathecal interleukin-6 as a potential predictive factor for vasospasm in subarachnoid hemorrhage. Neurosurgery 2007;60:828.

149. Wang Y, Zhong M, Tan XX, et al. Expression change of interleukin-8 gene in rabbit basilar artery after subarachnoid hemorrhage. Neurosci Bull 2007;23:151.

150. Bowman G, Bonneau RH, Chinchilli VM, et al. A novel inhibitor of inflammatory cytokine production (CNI-1493) reduces rodent post-hemorrhagic vasospasm. Neurocrit Care 2006;5:222.

151. Bowman G, Dixit S, Bonneau RH, et al. Neutralizing antibody against interleukin-6 attenuates posthemorrhagic vasospasm in the rat femoral artery model. Neurosurgery 2004;54:719.

152. Manning AM, Davis RJ. Targeting JNK for therapeutic benefit: from junk to gold? Nat Rev Drug Discov 2003;2:554.

153. Yatsushige H, Yamaguchi M, Zhou C, et al. Role of c-Jun N-terminal kinase in cerebral vasospasm after experimental subarachnoid hemorrhage. Stroke 2005;36:1538.

154. Cuzzocrea S. Shock, inflammation and PARP. Pharmacol Res 2005;52:72.

155. Satoh M, Date I, Nakajima M, et al. Inhibition of poly(ADP-ribose) polymerase attenuates cerebral vasospasm after subarachnoid hemorrhage in rabbits. Stroke 2001;32:225.

156. Pluta RM. Dysfunction of nitric oxide synthases as a cause and therapeutic target in delayed cerebral vasospasm after SAH. Neurol Res 2006;28:730.

157. Cosby K, Partovi KS, Crawford JH, et al. Nitrite reduction to nitric oxide by deoxyhemoglobin vasodilates the human circulation. Nat Med 2003;9:1498.

158. Weyerbrock A, Walbridge S, Pluta RM, et al. Selective opening of the blood-tumor barrier by a nitric oxide donor and long-term survival in rats with C6 gliomas. J Neurosurg 2003;99:728.

159. Pluta RM. Delayed cerebral vasospasm and nitric oxide: review, new hypothesis, and proposed treatment. Pharmacol Ther 2005;105:23.

160. Pluta RM, Dejam A, Grimes G, et al. Nitrite infusions to prevent delayed cerebral vasospasm in a primate model of subarachnoid hemorrhage. JAMA 2005;293:1477.

161. Gabikian P, Clatterbuck RE, Eberhart CG, et al. Prevention of experimental cerebral vasospasm by intracranial delivery of a nitric oxide donor from a controlled-release polymer: toxicity and efficacy studies in rabbits and rats. Stroke 2002;33:2681.

162. Pradilla G, Thai QA, Legnani FG, et al. Delayed intracranial delivery of a nitric oxide donor from a controlled-release polymer prevents experimental cerebral vasospasm in rabbits. Neurosurgery 2004;55:1393.

163. Pluta RM, Oldfield EH, Boock RJ. Reversal and prevention of cerebral vasospasm by intracarotid infusions of nitric oxide donors in a primate model of subarachnoid hemorrhage. J Neurosurg 1997;87:746.

164. Egemen N, Turker RK, Sanlidilek U, et al. The effect of intrathecal sodium nitroprusside on severe chronic vasospasm. Neurol Res 1993;15:310.

165. Inoue A, Yanagisawa M, Kimura S, et al. The human endothelin family: three structurally and pharmacologically distinct isopeptides predicted by three separate genes. Proc Natl Acad Sci U S A 1989;86:2863.

166. Sakurai T, Yanagisawa M, Inoue A, et al. cDNA cloning, sequence analysis and tissue distribution of rat preproendothelin-1 mRNA. Biochem Biophys Res Commun 1991;175:44.

167. Mascia L, Fedorko L, Stewart DJ, et al. Temporal relationship between endothelin-1 concentrations and cerebral vasospasm in patients with aneurysmal subarachnoid hemorrhage. Stroke 2001; 32:1185.

168. Seifert V, Loffler BM, Zimmermann M, et al. Endothelin concentrations in patients with aneurysmal subarachnoid hemorrhage. Correlation with cerebral vasospasm, delayed ischemic neurological deficits, and volume of hematoma. J Neurosurg 1995;82:55.

169. Hamann G, Isenberg E, Strittmatter M, et al. Absence of elevation of big endothelin in subarachnoid hemorrhage. Stroke 1993;24:383.

170. Yamaura I, Tani E, Maeda Y, et al. Endothelin-1 of canine basilar artery in vasospasm. J Neurosurg 1992;76:99.

171. Clozel M, Breu V, Burri K, et al. Pathophysiological role of endothelin revealed by the first orally active endothelin receptor antagonist. Nature 1993;365:759.

172. Zuccarello M, Boccaletti R, Romano A, et al. Endothelin B receptor antagonists attenuate subarachnoid hemorrhage-induced cerebral vasospasm. Stroke 1998;29:1924.

173. Matsumura Y, Ikegawa R, Suzuki Y, et al. Phosphoramidon prevents cerebral vasospasm following subarachnoid hemorrhage in dogs: the relationship to endothelin-1 levels in the cerebrospinal fluid. Life Sci 1991;49:841.

174. Cosentino F, McMahon EG, Carter JS, et al. Effect of endothelinA-receptor antagonist BQ-123 and phosphoramidon on cerebral vasospasm. J Cardiovasc Pharmacol 1993;8(Suppl 22):S332.

175. Kordestani RK, Counelis GJ, McBride DQ, et al. Cerebral arterial spasm after penetrating craniocerebral gunshot wounds: transcranial Doppler and cerebral blood flow findings. Neurosurgery 1997; 41:351.

176. Oertel M, Boscardin WJ, Obrist WD, et al. Posttraumatic vasospasm: the epidemiology, severity, and time course of an underestimated phenomenon: a prospective study performed in 299 patients. J Neurosurg 2005;103:812.

177. Dulkerian SJ, Kilpatrick L, Costarino AT Jr, et al. Cytokine elevations in infants with bacterial and aseptic meningitis. J Pediatr 1995;126:872.

178. Fassbender K, Ries S, Schminke U, et al. Inflammatory cytokines in CSF in bacterial meningitis: association with altered blood flow velocities in basal cerebral arteries. J Neurol Neurosurg Psychiatry 1996;61:57.

179. Fassbender K, Schminke U, Ries S, et al. Endothelial-derived adhesion molecules in bacterial meningitis: association to cytokine release and intrathecal leukocyte-recruitment. J Neuroimmunol 1997;74:130.

180. Mukai AO, Krebs VL, Bertoli CJ, et al. TNF-alpha and IL-6 in the diagnosis of bacterial and aseptic meningitis in children. Pediatr Neurol 2006;34:25.

181. Sethi S, Sharma P, Dikshit M. Nitric oxide- and oxygen-derived free radical generation from control and lipopolysaccharide-treated rat polymorphonuclear leukocyte. Nitric Oxide 2001;5:482.

182. van Deuren M, van der Ven-Jongekrijg J, Bartelink AK, et al. Correlation between proinflammatory cytokines and antiinflammatory mediators and the severity of disease in meningococcal infections. J Infect Dis 1995;172:433.

183. Pigott R, Dillon LP, Hemingway IH, et al. Soluble forms of E-selectin, ICAM-1 and VCAM-1 are present in the supernatants of cytokine activated cultured endothelial cells. Biochem Biophys Res Commun 1992;187:584.

184. Egge A, Waterloo K, Sjoholm H, et al. Prophylactic hyperdynamic postoperative fluid therapy after aneurysmal subarachnoid hemorrhage: a clinical, prospective, randomized, controlled study. Neurosurgery 2001;49:593.

185. Feigin VL, Rinkel GJ, Algra A, et al. Calcium antagonists in patients with aneurysmal subarachnoid hemorrhage: a systematic review. Neurology 1998;50:876.

186. Suarez JI, Shannon L, Zaidat OO, et al. Effect of human albumin administration on clinical outcome and hospital cost in patients with subarachnoid hemorrhage. J Neurosurg 2004;100:585.

187. Keyrouz SG, Diringer MN. Clinical review: prevention and therapy of vasospasm in subarachnoid hemorrhage. Crit Care 2007;11:220.

188. Rinkel GJ, Feigin VL, Algra A, et al. Circulatory volume expansion therapy for aneurysmal subarachnoid haemorrhage. Cochrane Database Syst Rev 2004:CD000483.

189. Hoh BL, Ogilvy CS. Endovascular treatment of cerebral vasospasm: transluminal balloon angioplasty, intra-arterial papaverine, and intra-arterial nicardipine. Neurosurg Clin N Am 2005;16:501.

190. Muizelaar JP, Zwienenberg M, Rudisill NA, et al. The prophylactic use of transluminal balloon angioplasty in patients with Fisher Grade 3 subarachnoid hemorrhage: a pilot study. J Neurosurg 1999;91:51.

191. Kinouchi H, Ogasawara K, Shimizu H, et al. Prevention of symptomatic vasospasm after aneurysmal subarachnoid hemorrhage by intraoperative cisternal fibrinolysis using tissue-type plasminogen activator combined with continuous cisternal drainage. Neurol Med Chir (Tokyo) 2004;44:569.

192. Klimo P Jr, Kestle JR, MacDonald JD, et al. Marked reduction of cerebral vasospasm with lumbar

drainage of cerebrospinal fluid after subarachnoid hemorrhage. J Neurosurg 2004;100:215.

193. Findlay JM, Kassell NF, Weir BK, et al. A randomized trial of intraoperative, intracisternal tissue plasminogen activator for the prevention of vasospasm. Neurosurgery 1995;37:168.

194. Pickard JD, Murray GD, Illingworth R, et al. Effect of oral nimodipine on cerebral infarction and outcome after subarachnoid haemorrhage: British aneurysm nimodipine trial. BMJ 1989;298:636.

195. Haley EC Jr, Kassell NF, Apperson-Hansen C, et al. A randomized, double-blind, vehicle-controlled trial of tirilazad mesylate in patients with aneurysmal subarachnoid hemorrhage: a cooperative study in North America. J Neurosurg 1997;86:467.

196. Kassell NF, Haley EC Jr, Apperson-Hansen C, et al. Randomized, double-blind, vehicle-controlled trial of tirilazad mesylate in patients with aneurysmal subarachnoid hemorrhage: a cooperative study in Europe, Australia, and New Zealand. J Neurosurg 1996;84:221.

197. Polin RS, Hansen CA, German P, et al. Intra-arterially administered papaverine for the treatment of symptomatic cerebral vasospasm. Neurosurgery 1998;42:1256.

198. Vajkoczy P, Horn P, Bauhuf C, et al. Effect of intra-arterial papaverine on regional cerebral blood flow in hemodynamically relevant cerebral vasospasm. Stroke 2001;32:498.

199. Kasuya H, Onda H, Sasahara A, et al. Application of nicardipine prolonged-release implants: analysis of 97 consecutive patients with acute subarachnoid hemorrhage. Neurosurgery 2005;56:895.

200. Vajkoczy P, Meyer B, Weidauer S, et al. Clazosentan (AXV-034343), a selective endothelin A receptor antagonist, in the prevention of cerebral vasospasm following severe aneurysmal subarachnoid hemorrhage: results of a randomized, double-blind, placebo-controlled, multicenter phase IIa study. J Neurosurg 2005;103:9.

201. Chaichana KL, Levy AP, Miller-Lotan R, et al. Haptoglobin 2-2 genotype determines chronic vasospasm after experimental subarachnoid hemorrhage. Stroke 2007;38:3266.

202. Dorsch NW. Cerebral arterial spasm–a clinical review. Br J Neurosurg 1995;9:403.

Biomarkers and Vasospasm After Aneurysmal Subarachnoid Hemorrhage

J. Dedrick Jordan, MD, PhD, Paul Nyquist, MD, MPH*

KEYWORDS

- Cerebral vasospasm • Subarachnoid hemorrhage
- Molecular basis of vasospasm
- Biological markers of vasospasm

Subarachnoid hemorrhage (SAH) from the rupture of saccular aneurysms (nontraumatic SAH) is a devastating and often fatal disease. Its incidence is 6 to 8 per 100,000 people years.[1] Even with the advancement and increased availability of neurosurgery and intensive care, the morbidity and mortality from aneurysmal SAH remains high. Prior to hospitalization, 12% of those with SAH die while approximately 40% of those surviving to hospitalization do not survive the first 30 days. These figures contribute to an estimated case-fatality rate of 25% to 50%.[2,3] The most common cause of death after survival of the initial hemorrhage is vasospasm. SAH is most frequently related to trauma. However, it is rarely a singular cause of fatal outcomes in traumatic brain injury and is not commonly associated with the medical complications of SAH, although this has been debated recently.[4] SAH from intracranial vascular rupture can be classified into two groups: those resulting from the rupture of a berry or saccular aneurysm, which represent 80% of nontraumatic SAH, and those associated with vascular malformations, such as arterial venous malformations, which represent 20% of all nontraumatic SAH.[2] The classical medical complications associated with SAH, such as vasospasm and cerebral salt wasting, are usually associated with the rupture of saccular aneurysms and are further discussed in this article.[5]

Vasospasm is the most common complication of SAH that leads to clinical deterioration. However, the molecular basis and pathophysiology are still poorly understood. Up to 70% of patients who survive SAH develop signs of vessel narrowing on transcranial Doppler ultrasound or angiography while clinically symptomatic vasospasm occurs in only 46% of those patients.[2,6,7] Rates of infarction after SAH are estimated to be approximately 25%.[8–11] Vasospasm can be defined both angiographically and clinically. Angiographic definition requires visualization of vessel narrowing in the affected vessel by angiography, while clinical vasospasm requires observation of the physical signs and symptoms of vasospasm. Classic symptoms of clinical vasospasm include altered levels of consciousness, confusion, focal motor symptoms, and new-onset aphasia. These symptoms typically develop over a period of hours to days and are referred to as delayed ischemic neurological deficits (DINDs).[2,12] In the early days of subarachnoid surgery, most of the delayed neurological deficits were attributed to progressive cerebral edema from the initial damage of the hemorrhage or from the surgery itself. However, as time passed, it has become clear

Johns Hopkins School of Medicine, 600 North Wolfe Street, Meyer 8-140, Baltimore, MD 21287-7840, USA
* Corresponding author.
E-mail address: pnyquis1@jhmi.edu

Neurosurg Clin N Am 21 (2010) 381–391
doi:10.1016/j.nec.2009.10.009

that DINDs are occurring independently of the initial hemorrhage or surgery.[12]

The proximal event leading to DIND still remains unclear. However, two facts are well established: (1) DIND is the result of tissue ischemia and represents a form of ischemic stroke and (2) DIND occurs in vascular territories where vasoconstriction has been documented angiographically. These observations strongly suggest a causal relationship between vascular constriction and ischemia, although in recent studies it has become less clear that the primary event causing ischemia and cell death is the constriction of the associated blood vessel.[13] It is possible that vascular constriction may be an epiphenomena or a contributing factor to parenchymal destruction and that the final ischemic event may be caused by other factors occurring directly within the parenchyma at the level of the neurovascular unit. This can be loosely supported by the results of trials, such as the Neurosurgery Cooperative Trial, which used the calcium channel blocker nicardipine, and the CONSCIOUS-1 Trial (Clazosentan to Overcome Neurological Ischemia and Infarction Occurring after Subarachnoid Hemorrhage–1 Trial), which tested the endothelin antagonist clazosentan.[14] While both nicardipine and clazosentan prevented vasospasm, neither was shown to prevent ischemia or DIND. Mechanical intervention with angioplasty, though successful in reversing the narrowing of the vessel, also failed to prevent DIND when performed at the onset of symptoms or prophylactically before the symptoms develop.[15] These interventions demonstrated efficacy in reducing the occurrence of angiographic vasospasm. However, they did not reduce the incidence of DINDs.[14,16]

The failure of new drugs and techniques to protect against DINDs has spurred research to isolate proteins that may affect the development of vasospasm. These proteins represent potential therapeutic targets as well as markers of vasospasm onset. The use of proteomics and translational research to understand vasospasm has a long history and understanding the current techniques can aid clinicians interested in furthering vasospasm research or in applying the newest clinical techniques to aid in the care of patients with vasospasm from aneurysmal SAH.

BASICS OF THE HUMAN PROTEOME

Human proteomics is the study of human proteins in the context of three realms: drug discovery, proteome mapping, and biologic understanding.[17] A number of new scientific techniques have been developed that allow for the identification of proteins from a number of human biologic tissues.[18] This material, usually collected in a specific clinical context, gives researchers a glimpse of the activity occurring as the direct result of disease. The study of proteomics in vasospasm and DIND could potentially help identify a variety of biomarkers from diverse tissue sources, including serum, cerebrospinal fluid (CSF), and extracellular parenchymal fluid. Vasospasm is a molecularly based phenomenon that involves complex cellular signaling. The identification of proteins associated with different stages of disease progression may enable the isolation of specific protein signals. The understanding of vasospasm through proteome analysis requires data collected in the setting of well-described clinical phenotypes.

The characterization of the human genome has produced a wave of information that has made it possible to estimate the number of genes contributing to the human proteome. Thus far, 19,438 genes have been identified with an additional 2188 predicted genes based on data from the completed human genome study. Thus far, 34,124 transcripts have been isolated, contributing to more than 100,000 proteins. Each gene can code for an estimated 10 to 20 different protein species. Thus the human proteome is vast with many potential targets.[17]

TISSUE SAMPLING

During the treatment of aneurysmal SAH, various parenchymal sites can be harvested for proteomic analysis. These include solid tissue, such as brain parenchyma; tissue approximating the vascular substructure, such as adventitia; and sections of vessel affected by aneurysmal rupture. Each of these tissue types requires sacrifice in the setting of surgical intervention and is rarely obtained in normal practice. More commonly acquired and easily accessible tissue types include blood, CSF, and extracellular fluid from cerebral microdialysis. Blood is a tissue with some characteristics of fluid. However it is actually a complex conglomerate more similar to that of a colloidal suspension. It potentially contains protein or genetic material from any compartment of the human body. Its proteome has not yet been completely characterized and is probably the largest of any tissue compartment in the body. The most commonly analyzed portion of human blood is serum and within it are tens of thousands of analytic targets. Injury or changes in any compartment of the human body are usually reflected in the proteome of blood. Thus blood is the most commonly accessed source for protein analysis in any clinical scenario.[18]

CSF and extracellular fluid are the next two most commonly tested sources of body fluid for protein analysis in the setting of SAH. CSF studies of proteins in the context of vasospasm are relatively common. The protein concentration of CSF is 400 times less than blood. About 2600 proteins have been identified in CSF at this time and a proteome map of CSF is available from several sources (http://www.expasy.ch/).[19,20] Extracellular fluid is often difficult to obtain as it requires the placement of a cerebral microdialysis catheter and yields only small amounts of fluid. However, its use is more frequent now as microdialysis catheters are increasingly placed for monitoring ischemic stress in the setting of brain injury. Studies looking at extracellular fluid in the setting of SAH and vasospasm are still limited while study of the extracellular fluid proteome is incomplete. A number of peptides have been identified by mass spectroscopy and these peptides represent 27 individual proteins. All of these proteins appear to represent proteins derived from CSF.[21–23]

Proteins isolated from blood exist in a background of great protein diversity represented by vast numbers of different protein types. It is estimated that 22 proteins represent 99% of the protein content of the blood. Thus, protein concentration in blood varies extensively, spanning 10 orders of magnitude. This dynamic range makes detection of a low concentration of small proteins specifically related to a single injury quite difficult. The dynamic range of mass spectroscopy, the most common means of identifying proteins in blood, is 2 orders of magnitude, not the 10 required to encompass the proteome. The situation is further complicated in that the proteins of highest interest tend to be those occurring at lower concentrations and are not the common constituents of blood. The solution to this problem requires both protein isolation and concentration with the goal of the purification and selection of specific components of blood.

The problem of dynamic range exists with CSF and extracellular fluid to a much lesser degree. The decreased number of proteins and the relative lower total concentration of protein lead to a decrease in the dynamic range and makes for more efficient protein isolation and concentration. However, there is still a wide dynamic range and the challenge of detecting proteins of interest in small samples with very low concentrations is still a major roadblock, particularly with the present technology.[18]

PROTEIN ISOLATION

The first stage of proteome analysis requires the isolation of individual proteins. The most commonly applied technique for protein isolation is two-dimensional gel electrophoresis. This technique uses a two-stage process, including pH immobilization with isoelectric focusing, followed by standard polyacrylamide gel electrophoresis. The proteins can then be visualized using special stains or immunoblotting techniques. Other important protein isolation technologies include affinity chromatography, ion-exchange chromatography, reversed-phase liquid chromatography, and capillary electrophoresis. Chromatography using all mediums is a popular method to isolate proteins. Such techniques as high-performance liquid chromatography are common and effective. Isotope-coded affinity tagging is another technique that modifies liquid or gas chromatography to isolate proteins. Isotope-coded affinity tagging incorporates a thiol-specific reactive group, with a radioactive marker containing an affinity tag, such as biotin. These markers bind to predetermined protein moieties in specific proteins, enabling isolation with traditional methods, such as high-performance liquid chromatography. Other gel-free proteomic technologies, such as capillary liquid chromatography and capillary electrophoresis, enable the isolation and identification of extremely small protein samples in a liquid or gas state.[24]

PROTEIN IDENTIFICATION

The time and effort required to identify proteins are determined in part by the abundance of the target of interest, as well as its purity, size, and stability during the purification process. The most commonly employed technique for definitive protein identification is mass spectrometry. Mass spectrometry employs protein ionization technology to produce ionized peptide fragments, from which mass-to-charge ratios are determined. Proteins are first eluted from a reversed phase column and then placed into the mass spectrometer. This is followed by chemical ionization and a mass-to-charge ratio determination for all of the individual peptides in the mixture of proteins. The tandem mass spectrometry technique is also frequently employed in protein identification. Individual ionized particles are isolated in time or space and then further fragmented by ionization. The resulting ionized products are further analyzed for their mass-to-charge ratio, resulting in a spectra, or collection, of masses for a given sample. The resulting spectra can then be compared to data from a large library of previously identified proteins. Most mass spectrometers can process approximately 7000 spectra per hour yielding identifiable proteins 10% of the time, enabling the identification of up to 700 to 1400 proteins an hour.[18]

Variations of quantitative mass spectroscopy methods have been developed, each with its own advantage and disadvantage.[25] The most common types are single or double mass spectroscopy, as previously discussed. However, this technique is limited in that it can isolate and identify only a few proteins from a given sample. Other mass spectroscopy techniques include electrospray ionization, which incorporates a coulombic pressure methodology to isolate single ionized columns of macromolecules in the setting of an aerosolized mixture. This enables greater protein isolation. Fourier transform ion cyclotron resonance mass spectrometry is another highly accurate mass spectroscopy technique. Especially suitable for samples with extremely low concentrations, this technique examines the cyclotron frequency of the charged macromolecule in a fixed magnetic field to determine mass-to-charge ratios.[26]

For high-throughput protein analysis, approaches to proteome analysis now combine protein isolation with protein identification via mass spectroscopy. These methods can be used in situations in which the tissue examined has a large dynamic range. Surface-enhanced laser desorption/ionization–time-of-flight (SELDI-TOF) mass spectrometry isolates proteins by using a stage that incorporates protein binding to a surface plate.[27] To selectively immobilize the target to the surface plate, this plate can be coated with antibodies or other substrates that interact with the sample. The surface is then energized with a laser and the ionized proteins are passed through an electric field and the time of flight is measured, which can be used to determine the mass-to-charge ratio. This method enables mass spectroscopy signaling and often direct protein identification.[26] This technology can be used to produce signatures that incorporate mass spectroscopy and time-of-flight ion analysis, which enables the identification of unique patterns that can be associated with specific diseases. These unique signatures have been used to identify specific disease states, such as cancer. One of the newer variants of SELDI is the matrix-assisted laser desorption/ionization–time-of-flight (MALDI-TOF) technique. This technique incorporates traditional SELDI technology with greater protein preparation, as the difference lies in the sample pretreatment. The protein is placed in a solid matrix instead of on a surface plate prior to ionization. This method makes it possible to more precisely control energy delivery. It also uses the characteristics of the matrix to enable better protein isolation through a high-throughput methodology that combines protein purification with precise protein identification.[26]

Other common methods of protein identification are enzyme-linked immunosorbent assay (ELISA) and luminex. These techniques use immunoprecipitation to isolate and purify proteins from various sources. ELISA is an older technique and often requires large quantities of proteins.[28,29] Each ELISA processing run requires recalibration and restandardization, which introduces variability. Furthermore, the volume of sample required is quite large and is typically an order of magnitude greater than that of other available technologies. Luminex uses newer technology and provides several benefits, including the ability to identify proteins from smaller samples, to run a larger number of samples within each batch and to reduce the variability between batches.

Protein microarrays are another method for protein isolation and identification.[30] These techniques employ a high-throughput methodology analyzing hundreds to thousands of samples at once. Arrays with specific markers for proteins or protein moieties are employed in a chip format. This technology enables the identification of thousands of proteins in a single chip and requires only microliters of sample.

Ultimately any protein isolated in sufficient quantity can be identified through protein sequencing. All methods employed in protein sequencing require highly purified samples in relatively large quantities. This approach is reserved for proteins and polypeptides that have not yet been characterized or for which precise characterization is needed for drug development or biological understanding.

BIOMARKERS AND MECHANISTIC APPROACHES TO VASOSPASM

The search for biomarkers in SAH and vasospasm has been proceeding for decades. A remarkably large literature focused on the analysis of biomarkers in the context of human tissue and SAH has been developed. At different times various techniques and theoretical perspectives have been employed. Each approach has been based on a theoretical understanding as to the underlying mechanisms of vasospasm. Different approaches have evolved with developments in molecular biology. The first and perhaps most successful mechanistic approach emphasizes moderators of inflammation.

Inflammation

Inflammation has become a focus of research in vasospasm as many observations have confirmed this direct link. It has been demonstrated that leukocytosis and fever are associated with worse outcomes in SAH.[31–33] Increased protein levels of several of the cellular adhesion molecules, including ICAM-1, VCAM-1, and the integrins, are associated with the development of vasospasm and worse clinical outcomes. Higher levels of these molecules have been measured in both the serum and CSF of patients who develop vasospasm.[34–40] Other inflammatory markers, including the cytokine interleukin (IL) 2 (IL-2), IL-2–receptor antagonists, and soluble CD8 have been sampled in the CSF of patients with SAH and vasospasm and are elevated as compared to controls. However, they are not predictive of vasospasm.[41] Furthermore, IL-6 and monocyte chemotactic protein–1 are higher in the CSF of patients who develop vasospasm.[42] IL-8 and E-selectin are inflammatory markers that have been measured in the ventricular cisterns of patients with ruptured and nonruptured aneurysms. IL-6 levels are significantly elevated in the blood of patients with SAH in general.[41,43,44] Complement has been measured using standard radioimmuno-assays in the serum and CSF of patients with vasospasm. These studies have demonstrated increased levels of the C3 and C4a components of the complement cascade in the early stages of SAH. These levels decline after the first few days.[45] Furthermore, CH50, C3, and C4 complement levels have been measured in serum of SAH patients and their levels have been predictive of vasospasm. After 5 to 10 days, however, serum complement levels were depleted in patients who went on to develop vasospasm.[46] Other mediators of inflammation, such as arachidonic acid metabolites, have also been examined. To date, no study has documented an association with prostacycline or thromboxane in any serological compartment.[2] However, 20-hydroxyeicosatetraenic acid, a metabolite of arachidonic acid, is elevated in the CSF of humans and animals with vasospasm.[47] Chitotriosidase, a human chitinase member of family 18 glycosyl-hydrolases and selectively secreted by activated macrophages, has been measured in the CSF and serum of humans with SAH. Mean CSF chitotriosidase levels were found to be higher on days 5 and 7 of SAH. The serum levels were higher than controls at all times in SAH patients although no relationship between symptomatic vasospasm and outcome was observed.[48]

Endothelial Activation

Endothelial activation is an important consideration in the setting of ischemic disease. Concentrations of soluble ICAM-1, soluble P-selectin, soluble E-selectin, and ED1-fibronectin are traditional markers of endothelial activation. Their levels have been sequentially measured throughout the course of treatment of patients with SAH. Concentrations of ICAM-1, soluble E-selectin, soluble P-selectin, ED1-fibronectin, von Willebrand Factor (vWf), and vWf propeptide have been measured in the serum of patients within 3 days of the onset of SAH to determine if any of the markers predict outcome. Early elevated vWf concentrations have been associated with poor outcome and the occurrence of ischemia. No other marker of endothelial activation has been associated with ischemia or poor outcome.[49] This positive association of raised vWf concentrations with DINDs may reflect a predisposition to further ischemic injury via the formation of microthrombi in the cerebral circulation secondary to endothelial activation. Further studies are needed to confirm these findings and to better understand the molecular basis of this relationship.

Hemoglobin Degradation

Undoubtedly the breakdown products of red blood cells and hemoglobin induce vasospasm as it has been well demonstrated that blood volume plays a role in the risk of vasospasm in animal models and in human observation studies.[50,51] It has also been shown that removal of the blood from the cisternal space facilitates a reduced risk of vasospasm.[13] Deoxyhemoglobin is the most likely irritant triggering vasospasm. Oxyhemoglobin is the most vasoactive substance in subarachnoid blood and its concentration in CSF mirrors the time course of vasospasm.[52–54] Free radicals, formed as a result of the toxic effects of subarachnoid blood and hemoglobin degradation, have been hypothesized to mediate many aspects of the pathophysiology of vasospasm. Emerging research implicates lipid peroxidation in addition to hemoglobin degradation byproducts in triggering vasospasm.[55] The hydroxide generated in the process of lipid peroxidation acts as a vasoconstrictor and, furthermore, 15-hydroperoxyeicosatetraenoic acid (15-HPETE) and other lipid byproducts initiate vasospastic physiology. Their CSF levels have been associated with an increased risk of vasospasm.[56] Measurements of cholesteryl ester hydroperoxides (CEOOH), which are generated during lipid peroxidation in plasma, may provide prognostic value. Plasma levels of CEOOH are elevated and peak 5 days after the onset of SAH. Furthermore, increased levels of CEOOH are associated with an increased mortality, are associated with an increased risk of vasospasm, and correlate with clinical outcome scales.[57]

Calcium Metabolism

Vasospasm and vasoconstriction are abnormal prolonged contractions of the smooth muscles of the vasculature, resulting in the sustained narrowing of the artery. Calcium plays a central and integral role in this process.[2,58] The contraction of the vessel walls involves the release of cytosolic calcium from a cellular reservoir, which leads to the contraction of smooth muscle in a sustained manner for prolonged periods. This can occur in a calcium dependent or independent manner. Many people have suggested that vasospasm stems from continuous elevation of cytosolic calcium, which causes sustained contraction of smooth muscle cells.[59] CSF levels of intracellular species of proteins that bind calcium are lower in individuals with symptomatic vasospasm.[60] Additionally, increased phosphorylation of key enzymes regulating cytosolic calcium reserves could also contribute to vasoconstriction in the setting of vasospasm.[61–64] The roles of protein kinase C–, calponin-, and caldesmon-based mechanisms, as well as mechanisms mediated through mitogen-activated protein kinase, have been examined.[44,65,66] To date, no proteomic approach has been applied to detect changes in the serum, CSF, or extracellular fluid level of any of these proteins. Levels of such proteins as calponin and caldesmon are potential markers of increased vasoconstriction mediating the prolonged contraction of smooth muscle. Phosphory-lated-phosphorylated myosin light chain kinase is another potential protein marker for prolonged and sustained constriction of smooth muscle cells and merits further study.

Nitric Oxide

Endothelial relaxing factors, such as nitric oxide (NO) or NO-containing compounds, play a central role in the mediation of vasoconstriction in vasospasm.[2] A variety of NO donors in humans and animals have demonstrated efficacy in the treatment of vasospasm and suggest that NO is a key player in vasoconstriction leading to clinical vasospasm.[67,68] NO is a diffusible free radical gas with a half-life of seconds. To date, no efficient method exists for precisely detecting and measuring NO in vivo. The findings of several studies reporting temporal changes in CSF total nitrite/nitrate (NOx) levels after SAH vary considerably. Many have focused on detection of its metabolites, yet even these are difficult to measure because of their

very short half-lives. The total nitrite/nitrate concentration has been determined by a vanadium-based assay with the colorimetric Griess reaction along with CSF oxyhemoglobin level as assessed by spectrophotometry. After an initial peak within the first 24 hours after SAH, CSF NOx decreases gradually and there is a significant correlation between CSF concentrations of NOx and levels of oxyhemoglobin. It has been demonstrated that patients with very good outcome have significantly lower CSF NOx than those with a worse outcome.[69]

Endothelin

Endothelin, a 21–amino acid polypeptide, is a potent vasoconstrictor and has been implicated in the pathophysiology of vasospasm. Endothelin 1 has been found to be elevated in the CSF of patients with vasospasm.[70,71] Two clinical trials have suggested efficacy for endothelin antagonists in the reduction of the observed vasoconstriction seen on angiograms. However, there was no significant reduction of DINDs.[14,72] Endothelin has been measured in the CSF and serum using a variety of methods and its level correlates closely with the time course of vasospasm in virtually all mediums measured.[71,73–75] Endothelin acts as the counterbalance to NO. However, its effects are long-acting than those of NO. Increases in endothelin's efficacy would have a profound effect on the duration and degree of vasoconstriction. Evidence related to endothelin could indicate that the transition of the artery of normal tone to its constricted state stems from a disruption of its normal physiologic state. A promising goal for the treatment of cerebral vasospasm would be to determine effective measures to regulate these two systems. Further basic and translational research is needed.

The Coagulation Cascade

SAH is associated with a consumptive coagulopathy. D-dimers and other fibrin split products are elevated in the serum and CSF of patients with SAH. Fibrin, fibrin degradation products, fibrinopeptide A (FPA), and other coagulant byproducts have been measured in the CSF of affected patients and these proteins act as markers of activation of the coagulation cascade. FPA has been selectively studied in patients with SAH with an initial elevation on days 0 to 1. However, this is followed by a subsequent decline over the ensuing days.[76] The mean level of FPA is higher in patients with higher Fischer grade SAH and this corresponds to the risk of vasospasm. Furthermore, a significant increase in the FPA level of patients with infarction has been observed. Patients with decreased blood clearance on computed tomography scan demonstrate a significantly higher rate of infarction and a higher level of FPA. These results suggest that the thrombin activity present in CSF correlates with increasing Fischer grade, faster clearance of blood on computed tomography scan, and the development of vasospasm.[76]

RECENT OBSERVATIONS

Recent advances in proteomics have yielded the discovery of new proteins that act as markers of brain injury in the setting of SAH and vasospasm. These approaches have identified new protein candidates and have aided in elucidating the molecular basis for vasospasm induced by SAH. Furthermore, these findings may provide new potential targets for the development of therapeutics and interventions aimed at preventing vasospasm. Research has focused on molecules that are markers for damage to different cellular components, such as neurons or axons. Recent analysis of the extracellular fluid from the frontotemporal lobes of a few SAH patients with vasospasm identified glyceraldehyde-3-phosphate as a protein candidate as a predictor of vasospasm. Several isoforms of glyceraldehyde-3-phosphate were elevated prior to the development of vasospasm while protein heat-shock cognate 71 kDa protein was decreased prior to vasospasm. These changes were observed at least 4 days prior to the onset of vasospasm.[77]

Neuronal Damage

Serum levels of S100-B and neuron-specific enolase have been examined in the setting of SAH. Levels of both of these proteins are known to correlate with outcome in head injury and stroke and are markers of neuronal injury. Oertel and colleagues[75] conducted a study to determine if the serum levels of S-100B and neuron-specific enolase could predict the development of vasospasm and outcome within the first 3 days after SAH. S-100B levels were significantly higher in those patients who did not develop vasospasm and also significantly higher in those patients who died, compared to those who survived no matter if their outcome was unfavorable or favorable. For the first 3 days after SAH, measurements of S-100B were identified as potential markers useful to predict death and the onset of vasospasm but did not distinguish favorable versus unfavorable outcomes for survivors.

Astrocytic Damage

Serum glial fibrillary acidic protein (s-GFAP) is a protein produced by the astrocytes. It is thought to be a marker of the degradation of the blood-brain barrier as well as damage to astrocytes. Knowing that s-GFAP concentrations are increased after stroke, Nylen and colleagues[78,79] prospectively collected serum samples of patients with SAH to determine if levels would correlate with brain injury and clinical outcomes. Serum samples were obtained over a 2-week interval from 116 adults after aneurysmal SAH and analyzed for s-GFAP levels. Increased s-GFAP levels were seen in 81 of these 116 patients. The maximum measured s-GFAP levels correlated with World Federation of Neurological Surgeons scale on arrival as well as on days 10 to 15. Maximum s-GFAP levels were increased in the patient group with radiological signs of focal lesions in the acute setting or at 1-year follow-up, compared with the group without focal lesions. Most importantly, maximum s-GFAP correlated with a worse clinical outcome.

Axonal Damage

Axonal damage occurs in the setting of SAH and serological protein markers specific for damage to the axons have been detected in patients with SAH. Patients with SAH have secondary axonal degeneration, which may adversely affect their outcome. Therefore, studies were aimed to determine if concentrations of axonal proteins, such as the neurofilament heavy chain (NfH) SMI35, are altered in SAH and whether these levels correlate with clinical outcome. Ventricular CSF was collected daily for up to 14 days in a longitudinal study of patients with aneurysmal SAH and the NfH SMI35 was quantified. The primary outcome measure was the Glasgow Outcome Score at 3 months. Of 148 samples from patients with SAH, pathologically high NfH levels in the CSF were found in 78 (52.7%) samples, compared with 20 (5%) of 416 samples from the reference population. A pathological increase in NfH was observed in all patients with a bad outcome. This increase typically became significant 7 days after the hemorrhage. The result was confirmed by analyzing the individual mean NfH concentrations in the CSF, and was reinforced by the inverse correlation of NfH in the CSF with the Glasgow Outcome Score.[80]

SUMMARY

Proteomics now offers an array of advanced technologies that enable the identification of small quantities of proteins from small samples. As these technologies are further developed, a major challenge will be to address the issue of dynamic variability. Other important factors hampering protein identification are the limitations of techniques for the sequestration and concentration of proteins of interest. Such techniques as two-dimensional gel electrophoresis and chromatography of all types are now becoming the focus of efforts to improve protein concentration and separation. Other technological breakthroughs, such as SELDI, MALDI, and protein microarrays, will play roles in the proteomics of vasospasm and help to more easily isolate and identify key proteins involved in vasospasm after SAH.

Prior to the isolation and purification of proteins, one must ensure that the compartment chosen for obtaining samples is the most biologically plausible. Different proteins from different tissue and cellular compartments can help identify proteins that are strongly related to very specific pathological processes, such as vasospasm. These proteins could be nuclear proteins derived from the nucleus of damaged cells and representing signaling characteristics specifically associated with the development of vasospasm. They could be proteins from the axons of cells representing axonal damage from prolonged ischemia. Other compartments include the vascular endothelium, the subintimal zone, and the muscularis layer. All of these are sites represent potential sources of proteins of interest that may be biomarkers or therapeutic targets in the setting of vasospasm.

Although the field of proteomics has achieved the goal of enabling the isolation and identification of targets from small samples, an even more important goal is the perfection of technology to ensure the proper sample selection from a biologically precise and generalized source. To achieve this requires the optimal design of clinical and translational studies aimed specifically at identifying protein substrates in the correct clinical setting. For SAH, this has been a major effort in recent years. The most import variable in any clinical study involves appropriate phenotype identification. In vasospasm, the use of transcranial Doppler and angiography is unlikely to become the gold standard for identification of symptomatic individuals. The gold standard continues to be the sharp eye of the experienced clinician who identifies patients with clinical changes directly attributable to vasospasm and who confirms the diagnosis by other modalities, such as transcranial Doppler and angiography. The appropriate clinical classification of patients with symptomatic vasospasm is the most important feature of phenotypic identification in this disease. This can be difficult in the setting of a complex brain injury surrounding SAH where other potential causes of neurological clinical decline exist.

It is also important to consider the timing of disease when investigating tissue sources as a means of studying this disease. Comparing samples from different days and their changing patterns of protein expression can help elucidate different aspects of a multistep biological process that initiates over the first 3 days after exposure to the initial SAH and progresses to disease expression over the ensuing 14 days. Such proteins as endothelin or other factors affecting endothelial activation may not be elevated until the patient is symptomatic. Such proteins as cellular adhesion factors are often activated early on in the first 3 days prior to the onset of clinical symptoms. However, this may prepare the vessels for further pathological changes seen during the next 2 weeks.

Proteomics have already played a role in the understanding of the pathophysiology of vasospasm in the setting on nontraumatic SAH. As technology improves and clinical experience heightens the sophistication of our understanding of this disease, the scientific yields from proteomics will only expand. It is likely that, as these technologies are further developed, we will develop a series of biomarkers that signify the onset and progression of vasospasm as well as molecules that can be effective therapeutic targets for future drug discovery.

REFERENCES

1. Wardlaw JM, White PM. The detection and management of unruptured intracranial aneurysms. Brain 2000;123(Pt 2):205–21.
2. Kolias AG, Sen J, Belli A. Pathogenesis of cerebral vasospasm following aneurysmal subarachnoid hemorrhage: putative mechanisms and novel approaches. J Neurosci Res 2009;87(1):1–11.
3. Hop JW, Rinkel GJ, Algra A, et al. Case-fatality rates and functional outcome after subarachnoid hemorrhage: a systematic review [review]. Stroke 1997; 28(3):660–4.
4. Armonda RA, Bell RS, Vo AH, et al. Wartime traumatic cerebral vasospasm: recent review of combat casualties. Neurosurgery 2006;59(6):1215–25 [discussion: 1225].
5. Diringer MN. Management of aneurysmal subarachnoid hemorrhage [review]. Crit Care Med 2009; 37(2):432–40.
6. Solenski NJ, et al. Medical complications of aneurysmal subarachnoid hemorrhage: a report of the multicenter, cooperative aneurysm study. Participants of the Multicenter Cooperative Aneurysm Study. Crit Care Med 1995;23(6):1007–17.

7. Dorsch NW. Cerebral arterial spasm—a clinical review. Br J Neurosurg 1995;9(3):403–12.

8. Hijdra A, et al. Delayed cerebral ischemia after aneurysmal subarachnoid hemorrhage: clinicoanatomic correlations. Neurology 1986;36(3):329–33.

9. Hirashima Y, et al. The use of computed tomography in the prediction of delayed cerebral infarction following acute aneurysm surgery for subarachnoid haemorrhage. Acta Neurochir (Wien) 1995; 132(1–3):9–13.

10. Forssell A, et al. CT assessment of subarachnoid haemorrhage. A comparison between different CT methods of grading subarachnoid haemorrhage. Br J Neurosurg 1995;9(1):21–7.

11. Rabinstein AA, et al. Patterns of cerebral infarction in aneurysmal subarachnoid hemorrhage. Stroke 2005;36(5):992–7.

12. Zambranski J, Hamilton MG. Cerebral vasospams. In: Spetzler R, Carter L, editors. Neurovascular surgery. New York: McGraw-Hill; 1994. p. 583–601.

13. Suarez JI, Tarr RW, Selman WR. Aneurysmal subarachnoid hemorrhage. N Engl J Med 2006; 354(4):387–96.

14. Macdonald RL, et al. Clazosentan to overcome neurological ischemia and infarction occurring after subarachnoid hemorrhage (CONSCIOUS-1): randomized, double-blind, placebo-controlled phase 2 dose-finding trial. Stroke 2008;39(11): 3015–21.

15. Zwienenberg-Lee M, et al. Effect of prophylactic transluminal balloon angioplasty on cerebral vasospasm and outcome in patients with Fisher grade III subarachnoid hemorrhage: results of a phase II multicenter, randomized, clinical trial. Stroke 2008; 39(6):1759–65.

16. Haley EC Jr, Kassell NF, Torner JC. A randomized trial of nicardipine in subarachnoid hemorrhage: angiographic and transcranial Doppler ultrasound results. A report of the Cooperative Aneurysm Study. J Neurosurg 1993;78(4):548–53.

17. Moseley FL, et al. The use of proteomics to identify novel therapeutic targets for the treatment of disease. J Pharm Pharmacol 2007;59(5):609–28.

18. Issaq HJ, Xiao Z, Veenstra TD. Serum and plasma proteomics. Chem Rev 2007;107(8):3601–20.

19. Hoogland C, et al. The 1999 SWISS-2DPAGE database update. Nucleic Acids Res 2000;28(1):286–8.

20. Bairoch A, et al. The Universal Protein Resource (UniProt). Nucleic Acids Res 2005;33(Database issue):D154–9.

21. Mann M, Pandey A. Use of mass spectrometry-derived data to annotate nucleotide and protein sequence databases. Trends Biochem Sci 2001; 26(1):54–61.

22. Appel RD, Bairoch A. Post-translational modifications: a challenge for proteomics and bioinformatics. Proteomics 2004;4(6):1525–6.

23. Steen H, Mann M. The ABC's (and XYZ's) of peptide sequencing. Nat Rev Mol Cell Biol 2004;5(9): 699–711.

24. Ramstrom M, et al. Cerebrospinal fluid protein patterns in neurodegenerative disease revealed by liquid chromatography-Fourier transform ion cyclotron resonance mass spectrometry. Proteomics 2004;4(12):4010–8.

25. Righetti PG, et al. Proteome analysis in the clinical chemistry laboratory: myth or reality? Clin Chim Acta 2005;357(2):123–39.

26. Bergquist J, et al. Peptide mapping of proteins in human body fluids using electrospray ionization Fourier transform ion cyclotron resonance mass spectrometry. Mass Spectrom Rev 2002;21(1):2–15.

27. Merchant M, Weinberger SR. Recent advancements in surface-enhanced laser desorption/ionization-time of flight-mass spectrometry. Electrophoresis 2000;21(6):1164–77.

28. Lequin RM. Enzyme immunoassay (EIA)/enzyme-linked immunosorbent assay (ELISA). Clin Chem 2005;51(12):2415–8.

29. Lawlor K, Nazarian A, Lacomis L, et al. Pathway-based biomarker search by high-throughput proteomics profiling of secretomes. J Proteome Res 2009; 8(3):1489–503.

30. MacBeath G, Schreiber SL. Printing proteins as microarrays for high-throughput function determination. Science 2000;289(5485):1760–3.

31. McGirt MJ, et al. Leukocytosis as an independent risk factor for cerebral vasospasm following aneurysmal subarachnoid hemorrhage. J Neurosurg 2003;98(6):1222–6.

32. Maiuri F, et al. The blood leukocyte count and its prognostic significance in subarachnoid hemorrhage. J Neurosurg Sci 1987;31(2):45–8.

33. Oliveira-Filho J, et al. Fever in subarachnoid hemorrhage: relationship to vasospasm and outcome. Neurology 2001;56(10):1299–304.

34. Bavbek M, et al. Monoclonal antibodies against ICAM-1 and CD18 attenuate cerebral vasospasm after experimental subarachnoid hemorrhage in rabbits. Stroke 1998;29(9):1930–5 [discussion: 1935–6].

35. Polin RS, et al. Detection of soluble E-selectin, ICAM-1, VCAM-1, and L-selectin in the cerebrospinal fluid of patients after subarachnoid hemorrhage. J Neurosurg 1998;89(4):559–67.

36. Nissen JJ, et al. The selectin superfamily: the role of selectin adhesion molecules in delayed cerebral ischaemia after aneurysmal subarachnoid haemorrhage. Acta Neurochir Suppl 2000;76:55–60.

37. Nissen JJ, et al. Serum concentration of adhesion molecules in patients with delayed ischaemic neurological deficit after aneurysmal subarachnoid haemorrhage: the immunoglobulin and selectin superfamilies. J Neurol Neurosurg Psychiatr 2001; 71(3):329–33.

38. Mack WJ, et al. Outcome prediction with serum intercellular adhesion molecule-1 levels after aneurysmal subarachnoid hemorrhage. J Neurosurg 2002;96(1):71–5.

39. Mocco J, et al. Elevation of soluble intercellular adhesion molecule-1 levels in symptomatic and asymptomatic carotid atherosclerosis. Neurosurgery 2001;48(4):718–21 [discussion: 721–2].

40. Tanriverdi T, et al. Serum and cerebrospinal fluid concentrations of E-selectin in patients with aneurysmal subarachnoid hemorrhage. Braz J Med Biol Res 2005;38(11):1703–10.

41. Mathiesen T, et al. Increased interleukin-6 levels in cerebrospinal fluid following subarachnoid hemorrhage. J Neurosurg 1993;78(4):562–7.

42. Gaetani P, et al. Cisternal CSF levels of cytokines after subarachnoid hemorrhage. Neurol Res 1998; 20(4):337–42.

43. Gallia GL, Tamargo RJ. Leukocyte-endothelial cell interactions in chronic vasospasm after subarachnoid hemorrhage. Neurol Res 2006;28(7):750–8.

44. Laher I, Zhang JH. Protein kinase C and cerebral vasospasm. J Cereb Blood Flow Metab 2001; 21(8):887–906.

45. Kasuya H, Shimizu T. Activated complement components C3a and C4a in cerebrospinal fluid and plasma following subarachnoid hemorrhage. J Neurosurg 1989;71(5 Pt 1):741–6.

46. Kawano T, Yonekawa Y. Serum complements as indicator for predicting vasospasm and its severity after aneurysmal subarachnoid hemorrhage. Nippon Geka Hokan 1990;59(3):189–97.

47. Renic M, et al. Effect of 20-HETE inhibition on infarct volume and cerebral blood flow after transient middle cerebral artery occlusion. J Cereb Blood Flow Metab 2009;29(3):629–39.

48. Isman FK, et al. Cerebrospinal fluid and serum chitotriosidase levels in patients with aneurysmal subarachnoid haemorrhage: preliminary results. Turk Neurosurg 2007;17(4):235–42.

49. Frijns CJ, et al. Endothelial cell activation markers and delayed cerebral ischaemia in patients with subarachnoid haemorrhage. J Neurol Neurosurg Psychiatr 2006;77(7):863–7.

50. Zhang ZD, et al. Delayed clot removal and experimental vasospasm. Acta Neurochir Suppl 2001;77:33–5.

51. Fisher CM, Kistler JP, Davis JM. Relation of cerebral vasospasm to subarachnoid hemorrhage visualized by computerized tomographic scanning. Neurosurgery 1980;6(1):1–9.

52. Macdonald RL, Weir BK. A review of hemoglobin and the pathogenesis of cerebral vasospasm. Stroke 1991;22(8):971–82.

53. Nishizawa S, Laher I. Signaling mechanisms in cerebral vasospasm. Trends Cardiovasc Med 2005; 15(1):24–34.

54. Pluta RM. Delayed cerebral vasospasm and nitric oxide: review, new hypothesis, and proposed treatment. Pharmacol Ther 2005;105(1):23–56.

55. Macdonald RL, Weir BK. Cerebral vasospasm and free radicals. Free Radic Biol Med 1994;16(5): 633–43.

56. Cook DA, Vollrath B. Free radicals and intracellular events associated with cerebrovascular spasm. Cardiovasc Res 1995;30(4):493–500.

57. Polidori MC, et al. Increased levels of plasma cholesteryl ester hydroperoxides in patients with subarachnoid hemorrhage. Free Radic Biol Med 1997;23(5):762–7.

58. Horowitz A, et al. Mechanisms of smooth muscle contraction. Physiol Rev 1996;76(4):967–1003.

59. Tani E, Matsumoto T. Continuous elevation of intracellular Ca2+ is essential for the development of cerebral vasospasm. Curr Vasc Pharmacol 2004; 2(1):13–21.

60. Alexander SA, et al. Cerebrospinal fluid apolipoprotein E, calcium and cerebral vasospasm after subarachnoid hemorrhage. Biol Res Nurs 2008; 10(2):102–12.

61. Harada T, et al. The time course of myosin light-chain phosphorylation in blood-induced vasospasm. Neurosurgery 1995;36(6):1178–82 [discussion: 1182–3].

62. Sun H, et ál. Myosin light chain phosphorylation and contractile proteins in a canine two-hemorrhage model of subarachnoid hemorrhage. Stroke 1998; 29(10):2149–54.

63. Chrissobolis S, Sobey CG. Evidence that Rho-kinase activity contributes to cerebral vascular tone in vivo and is enhanced during chronic hypertension: comparison with protein kinase C. Circ Res 2001;88(8):774–9.

64. Chrissobolis S, et al. Role of inwardly rectifying K(+) channels in K(+)-induced cerebral vasodilatation in vivo. Am J Physiol Heart Circ Physiol 2000;279(6): H2704–12.

65. Aoki K, et al. Role of MAPK in chronic cerebral vasospasm. Acta Neurochir Suppl 2001;77:55–7.

66. Aoki K, et al. Role of MAPK in chronic cerebral vasospasm. Life Sci 2002;70(16):1901–8.

67. Pluta RM, Oldfield EH, Boock RJ. Reversal and prevention of cerebral vasospasm by intracarotid infusions of nitric oxide donors in a primate model of subarachnoid hemorrhage. J Neurosurg 1997; 87(5):746–51.

68. Pradilla G, et al. Delayed intracranial delivery of a nitric oxide donor from a controlled-release polymer prevents experimental cerebral vasospasm in rabbits. Neurosurgery 2004;55(6):1393–9 [discussion: 1399–400].

69. Rejdak K, Petzold A, Sharpe MA, et al. Cerebrospinal fluid nitrite/nitrate correlated with

oxyhemoglobin and outcome in patients with subarachnoid hemorrhage. J Neurol Sci 2004; 219(1–2):71–6.

70. Seifert V, et al. Endothelin concentrations in patients with aneurysmal subarachnoid hemorrhage. Correlation with cerebral vasospasm, delayed ischemic neurological deficits, and volume of hematoma. J Neurosurg 1995;82(1):55–62.

71. Kastner S, et al. Endothelin-1 in plasma, cisternal CSF and microdialysate following aneurysmal SAH. Acta Neurochir (Wien) 2005;147(12):1271–9 [discussion: 1279].

72. Shaw MD, et al. Efficacy and safety of the endothelin, receptor antagonist TAK-044 in treating subarachnoid hemorrhage: a report by the Steering Committee on behalf of the UK/Netherlands/Eire TAK-044 Subarachnoid Haemorrhage Study Group. J Neurosurg 2000;93(6):992–7.

73. Zimmermann M, et al. Prevention of cerebral vasospasm after experimental subarachnoid hemorrhage by RO 47-0203, a newly developed orally active endothelin receptor antagonist. Neurosurgery 1996;38(1):115–20.

74. Pluta RM, et al. Source and cause of endothelin-1 release into cerebrospinal fluid after subarachnoid hemorrhage. J Neurosurg 1997;87(2):287–93.

75. Oertel M, et al. S-100B and NSE: markers of initial impact of subarachnoid haemorrhage and their relation to vasospasm and outcome. J Clin Neurosci 2006;13(8):834–40.

76. Kasuya H, Shimizu T, Okado T, et al. Activation of the coagulation system in the subarachnoid space after subarachnoid haemorrhage: serial measurement of fibrinopeptide A and bradykinin of cerebrospinal fluid and plasma in patients with subarachnoid haemorrhage. Acta Neurochir (Wien) 1988;91:120–5.

77. Maurer MH, et al. Identification of early markers for symptomatic vasospasm in human cerebral microdialysate after subarachnoid hemorrhage: preliminary results of a proteome-wide screening. J Cereb Blood Flow Metab 2007;27(10):1675–83.

78. Nylen K, et al. CSF-neurofilament correlates with outcome after aneurysmal subarachnoid hemorrhage. Neurosci Lett 2006;404(1–2):132–6.

79. Nylen K, et al. Serum glial fibrillary acidic protein is related to focal brain injury and outcome after aneurysmal subarachnoid hemorrhage. Stroke 2007; 38(5):1489–94.

80. Petzold A, et al. Axonal pathology in subarachnoid and intracerebral hemorrhage. J Neurotrauma 2005;22(3):407–14.

Index

Note: Page numbers of article titles are in **boldface** type.

A

Acetaminophen, for fever, 328
Adrenomedullin, in cerebral salt-wasting syndrome, 343–344
Adult respiratory distress syndrome, 332
Age considerations, 222, 227, 236–237
Alcohol consumption, 237–238
Aldosterone imbalance, in cerebral salt-wasting syndrome, 340–341
Anemia, 328–329
Aneurysmal subarachnoid hemorrhage
  aneurysm size and location in, 223, 238
  cerebral salt wasting in, 333, **339–352**
  clinical features of, 381
  cost of, 239–242
  diagnosis of, 224–225, 305–312
  epidemiology of, **221–233,** 247, 381
  grading of, 225–226, 236, 238–239
  imaging of, **305–323**
  multilobed, 256–257
  nontreated, 225
  outcome of, 235–239
  pathophysiology of, 382
  prognosis for, 227–228
  risk factors for, 235–239, 247
  screening for, 241
  treatment of
    complications of, 237, **325–338**
    endovascular, **271–280**
    hydrocephalus after, 255–256, **263–271**
    noninvasive, **305–323**
    surgical, **247–261**
    timing of, 226–227, 248
    vasospasm after. *See* Vasospasm.
  versus nontraumatic nonaneurysmal subarachnoid hemorrhage, 224–225
Angiography
  computed tomography
    for aSAH, 224, 308–310
    for vasospasm, 282, 292–293, 315–316
  digital subtraction
    for aSAH, 224, 253
    for vasospasm, 292, 356
  fluorescent, 253
  magnetic resonance
    for aSAH, 224, 310–312
    for vasospasm, 293, 318
Angioplasty, transluminal balloon, for vasospasm, 287–288, 357

Angiotensin imbalance, in cerebral salt-wasting syndrome, 340–341
Anterior parasagittal craniotomy, 250–251
Antiinflammatory agents, for vasospasm prevention, 368–369
Antiplatelet agents, 275–277
Arctic Sun temperature management system, for fever, 328
Arrhythmias, 331
aSAH. *See* Aneurysmal subarachnoid hemorrhage.
Aspirin, 275–277, 356
Astrocytic damage, in vasospasm, 387
Atrial natriuretic peptide, in cerebral salt-wasting syndrome, 342–343
Axonal damage, in vasospasm, 387

B

Bacteremia, 333
Balloon angioplasty, transluminal, for vasospasm, 287–288, 357
Balloon-assisted liquid polymer embolization, 272
Basilar artery
  aneurysm of, 223
  vasospasm of, 298
Bicaudate index, for hydrocephalus, 264–265
Biomarkers
  for aSAH, 239
  for vasospasm, 368, **381–391**
    astrocytic damage, 387
    axonal damage, 387
    calcium metabolism, 386
    coagulation cascade, 386–387
    endothelial activation, 385
    endothelin, 386
    hemoglobin degradation, 385–386
    identification of, 383–384
    inflammation, 384–385
    isolation of, 383
    neuronal damage, 387
    nitric oxide, 386
    proteomics of, 382
    tissue sampling for, 382–383
Blood, vasospasm biomarkers in, 382–383
Blood stream infections, 333
Blood transfusions, 328–329
Body mass index, high, aneurysm risk in, 224
Brain Attack Surveillance in Corpus Christi project, 227

Neurosurg Clin N Am 21 (2010) 393–398
doi:10.1016/S1042-3680(10)00009-4

Moving?

Make sure your subscription moves with you!

To notify us of your new address, find your **Clinics Account Number** (located on your mailing label above your name), and contact customer service at:

Email: journalscustomerservice-usa@elsevier.com

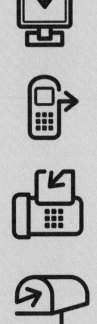

800-654-2452 (subscribers in the U.S. & Canada)
314-447-8871 (subscribers outside of the U.S. & Canada)

Fax number: 314-447-8029

Elsevier Health Sciences Division
Subscription Customer Service
3251 Riverport Lane
Maryland Heights, MO 63043

*To ensure uninterrupted delivery of your subscription, please notify us at least 4 weeks in advance of move.

Printed and bound by CPI Group (UK) Ltd, Croydon, CR0 4YY

03/10/2024

01040359-0017